Cost-Eff
Diagnostic Imaging

Zachary D. Grossman, MD, FACR
Chairman, Department of Radiology
The Roswell Park Cancer Institute
Professor of Radiology and Nuclear Medicine
State University of New York School of Medicine and Biomedical
Sciences at Buffalo
Buffalo, New York

Douglas S. Katz, MD
Director of Body CT
Vice Chair, Department of Radiology
Winthrop-University Hospital
Professor of Clinical Radiology
State University of New York at Stony Brook
Stony Brook, New York

Ronald A. Alberico, MD
Director of Neuroradiology and Head/Neck Imaging,
The Roswell Park Cancer Institute
Director of Neuroradiology and Head/Neck Imaging
Women and Children's Hospital of Buffalo
Associate Professor of Clinical Radiology
Assistant Professor of Clinical Neurosurgery
State University of New York School of Medicine and Biomedical
Sciences at Buffalo
Buffalo, New York

Peter A. Loud, MD
Director of Body Imaging
Director of Ultrasound
The Roswell Park Cancer Institute
Associate Professor of Clinical Radiology
State University of New York School of Medicine and Biomedical
Sciences at Buffalo
Buffalo, New York

Jonathan S. Luchs, MD
Director of Musculoskeletal Radiology
Medical Director, Winthrop Radiology Associates, P.C.
Winthrop-University Hospital
Assistant Professor of Clinical Radiology
State University of New York at Stony Brook
Stony Brook, New York

Ermelinda Bonaccio, MD
Director of the Mammography Center
The Roswell Park Cancer Institute
Buffalo, New York

Cost-Effective Diagnostic Imaging:
The Clinician's Guide

4th edition

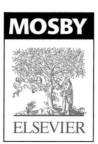

MOSBY

ELSEVIER

MOSBY
ELSEVIER

An Affiliate of Elsevier
1600 John F. Kennedy Boulevard
Suite 1800
Philadelphia, Pennsylvania 19103

COST-EFFECTIVE DIAGNOSTIC IMAGING: ISBN-13: 978-0-323-03283-4
THE CLINICIAN'S GUIDE, FOURTH EDITION ISBN-10: 0-323-03283-4
Copyright © 2006, Mosby, Inc., an affiliate of Elsevier.

NOTICE

Medicine is an ever-changing field. Standard safety precautions must
be followed, but as new research and clinical experience broaden our
knowledge, changes in treatment and drug therapy may become
necessary or appropriate. Readers are advised to check the most current
product information provided by the manufacturer of each drug to be
administered to verify the recommended dose, the method and
duration of administration, and contraindications. It is the
responsibility of the treating physician, relying on experience and
knowledge of the patient, to determine dosages and the best treatment
for each individual patient. Neither the Publisher nor the editors
assume any liability for any injury and/or damage to persons or
property arising from this publication.

The Publisher

ISBN-13: 978-0-323-03283-4
ISBN-10: 0-323-03283-4

Editor: *Rolla Couchman*
Editorial Assistant: *Dylan Parker*
Publishing Services Manager: *Joan Sinclair*
Designer: *Steven Stave*
Marketing Manager: *Laura Meiskey*

Printed in China.
Last digit is the print number: 9 8 7 6 5 4 3 2 1

To my family,
To my wonderful colleagues at Roswell Park,
  And in loving memory of
    Susan Ronnie Grossman

ZDG

To my former, currrent, and future residents in diagnostic radiology and to the former, current, and future clinical housestaff at Winthrop-University Hospital, all of whom maintain my interest in academic radiology and in academic medicine.

DSK

With unending love and appreciation to my beautiful wife, Nancy; to my children, Amy and Sarah; and to my parents, Ruth and Alden.

PL

To my wife and best friend, Michelle, and to my wonderful sons, Spencer and Zachary.

JL

To my parents, Mary and Joseph, and my husband, Keith, for their constant love and support, and to my sons, Henry and Spencer, for making it all worthwhile.

EB

Preface

What Cost-Effective Diagnostic Imaging Really Means

Cost-effective diagnostic imaging does not mean doing the cheapest test first! For two generations, skull films were taken after head trauma; millions of dollars were wasted on this inexpensive imaging study, which does not address the central clinical issue of head trauma: Is the brain injured?

Cost-effective diagnostic imaging does not necessarily mean doing the most accurate test first! Magnetic resonance (MR) imaging of the long bones is virtually 100% sensitive and 100% specific for fractures, whereas standard x-rays are occasionally falsely negative (and rarely falsely positive), yet the huge cost differential between MR per exam (more than $500 for the tibia and fibula) and bone radiographs ($28 for the tibia and fibula) makes MR cost ineffective as a screen for fractures.

Cost-effective imaging is a well-thought-out balance between the most accurate and often most expensive tests and the less accurate, less expensive tests. It is easy to see that no purpose is served by inexpensive initial procedures that are inaccurate or irrelevant (like skull films after head trauma) or by expensive tests that are only slightly more accurate than much cheaper exams (like initial magnetic resonance imaging for long bone fractures). Only after considerable reflection, however, does one conclude that, in certain instances, moderately priced tests with intermediate accuracy are more expensive in the long run than expensive tests that are invariably conclusive. However, moderately expensive tests that are highly accurate should always precede expensive tests whose accuracy is only slightly greater.

How is the clinician to choose among imaging exams?

- **Clearly, the choice of diagnostic studies, problem by problem, requires knowledge of imaging that is beyond the scope of the already overburdened primary physician, not to mention the medical student, resident, physician's assistant, and nurse practitioner.**
- **Clinical specialists are best informed only about their particular area of expertise and because diseases affect multiple organ systems and the pace of imaging development has been breathtaking, even clinical specialists are often out of touch with the best imaging protocols that apply to their patients.**
- **Radiology itself is so subspecialized that even radiologists are often uninformed about the effectiveness (and costs!) of imaging procedures outside of their own area!**

We hope and expect that this little book will painlessly help the clinician make appropriate choices. Let us know what you think.

Acknowledgments

First and foremost, the lead author thanks Dr. Janine Milligan, who, in her second year of medical school, spied a dusty, half-forgotten copy of the third edition (Mosby, 1995) and after thumbing through it persuaded the author to contact Elsevier about a fourth edition. Without Janine, this edition would not exist. Subsequently, she made invaluable corrections and suggestions for multiple chapters. I am in her debt.

Expert help on individual Chapters was provided by Sharmila Dorbala MD, FACC, Associate Director of Nuclear Cardiology, The Harvard Medical School, Boston, Massachusetts (Myocardial Ischemia/Coronary Artery Disease); Charles (Chuck) E. Ray, MD, Director of Interventional Radiology, the Denver Health Medical Center, Denver, Colorado (Renovascular Hypertention); Garin Tomaszewski, MD, Director of Interventional Radiology, The Roswell Park Cancer Institute, Buffalo, New York, (GI Bleeding); and Dominick Lamonica, MD, Director of Nuclear Medicine, The Roswell Park Cancer Institute (Intractable Epilepsy). Monica Jain, MD, was a full co-author of chapter 55 while she was a third-year radiology resident at the Winthrop-University Hospital. Mr. John Warner, CNMT, Chief Technologist in Nuclear Medicine at The Roswell Park Cancer Institute, and Alan Litwin, MD, Radiologist (Body Imaging) at Roswell Park, provided invaluable help in image selection, processing, and transmission.

Dr. Dorbala's in-depth knowledge of cardiology, nuclear medicine, and all phases of cardiac imaging was especially crucial.

Dr. Christine Van Cot made valuable suggestions for multiple chapters, particularly Skeletal Metastases, while a fourth-year student.

My remarkable assistant, Ms. Kathleen Koblich, helped me prepare the manuscript and tolerated my computer illiteracy with aplomb.

My dear friend and associate, Jack LaShomb, Administrator of the Department of Radiology at The Roswell Park Cancer Institute, provided endless help in terms of "cost data," and without his overall support and encouragement the project could not have been completed.

Finally, I would like to acknowledge my debt to clinicians everywhere who strive to use imaging technology in the most efficient way for the sake of their patients; I hope that this little book supports their efforts.

Introduction

One of the remarkable paradoxes in contemporary American medicine is the presence of a vague but definite malaise surrounding radiologic diagnosis at a time of unparalleled excitement and accomplishment in the development of imaging hardware and techniques. . . . Too many available choices—especially if imperfectly understood—create confusion and anxiety in the chooser . . .

The clinical service . . . enters the radiologic "supermarket," whose shelves are increasingly filled with exotic and expensive studies, and orders tests. . . . It is no indictment of clinical services to say that confusion surrounds the imaging workup.

—R. S. Heilman[1]

HOW TO USE THIS BOOK

Cost-Effective Diagnostic Imaging: The Clinician's Guide has been designed as a practical working manual—a brief text containing state-of-the-art information in the form of clear, cogent imaging protocols that cover important medical and surgical problems. Clinical problems are analyzed in terms of the most cost-effective, direct, and efficient route to diagnosis. Each chapter stands alone: Although there is extensive cross-referencing, **no chapter requires knowledge of a previous chapter.** The book should be consulted on a problem-by-problem basis—"in the heat of battle." Clinicians with a lot of time on their hands might consider a cover-to-cover reading, but we frankly do not recommend that approach, which would prove taxing to even the most retentive and disciplined mind.

We have selected problems whose workup is dominated by imaging and in general avoided detailed discussion of physical diagnosis and nonimaging diagnostic exams, particularly laboratory tests. Clinicians do not need to be taught clinical medicine by radiologists, and such material is exhaustively covered and readily available in major medical and surgical texts, which devote far too little space to modern imaging! Nonetheless, we cannot avoid touching on a few key laboratory exams, like D-dimer in the workup of pulmonary embolus.

This book **does not** replace or supersede consultation with the radiologist or nuclear imager; in fact, we encourage such consultation. We stress throughout that communication is the surest means of defining the best imaging solution to a clinical problem. Although our protocols cover many variations and contingencies that affect the imaging workup, unique circumstances that are best approached through discussion between the imager and the clinician(s) inevitably will arise. Such communication is most effective when **both** parties are well informed about the options under consideration.

PROCEDURE "COSTS"

Our belief is that cost-effective imaging is fostered by knowledge of what imaging procedures actually cost, at least in relative terms. Therefore, at the beginning of each chapter we have designated the relative cost of the tests that relate to the problem at hand, using the shorthand devised for restaurant or travel guides. The lowest-cost procedures are designated by a single dollar sign (**$**), the highest by six dollar signs. (**$$$$$$**).

By way of specifics, clinicians will be interested to know that old-fashioned plain films ("X-rays") are least expensive ($35 to $150, depending on the number of films and projections in the examination); ultrasound (US) costs more than plain films (about $100); computed tomography (CT or "CAT scan") costs between $250 and $375 (depending on the region examined and the need for contrast medium or "dye"); magnetic resonance imaging (MR or MRI) can be twice as expensive as CT (depending on the need for a basic or a complex study); most conventional nuclear medicine scans cost about the same as CT, whereas others that use exotic radionuclides are much higher; positron emission tomography (PET) is a quantum jump higher ($2200); and certain complex interventional procedures are even more expensive than PET. **THUS,** we have designated plain films as **$**, US as **$$**, CT as **$$$**, most nuclear medicine as **$$$**, MRI **$$$$**, PET as **$$$$$**, and a few interventional procedures as **$$$$$$**.

Here we differentiate between **charges**—i.e., what appears on the bill sent by the radiologist and his or her institution—and what is actually **paid**. In other words, a particular hospital or private radiology practice may bill $1000 for a particular study, but the insurance company or "third party payer" may pay only $500. **Thus, the "cost" of the procedure, to the healthcare system, is in fact $500.** Because different third party payers **reimburse different amounts for the same procedure,** we have used the actual 2005 reimbursements by the largest payer of all, the United States government, through Medicare. These figures reflect **the total reimbursement for a given procedure,** "professional" (the radiologist), "technical" (the institution), and any other factors (e.g., radiopharmaceuticals, stents, catheters, contrast medium, etc.).

GENERAL CONSIDERATIONS

We assume throughout that modern equipment and expertise are available. Where special technology will significantly affect the choice of an exam, we explain and emphasize that requirement.

Although familiarity with imaging techniques is not a prerequisite for understanding individual chapters, the following basic, practical information is included for those who wish to acquaint themselves with the general terminology and methods of modern imaging.

COMPUTED TOMOGRAPHY

Computed tomography (CT) is a radiographic method; however, the x-ray beam is fired through the patient from many angles to generate each image. The x-rays of standard radiography are detected by film, but for CT they strike radiation detectors, which produce a minute electrical impulse proportional to the intensity of the x-ray beam. The electrical current is quantitated numerically ("digitized") and computer stored. (Standard x-ray films, of course, record the effect of x-rays on film as film "blackening.") Unlike standard radiography, CT images can be manipulated and analyzed with the aid of a computer. Sets of photographically optimized images can be subsequently recorded on film for display on standard x-ray film view boxes or interpreted directly from computer monitors.

The standard imaging plane of CT is "axial," and its view of the body is analogous to looking at a slice of bread. From its creation in the early 1970s until the mid-1990s, CT scanners created one slice at a time, after which the patient was moved and another slice was created ("stop and shoot mode"); since the late 1990s, virtually all scanners have operated in the "helical" or "spiral" mode—the table holding the patient moves continuously, while the x-ray tube and its detectors (the "gantry") rotate continuously. Helical CT scanners create a seamless data set without the discontinuities of "stop and shoot" systems. Moreover, newer units fire the beam concurrently at multiple detectors (multidetector CT, or MDCT). These machines create 4, 8, 16, or even 64 slices concurrently in the helical mode, resulting in phenomenal acquisition speed. Motion blur is virtually eliminated. Sixty-four–detector machines will become commonplace by the end of 2006, enabling the clear visualization of blood vessels, even those in constant motion like the coronary arteries, after a **peripheral intravenous bolus injection of contrast medium**—no coronary artery catheterization required! This method is termed **CT angiography,** or CTA.

The ability of CT to display slices of anatomy without superimposition is the principal basis for its superiority to standard radiography. Moreover, data quantitation and increased sensitivity of the radiation detectors, as opposed to film, result in greater sensitivity to small density changes. **In other words, CT can detect slight variations in tissue density when standard X-rays do not; the gain in sensitivity is more than 100-fold. For example, renal stones that are "radiolucent" on an abdominal film are often radiodense on CT.** The virtually seamless, motion-free axial images of MDCT are easily "reformatted" into sagittal or coronal planes.

In modern radiologic practice, most chest, abdominal, and pelvic CT studies require intravenous contrast medium and pelvic/abdominal studies require both intravenous and oral contrast media, the latter ingested about one hour before the scan, the former delivered as an intravenous bolus during the scan. The oral contrast medium opacifies bowel to differentiate it from other abdominal densities, and the intravenous contrast medium defines blood vessels and all lesions that are vascular or partly vascular (tumors, inflammations, etc.).

Because CT was originally termed "computed axial tomography" or "computer assisted tomography," the acronyms "CAT" and "CAT scan" appear in portions of the medical literature. Universally, radiologists prefer "CT." **Because all CT units in the United States are now helical (the preferred description to "spiral"), we use the term "CT" to indicate "helical CT." Moreover, MDCT is so ubiquitous at the time of this (fourth) edition that we use the shorter term "CT" to also indicate MDCT.**

CT is never a bedside examination.

SONOGRAPHY OR ULTRASOUND

To generate ultrasound (US) or sonographic images, a hand-held transducer passes over the skin, gliding along a thin film of acoustical gel applied at the start of the exam. Any skin lesions, surgical dressings, drains, or wounds may interfere with sonography; the sonographer must circumvent these impediments, and sometimes the study is technically limited or completely unfeasible.

The high-frequency sound waves of sonography emanate from the handheld transducer and bounce off of internal structures. The returning sound beam ("echo") is detected by the transducer and converted into an image by computer. The contours of many internal structures are well defined by US, and a lesion's ability to reflect echoes (its "echogenicity") is often characteristic.

Sonography delivers no ionizing radiation. Although its complete effects are not fully known, most authorities agree that any risk is minimal compared with that of standard radiography, CT, or nuclear imaging. **Thus, sonography is particularly valuable for the study of children, pregnant women, and women of childbearing age.**

Unlike ionizing radiation, the sound-wave frequencies of diagnostic ultrasound cannot penetrate bone and gas. Thus, US of the brain after the fontanels have closed is feasible only after craniotomy, and ultrasound of aerated lungs is not possible. Moreover, intestinal gas is an impediment to viewing portions of the abdomen and portions of the liver and spleen under the ribs may be inaccessible.

Conventional US, like CT, defines the structure of organs. However, color Doppler US technology assesses organ perfusion. Perfusion data are particularly useful for differentiating ischemic lesions, such as testicular torsion, from inflammatory lesions like epididymitis. "Power" Doppler is more sensitive as a measure of blood flow.

Synonyms for sonography include *ultrasound, ultrasonography, medical sonography, "sono,"* and *"echo."* **In many institutions, US can be a bedside examination**.

NUCLEAR IMAGING

Unlike radiography and CT, which transmit x-rays **through** the patient's body, nuclear images are created from gamma rays emitted **by** the patient's body; these gamma rays originate from radiopharmaceuticals previously delivered orally or intravenously. Thus, nuclear imaging is sometimes called "emission imaging," as opposed to radiographic "transmission imaging."

Nuclear images (scans) are almost completely non-invasive, and they usually—but not always—deliver less radiation than standard x-rays or CT. The occasional morbidity and rare mortality associated with radiographic contrast media are virtually unknown with nuclear pharmaceuticals (radiopharmaceuticals), **which are subpharmacologic in dose.**

Because nuclear imaging utilizes organ- or system-specific radiopharmaceuticals, **the technique excels in functional assessment;** bone-seeking agents accumulate in the skeleton according to osseous blood flow and metabolism rather than according to architectural change; renal scans assess glomerular filtration rate and effective renal plasma flow, as well as renal size and contour. However, in most instances, the structural or anatomic information provided by nuclear studies is inferior to that of standard radiography, CT, magnetic resonance imaging, and US.

Radionuclide imaging uses many isotopes with different half-lives and gamma-ray energies, but by far the most common isotope is technetium-99m (Tc-99m). Radioisotopes can be bound to many chemicals whose structures determine the in vivo distribution of the resulting radiopharmaceutical compounds. Tc-99m is a component of many radiopharmaceuticals with different biodistributions. Therefore, from the standpoint of nuclear imagers, "a technetium scan" has little meaning: Is a Tc-99m-HIDA (hepatobiliary iminodiacetic acid) study for the gallbladder intended, or perhaps a Tc-99m-methylene diphosphonate (MDP) scan for the skeleton? Because one cannot expect the busy clinician to keep track of the many radiopharmaceuticals available, most nuclear medicine departments urge that the scan be ordered according to the system under study for a given tentative diagnosis; thus an ideal requisition would read, "bone scan, rule out bone metastases" or "gallbladder scan, rule out acute cholecystitis."

The standard instrument for acquiring nuclear images is the gamma scintillation camera (gamma camera). This device detects the gamma rays emitted by a radiopharmaceutical inside the patient and displays its distribution and intensity as a "scan."

Synonyms for radionuclide imaging include *nuclear medicine, nuclear imaging, isotope imaging, nuclear medicine imaging, scintigraphy, gamma scintigraphy, nuclear scanning, nuclear medicine scanning, isotope scanning,* and *radionuclide scanning.* Although portable scanners were in vogue many years ago, in current practice, nuclear imaging is almost never a portable, bedside examination.

A variation of nuclear imaging, called *single photon emission computed tomography* (SPECT), has become widely available. Standard radionuclides are used with SPECT to generate images in "slices," much like those of CT. SPECT markedly increases the sensitivity of nuclear scanning but almost always increases its cost.

The most dramatic and revolutionary outgrowth of nuclear imaging is PET (positron emission tomography). PET requires a camera that detects pairs of 511 Kev photons produced by the annihilation reaction that occurs when positrons are emitted from certain cyclotron-produced radionuclides. This originally exotic technology has recently become mainstream, **driven by improved camera technology and widespread availability of a key molecule, FDG (fluorodeoxyglucose) labeled with the positron emitter, fluorine-18. FDG mimics the biodistribution of ordinary glucose**—to a point; it is accumulated by tissues that use glucose in proportion to their glucose metabolism, but it never completes the Krebs cycle and remains forever trapped in the cell. **Combined PET technology and FDG can identify sites of high glucose metabolism—especially tumors, the more malignant and faster-growing the better!** Also, PET images are by nature tomographic—that is, they are "slice data" of much higher spatial resolution than conventional nuclear imaging. **Extensive studies have proven that tumor response to chemotherapy can be better monitored by**

FDG uptake than by tumor size, so many chemotherapy patients will probably soon be monitored by FDG-PET, at first in combination with CT and then perhaps in lieu of CT.

Because only FDG is now both widely available and FDA approved, the term "FDG-PET" has become synonymous—especially among clinicians—with "PET," but we recommend calling each PET exam what it actually is; thus, "FDG-PET" should be called "FDG-PET"! This recommendation is not for the sake of nitpicking; rather, it is motivated by recent advances in the chemistry of "molecular imaging"—**new molecules labeled with fluorine-18 will soon be available**—e.g., fluorinated thymidine (FLT). **The uptake of FLT by a cell mirrors its DNA synthesis,** and the effect of chemotherapy can be more sensitively monitored by uptake of FLT (by FLT-PET) than by assessing change in tumor size (by CT) or even glucose uptake (by FDG-PET). Other powerful molecular probes are under development, including a compound labeled with Cu-60 that adheres only to hypoxic tissue (the most chemotherapy- and radiotherapy-resistant portion of a tumor, which is most likely to regrow and therefore merits a "boosted" radiation dose). Thus, **multiple types of PET scans will be available within 5 years,** and precision in terminology now will avoid confusion later. **FDG-PET is only the tip of the iceberg, and the future of PET will be no less than explosive**.

PET/CT

The functional information of FDG-PET is greatly augmented by correlation with the anatomic information of CT. Originally, the correlation simply meant studying the two exams side by side; later, image "fusion" technology was developed so that the two types of images could be seen on top of each other as an overlay. Because the two exams were generated by **different machines at different times,** some error in line up, called *misregistration*, was inevitable. To eliminate most of the misregistration, PET scanners and CT scanners were combined into single hybrid units that generate both studies in sequence, on the same table, with the patient in the same position. The CT created for the purpose of image overlay, however, is most often **NOT equivalent to a conventional diagnostic CT**, because intravenous contrast medium is usually not used. **THEREFORE, ALL CLINICIANS SHOULD UNDERSTAND THAT A PATIENT WHO REQUIRES A DIAGNOSTIC CT *AND* A PET WILL PROBABLY NEED A SEPARATE FULLY DIAGNOSTIC CT, EVEN IF THE PET IS OBTAINED ON A HYBRID PET/CT UNIT. (At the time of this writing, however, new PET/CT protocols are under development, so that some oral and intravenous radiographic contrast medium can be administered, upgrading the CT portion of a PET/CT almost to conventional diagnostic CT levels.)**

ANGIOGRAPHY/INTERVENTIONAL RADIOLOGY (IR)

Conventional angiography involves injection of radiographic contrast medium directly into a blood vessel during rapid-sequence filming. To deliver contrast medium to a desired site—for example, the superior mesenteric artery or carotid artery—a catheter is introduced percutaneously, typically via the femoral artery or vein, and is advanced to the appropriate blood vessel. Angiography is thus more invasive than CT, US, magnetic resonance imaging, or nuclear imaging.

Angiography, particularly arteriography, carries a small, but significant, risk of potentially serious complications, including hemorrhage, vascular perforation, embolism, thrombosis, organ infarction, reaction to contrast medium, and even death. Angiograms, of course, are riskier in patients with bleeding diatheses, so an attempt to normalize—or at least stabilize—the clotting profile, in concert with the angiographer, may be necessary.

Most angiographic studies, including arteriograms, are safely performed on outpatients. **CTA produced by MDCT has largely replaced conventional catheter**

angiography for diagnostic purposes because the images of CTA are usually diagnostic. However, catheter angiography is critical in all cases where repair or transcatheter therapy is contemplated, and in some specialized areas it remains the gold standard for diagnostic purposes.

A wide variety of specialized catheters, needles, and other devices for intervention and therapy is available. **In many instances, these procedures are safer, more effective, and less costly than corresponding surgical alternatives**. Interventional procedures that have gained widespread acceptance include CT- or ultrasound-guided biopsies of virtually every organ caudal to the skull base, dilatation of stenotic vessels (percutaneous angioplasty), dilatation of biliary strictures, biliary drainage and calculus removal, nephrostomy tube placement, and abscess drainage. Transcatheter placement of a stent to maintain patency is a common procedure, once a blood vessel is dilated. Delivery of drugs and embolic material to specific sites through a catheter is also feasible. The newest item in the IR arsenal is radio frequency ablation (RFA), a procedure involving the guided percutaneous puncture of a tumor and insertion of a probe, followed by ablation of the tumor with radio frequency energy emitted by the end of the probe.

MAGNETIC RESONANCE IMAGING

Magnetic resonance imaging (MRI) uses signals emitted by the patient's body when placed in a strong magnetic field and perturbed by tiny pulses of radio frequency energy; a computer processes the signals into images. The MR "scanner" operates by varying magnetic fields and delivering pulses of energy at particular radio frequencies and particular time intervals. Because these fields and energy pulses are independent of patient orientation, MR images can be obtained in any plane; typically, they are axial, sagittal, or coronal. Like CT, MR visualizes a slice of anatomy whose thickness can be varied according to the body part examined and the purpose of the study.

MR reflects the distribution of hydrogen atoms in the body and their molecular surroundings. Although a more detailed discussion is beyond the scope of this book, two different types of images are produced routinely: T1-weighted and T2-weighted. Tl-weighted images tend to show greater anatomic detail, whereas T2-weighted images often highlight specific pathologic processes to a greater degree.

MR devices look like elongated CT scanners. They include a tubular magnet into which the patient is placed. Although the "tube" is open on both ends, some patients experience anxiety in such confined circumstances, and occasionally claustrophobic patients refuse the study. Newer "open bore architecture" units are much less confining, and even in units of standard design thoughtful adaptations (sedation, headphones with music, exam prone rather than supine, **anxiolytic drugs,** etc.) can make the study compatible for all but the most anxious patients. The magnetic field is of such strength that any local ferromagnetic material is affected; thus, patients with conventional life-support equipment or monitoring devices must not enter the field, lest the equipment be rendered nonfunctional or be pulled into the magnet. However, newer MR-compatible life-support systems are now available**. A PACEMAKER IS AN ABSOLUTE CONTRAINDICATION TO MAGNETIC RESONANCE IMAGING**. Patients with any cerebral aneurysm clips should not undergo MR because of the possibility that clip motion will disrupt the cerebral vasculature. Furthermore, ferromagnetic materials can disturb the field and interfere with the imaging process.

MR angiography (MRA) defines blood vessels, sometimes with the aid of gadolinium-based contrast media. Like CTA, MRA uses only a peripheral intravenous injection, yet major blood vessels can be visualized. Currently, MRA is inferior to CTA, as well as more time consuming, but many investigators believe that in the next decade MRA will surpass CTA. Because MRA delivers no ionizing radiation, it would then have a distinct advantage from a safety standpoint.

MR is never a portable examination, but some neuro-surgical suites have installed intraoperative MR units, **so that the neurosurgeon can actually see inside of the brain during surgery!**

CONTRAST MATERIAL OR CONTRAST MEDIUM: WHAT THE CLINICIAN NEEDS TO KNOW

Radiographic contrast media for intravenous use are organic molecules containing iodine. The iodine produces "contrast" by blocking x-rays. As it is excreted by the kidneys, contrast medium allows visualization of the urinary tract; in patients with normal renal function, negligible amounts are excreted through the biliary system and gut. In addition to its use in imaging the urinary tract, intravenous contrast medium is crucial for many radiographic exams, including CT of the abdomen, head, and chest, as well as all CTA and catheter angiography. **Because intravenous contrast medium enhances the visualization of many lesions, "CT enhanced with intravenous contrast medium" is usually termed *enhanced CT*. In this text we also refer to "MR enhanced with intravenous contrast medium" as *enhanced MR*.** Synonyms for contrast medium include *contrast material, contrast agents*, and, colloquially, *"dye."*

Advanced renal failure is a contraindication to radiographic contrast media, but mild chronic renal failure (creatinine approximately less than 2.0) is usually compatible with iso-osmolar contrast medium (e.g., Visipaque), if combined with judicious hydration and monitoring. In all cases, oral medications containing metformin hydrochloride (Glucophage, Glucovance) should be discontinued 12 hours before the exam and avoided for at least 48 hours afterward. Contrast medium is also relatively contraindicated in multiple myeloma, pheochromocytoma, and sickle cell disease. Of course, a strong history of a previous adverse reaction to contrast medium is a contraindication, although if the exam is absolutely necessary, pretreatment with steroids and diphenhydramine may be considered. In all cases of relative contraindication, the radiologist should be contacted personally.

MR contrast media, unlike radiographic contrast media, are gadolinium based rather than iodine based. Although generally safe even in the presence of renal failure, they can rarely be associated with adverse reactions and even death. Neuroradiologists, who are known for idiosyncratic colloquial terms—e.g., an enhancing lesion of uncertain etiology in the brain is sometimes actually called a "UBO" (unidentified bright object)—like to call a gadolinium-enhanced study "with gad."

Any organization or institution that administers either iodine-based or gadolinium-based contrast materials intravenously should be fully prepared for resuscitative efforts and emergency life support.

RISKS OF IONIZING RADIATION

Half of the ionizing radiation dose received by the United States population is due to medical diagnostic or therapeutic irradiation. The risks from this radiation exposure are very low but very real. They include genetic defects, carcinogenesis, and developmental defects in exposed fetuses. For all but moderately high rates of exposure to fetuses, the risks are exceedingly small when compared with spontaneous rates of mutation, cancer, and birth defects. There is general agreement that the benefits from appropriately ordered diagnostic exams far outweigh the risks. If a diagnostic exam is really needed, the fact that radiation exposure will occur should not override clinical judgment.

A WORD ABOUT CITED LITERATURE

In keeping with the brief, concise nature of this book, we have limited "references" to lists of "additional reading."

REFERENCE

1. Heilman RS: What's wrong with radiology. N Engl J Med 1982;306:447–449.

Contents

Part *I*

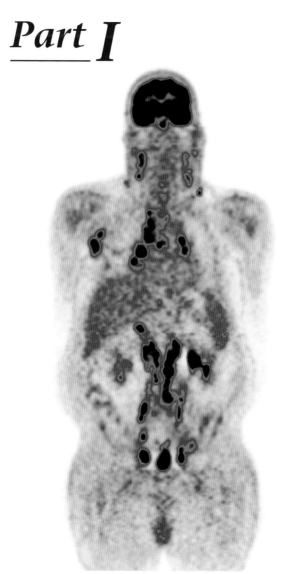

Gastrointestinal

Gallstones/Acute Cholecystitis

INTRODUCTION

Gallstones are common, affecting approximately 10% of adults in the United States. In western countries most stones are primarily cholesterol, whereas in Asia they are mostly bile pigment. Gallstones are more common in women and in the elderly.

The vast majority of acute cholecystitis is caused by a stone obstructing the cystic duct. The best initial study to assess right upper quadrant pain is ultrasound (US)—because it is the most accurate method for detecting gallstones, easily localizes the gallbladder to confirm the site of pain, and also can define abnormalities in the right kidney, liver, or head of the pancreas, which can mimic the clinical picture of acute cholecystitis. Other imaging modalities, including the nuclear technetium 99m (Tc-99m)–hepatobiliary iminodiacetic acid (HIDA) scan, which evaluates cystic duct patency, and computed tomography (CT), which can define alternate causes of pain or complications of cholecystitis, play an important role if US is not definitive.

A more challenging but uncommon dilemma is **acute acalculous cholecystitis,** in which the gallbladder is inflamed **but the cystic duct is not necessarily obstructed.** In such cases, US can strongly suggest acute cholecystitis (point tenderness, pericholecystic edema, gallbladder wall thickening), **yet HIDA may reveal a patent cystic duct.** (The cystic duct can be patent or obstructed depending on the degree of duct wall edema.)

Relative Costs: Abdominal US, **$$**; HIDA, **$$**.

3

▌PLAN AND RATIONALE

STEP 1: ULTRASOUND (US)

Ideally, patients should fast for 6 to 8 hours before US. The gallbladder then fills with bile, and gallstone detection is optimal. If the presence or absence of gallstones is the issue, without the setting of acute pain, and US is negative, then stones are virtually excluded, and the workup ends.

In the setting of acute right upper quadrant pain, US virtually always localizes the gallbladder; therefore, the sonographer can determine whether abdominal tenderness is localized specifically to that organ. This "sonographic Murphy's sign" is extremely valuable. (The sonographer asks the patient to localize the site of maximum tenderness and places the US probe there to confirm that it overlies the gallbladder.) Calculi, pericholecystic fluid, and gallbladder wall thickening can also be defined. Because the acutely inflamed gallbladder is typically distended, detection of a collapsed gallbladder is a useful negative predictive finding. When calculi and a positive sonographic Murphy's sign coexist, acute cholecystitis is extremely likely, and the imaging workup ends.

Sometimes, however, only one or two suggestive findings are present, along with a confusing clinical picture; in these circumstances, HIDA can be an effective follow-up.

> **Thus, when US and the clinical picture are equivocal:**

STEP 2: NUCLEAR TECHNETIUM 99M–HEPATOBILIARY IMINODIACETIC ACID (TC-99M-HIDA) SCAN

After intravenous injection, HIDA is cleared from the circulation and rapidly excreted by the liver into the biliary tree, filling the gallbladder by retrograde passage through the cystic duct and entering the duodenum via the common duct. Injection of intravenous morphine is often part of the procedure to encourage gallbladder filling; morphine constricts the sphincter of Oddi, increasing back pressure in the duct system and forcing HIDA retrograde into the gallbladder if the cystic duct is patent.

HIDA can establish whether the cystic duct is patent, **because gallbladder filling proves cystic duct patency. Cystic duct patency is very strong evidence against acute obstructive cholecystitis, because cystic duct obstruction by a stone is the hallmark of that condition.** (False positive studies may occur in chronic cholecystitis or in patients who are fasting or are on hyperalimentation, because in these circumstances the gallbladder is often filled with thick bile or sludge, which prevents HIDA from entering.) Although HIDA has higher sensitivity and specificity than US for acute cholecystitis, it does not evaluate other potential causes of right upper quadrant pain and is therefore less useful in many acute situations.

If US suggests acute cholecystitis and HIDA fails to fill the gallbladder, acute obstructive cholecystitis is highly likely, and the workup ends.

If US suggests acute cholecystitis **and HIDA fills the gallbladder,** cystic duct patency is proven, and acute **obstructive** cholecystitis is excluded. **The imaging workup ends, but the unlikely possibility of acalculous nonobstructive acute cholecystitis remains; the diagnostic decision is then a clinical one.**

SUMMARY AND CONCLUSIONS

1. US is the examination of choice to evaluate a patient for gallstones.
2. The initial study of choice for suspected acute cholecystitis is US, because the usual clinical situation calls for an **imaging survey of the right upper quadrant.**
3. If sonographic and clinical findings strongly support the diagnosis of acute cholecystitis, further imaging is usually unnecessary.

4. If the diagnosis is equivocal after US, HIDA is appropriate to establish whether the cystic duct is patent. A patent cystic duct excludes obstructive acute cholecystitis.
5. A diagnosis of acalculous nonobstructive cholecystitis can be challenging and often relies on a combination of sonographic/scintigraphic/clinical findings in a high-risk patient.

ADDITIONAL COMMENTS

- The fact that US delivers no ionizing radiation is particularly important in the context of gallbladder stones/chronic cholecystitis, because many patients studied for this problem are young or middle-aged women, whose ovaries should be spared any avoidable radiation burden.
- Some studies have indicated that delayed gallbladder filling with HIDA is a reliable sign of **chronic** cholecystitis, and such a finding may be reported during a HIDA study for suspected **acute** cholecystitis.
- US can also determine whether the bile ducts are dilated and can often define choledocholithiasis, but sensitivity may be limited by incomplete visualization of the extrahepatic ducts. This issue arises in many cases of jaundice.
- Abdominal CT is the best modality to evaluate suspected complications of cholecystitis, such as perforation or abscess, and to confirm a suspected diagnosis of emphysematous cholecystitis. CT or US can guide the radiologist during abscess drainage or cholecystostomy tube placement when immediate surgery is contraindicated.
- Although US is the examination of choice to establish the presence or absence of gallbladder stones, other imaging techniques can sometimes identify stones, including CT and even plain films.

■ SUGGESTED READING

Bortoff GA, Chen MY, Ott DJ, et al: Gallbladder stones: imaging and intervention. Radiographics 2000;20:751–766.

Bree RL, Ralls PW, Balfe DM, et al: Evaluation of patients with acute right upper quadrant pain. American College of Radiology. Appropriateness Criteria. Radiology 2000;215(Suppl):153–157.

Freitas JE: Cholescintigraphy. In Ell PJ, Gambhir SS (eds): Nuclear Medicine in Clinical Diagnosis and Treatment, 3rd ed. Philadelphia, Churchill Livingstone, 2004, pp 1657–1684.

Hanbidge AE, Buckleer PM, O'Malley ME, Wilson SR: Imaging evaluation for acute pain in the right upper quadrant. Radiographics 2004;24:1117–1135.

Laing FC: The gallbladder and bile ducts. In Rumack CM, Wilson SR, Charboneau JW (eds): Diagnostic Ultrasound, 2nd ed. St. Louis: Mosby, 1998, pp 175–223.

Mariat G, Mahul P, Previt N, et al: Contribution of ultrasonography and cholescintigraphy to the diagnosis of acute acalculous cholecystitis in intensive care unit patients. Intensive Care Med 2000;26:1658–1663.

Biliary Tract Obstruction/Hepatic Dysfunction

INTRODUCTION

Ultrasound (US), computed tomography (CT), and magnetic resonance (MR) imaging are key to the initial workup of patients **with suspected biliary tract obstruction** and also apply to the evaluation of patients with hepatic dysfunction **unrelated to biliary tract obstruction.**

Jaundice, with or without right upper quadrant pain, often results from biliary tract obstruction. In the presence of jaundice, **the goal of diagnostic imaging is to establish whether obstruction is present, and, if so, why**. Obstructing biliary tract stones usually pass distally to the sphincter of Oddi or to the common bile duct (CBD) at the level of the pancreas, but tumors of the pancreas/ampullary region can also cause biliary tract obstruction (see also **CHAPTER 5, Pancreatic Mass**), as can nonmalignant strictures. The **extrahepatic ducts** are more compliant than the **intrahepatic ducts** (no surrounding support from adjacent liver tissue) and therefore dilate sooner after obstruction than do the intrahepatic ducts.

In patients **with hepatic dysfunction but without suspected ductal dilation,** imaging can confirm the presence of fatty infiltration and estimate its extent, sometimes demonstrate findings consistent with acute hepatitis, identify cirrhosis and/or its complications, and guide a liver biopsy.

Generally, the workup starts with US, but additional testing is usually required if ductal dilation is identified.

Relative Costs: US, **$$**; CT, **$$$**; MR/MRCP, **$$$$**; EUS, **$$$$**; Tc-99m-HIDA, **$$**; ERCP, **$$$$**.

PLAN AND RATIONALE

When biliary tract obstruction is suspected:

STEP 1: ULTRASOUND (SONOGRAPHY, US)

US is the best initial examination for suspected biliary tract obstruction.

The intrahepatic ducts, gallbladder, CBD, and pancreas can be visualized (although definition of the pancreas and the distal CBD is variable and often limited, due to overlying bowel gas/soft tissue).

If sonography reveals normal ducts, the workup usually ends.

Rarely, clinical evidence suggests ongoing obstruction in the presence of sonographically **normal ducts;** this pattern usually results from **very recent obstruction; the ducts may not have had sufficient time to dilate.** In this event, the simplest approach is to repeat US after 24 to 48 hours; however, CT (see **Step 2,** below), MR cholangiopancreatography (MRCP), or HIDA (see **ADDITIONAL COMMENTS**) sometimes apply.

If US suggests that ductal dilation and probably obstruction are present (taking into account the patient's age, the presence of intrahepatic versus extrahepatic dilation, and whether the patient has had a cholecystectomy), **an attempt is made to determine the cause of the obstruction**. Although sonography's sensitivity for determining **a specific cause** of obstruction is lower than its sensitivity for defining ductal dilation, in some patients CBD stone(s) (which occur[s] in up to 18% of patients with symptomatic gallstones), a pancreatic head region tumor, or another obstructing lesion may be identified.

If US fails to identify a specific cause of biliary dilation and, likely, obstruction, MRCP or CT is next.

STEP 2: MAGNETIC RESONANCE CHOLANGIOPANCREATOGRAPHY (MRCP) OR COMPUTED TOMOGRAPHY (CT)

The choice of MRCP or contrast-enhanced CT depends upon specific sonographic findings combined with clinical information. For example, in a patient with sonographically proven gallstones and/or cholecystitis, with dilated bile ducts and clinical suspicion of a CBD stone (but without a definite stone seen on sonography, which is typically the case), MRCP is next. If no specific underlying etiology is likely, either CT or MRCP is appropriate, with a decision weighted toward MRCP if the concern is **probably ductal,** and toward CT if **the pancreas itself is more suspect.**

MRCP is the best noninvasive imaging test for evaluation of the bile ducts and the pancreatic duct. Breath-held, heavily "T2-weighted" images are generated, without contrast medium. The accuracy of MRCP for diagnosis or exclusion of a CBD stone is very high, approaching that of endoscopic retrograde cholangiopancreatography (ERCP), and its accuracy for stricture identification is also excellent. The pancreatic study is often combined with images of the remainder of the abdomen.

Contrast-medium–enhanced CT is the optimal noninvasive method for evaluation of the pancreas itself. We generally prefer CT to even the best MRCP, because CT defines the pancreas and adjacent structures (especially blood vessels) in exquisite detail. However, when the iodinated contrast medium of CT is contraindicated (see the **INTRODUCTION** to this book), when the etiology of the obstruction is **completely unclear,** or when an obstructing CBD stone is suspect, MRCP is a better choice.

If all noninvasive imaging has failed to explain the ductal dilation, then **direct guided cannulation of the biliary and pancreatic ducts with ERCP and visualization with endoscopic US remain as options.**

STEP 3: ENDOSCOPIC ULTRASOUND (EUS)/ENDOSCOPIC RETROGRADE CHOLANGIOPANCREATOGRAPHY (ERCP)

EUS: Under conscious sedation, a gastroenterologist introduces a specialized endoscope containing a high-frequency transducer, from which ultrasound penetrates the stomach and duodenum, permitting detailed evaluation of the CBD and the pancreas. **EUS is the most sensitive imaging examination for pancreatic head region tumors.** The high-frequency transducer defines details of the retroperitoneum that are impossible to see through the skin of the anterior or posterior abdomen during standard transabdominal US. Biopsies are possible through ports in the scope.

ERCP: Under conscious sedation, the bile ducts and the pancreatic duct are cannulated and filled with contrast medium injected through an endoscope introduced trans-orally and placed in the duodenum. The procedure is performed by a skilled gastroenterologist under fluoroscopic control, usually in a radiology department. The site of obstruction is identified and its cause often defined (e.g., CBD stone) or inferred (e.g., focal high-grade stricture of the CBD or narrowed pancreatic ducts from pancreatic tumor). An obstructing CBD stone can sometimes be extracted on the spot.

EUS and ERCP are performed separately, but they are complementary in some patients. **ERCP demonstrates ductal anatomy and enables procedures such as papillotomy, stone extraction, stent placement, and ductal brushings, whereas EUS examines the pancreatic ducts and the surrounding anatomy, including the CBD and pancreatic ducts,** and enables biopsy of a focal pancreatic abnormality. **The choice and sequence of procedures should be determined by the gastroenterologist together with the radiologist, reviewing all imaging studies and clinical data together.**

When hepatic dysfunction *without* biliary tract obstruction is suspected:

Suspected Diffuse Fatty Liver

A frequent source of concern is the patient with relatively mild liver malfunction and presumptive diffuse fatty infiltration. **Ultrasound is sensitive and specific for this common problem and categorizes the extent of fatty infiltration, based on echogenicity (the degree of ultrasound reflection) of the liver.** In severe fatty infiltration, for example, the anterior liver is very "bright," and the posterior liver is completely obscured. (Fatty infiltration of the liver has assumed increased importance lately, as its relationship to the development of non-alcoholic chronic hepatitis and cirrhosis in some individuals has been recognized.)

Suspected Acute Hepatitis

Although acute hepatitis is usually a clinical/laboratory diagnosis, occasionally a radiologist may suggest it on US performed for right upper quadrant pain. Sometimes the US was ordered to exclude concurrent biliary dilation, estimate hepatic size, search for associated abdominal processes (such as splenomegaly, gallbladder disease, and ascites), or to exclude other causes of pain.

Known or Suspected Cirrhosis

US, CT, and MR are all effective in the study of suspected cirrhosis (Fig. 2-1).

US is often the first study performed, because it is inexpensive and universally available and delivers no ionizing radiation, so that it can be repeated serially. Primary findings consistent with cirrhosis include nodularity of the liver surface and heterogeneous parenchymal "echotexture"; ancillary findings, especially when portal hypertension is also present, include ascites, varices, and splenomegaly. **Foci of hepatocellular carcinoma can also be identified in some patients.**

CT and MR have unique advantages and disadvantages for this evaluation, and both can demonstrate the

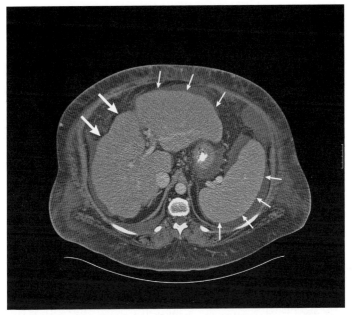

Figure 2-1. Abdominal CT in a 57-year-old woman with cirrhosis. The liver has a nodular contour (*two large arrows*). The left hepatic lobe is enlarged (*three arrows*), and there is ascites. Also, the spleen (*four arrows*) is mildly enlarged.

findings seen by US. Both effectively screen for suspected hepatocellular carcinoma, although there is much controversy regarding their advantages, disadvantages, and techniques. Even the issue of optimum contrast medium (i.e., gadolinium-based compounds versus iron-particle–based media) for MR remains unresolved; the spirited dialogue on this subject alone could fill this volume.

Guided Liver Biopsy (see also CHAPTER 60, Percutaneous Guided Biopsy and Imaging-Guided Therapy)
When biopsy is indicated, the procedure is usually imaging guided (CT or US), performed by a radiologist, a hepatologist/gastroenterologist, or both. Typically, a biopsy "gun" obtains core samples for histopathology.

SUMMARY AND CONCLUSIONS

1. When biliary obstruction is suspected, **US is the recommended initial examination.** If findings are negative, the workup for biliary obstruction usually ends, unless the obstruction may be **extremely early,** in which case US can be repeated in 24 to 48 hours. When US reveals or even suggests biliary duct dilation, **additional imaging is usually required to determine the underlying cause and facilitate appropriate treatment.**

2. After US demonstrates biliary dilation, CT or MRCP can help determine the cause.

3. **MRCP is the noninvasive imaging test of choice for a suspected common duct stone. The authors consider CT the noninvasive imaging test of choice for suspected pancreatic cancer, including tumors involving the pancreatic head region (see also CHAPTER 5, Pancreatic Mass).**

4. **The next step in the workup for biliary obstruction/dilation is ERCP and/or EUS. These relatively invasive tests can make the diagnosis and permit both biopsy and various curative therapies.**

5. US is the best initial test for suspected fatty infiltration of the liver.

6. **US, CT, and MR can all apply to the diagnosis of cirrhosis and its suspected complications, especially hepatocellular carcinoma.** However, the precise role and the techniques of each are the subject of enormous controversy in the imaging and clinical literature.

7. Imaging guidance, usually with sonography but sometimes with CT, is very helpful for performing a safe and atraumatic liver biopsy in patients with suspected or known diffuse hepatic disease.

Imaging guidance avoids injury to major intrahepatic blood vessels, the adjacent lung, and other organs.

ADDITIONAL COMMENTS

- In the **occasional** patient for whom clinical evidence suggests mild biliary obstruction but US findings are normal or equivocal (e.g., in a post-cholecystectomy patient who may have **mild** biliary dilation, especially of the CBD), a nuclear technetium 99m (Tc-99m)–hepatobiliary iminodiacetic acid (HIDA) scan is appropriate. After intravenous injection of the agent, HIDA is cleared from the circulation by the liver and excreted into the biliary tree. Prompt visualization of the duodenum proves that the CBD is patent, and the workup usually ends.

    Failure of HIDA to enter the duodenum (unless there is marked hepatic malfunction, which prevents accumulation and excretion of the pharmaceutical by the liver) confirms obstruction. A repeat sonogram is often considered a better alternative, because the sonogram is not dependent upon good hepatic function. The underlying logic of US or MRCP for this problem is that biliary dilation usually correlates with obstruction, but in **RARE** cases in which this is not believed to be the case, a HIDA scan, which is a physiologic rather than an anatomic test, can be helpful.

- A HIDA scan is also the test of choice for confirming or disproving a suspected bile leak following cholecystectomy or partial hepatic resection (see also **CHAPTER 4, Bile Leak**). In cases in which ERCP cannot be performed or fails (most often in patients who have had prior surgery and altered anatomy, such as a biliary bypass procedure) and substantial biliary obstruction is confirmed on CT, US, or MRCP, percutaneous transhepatic cholangiography (PTC) may confirm obstruction and also decompress the obstructed bile ducts.

    PTC involves percutaneous needle puncture of the liver through the abdominal wall, followed by injection of contrast medium into an intrahepatic duct, filling and defining the ducts proximal to an obstruction. PTC with a thin needle is quite safe, and the interventional radiologist can then place a variety of percutaneous drainage catheters, dilate strictures, and place ductal stents to bypass various types of obstruction.

- MRCP appears to be an accurate test for the evaluation and follow-up of patients with known sclerosing cholangitis, but the accuracy for early diagnosis remains unknown.

- If cholangiocarcinoma is suspected based on initial imaging studies or on the patient's history (e.g., new stricture in a patient with sclerosing cholangitis), confirming the diagnosis is a challenge. A variety of approaches may be used, including close comparison with prior imaging studies, use of delayed CT or MR images (some cholangiocarcinomas, because of their fibrotic nature, pick up contrast medium and retain it on delayed images, making them more visible), and biopsy (especially by ERCP, whenever possible).

- MR can define the presence and extent of abnormal hepatic iron deposition, but usually MR does not substitute for biopsy.

- Even with state-of-the-art CT and MR, establishing the presence or absence of a pancreatic head region tumor (as opposed to ductal stricture or chronic pancreatitis) can be surprisingly difficult. EUS with biopsy is especially helpful in this situation.

- Although CT is **not** the test of choice for prospective diagnosis of a CBD stone, CT can sometimes establish the diagnosis, particularly when the density of the stone is sufficient; its accuracy is significantly lower than that of MRCP and ERCP.

- CT and MR can also establish the diagnosis of fatty infiltration of the liver.

- Intravenous contrast medium for sonography, not presently approved for use in the United States, is used elsewhere to improve detection and characterization of liver masses.

▌SUGGESTED READING

Baron RL, Gore RM: Diffuse liver disease. In Gore RM, Levine MS (eds): Textbook of Gastrointestinal Radiology. WB Saunders, Philadelphia, 2000, pp 1590–1630.

Carr-Locke DL: Overview of the role of ERCP in the management of diseases of the biliary tract and the pancreas. Gastrointest Endosc 2002;56(6 Suppl):S157–S160.

Fulcher AS: MRCP and ERCP in the diagnosis of common bile duct stones. Gastrointest Endosc 2002;56(6 Suppl):S178–S182.

Hartman EM, Barish MA: MR cholangiography. MRI Clin North Am 2001;9:841–855.

Hawes RH: Diagnostic and therapeutic uses of ERCP in pancreatic and biliary tract malignancies. Gastrointest Endosc 2002;56(6 Suppl): S201–S205.

Ko CW, Lee SP: Epidemiology and natural history of common bile duct stones and prediction of disease. Gastrointest Endosc 2002;56 (6 Suppl):S165–S169.

Mark DH, Flamm CR, Aronson N: Evidence-based assessment of diagnostic modalities for common bile duct stones. Gastrointest Endosc 2002;56(6 Suppl):S190–S194.

Mortele KJ, Ji H, Ros PR: CT and magnetic resonance imaging in pancreatic and biliary tract malignancies. Gastrointest Endosc 2002;56(6 Suppl):S206–S212.

Hepatic Masses/ Hepatic Metastases

INTRODUCTION

Hepatic masses may be benign or malignant. Therapy requires an accurate diagnosis, which in turn relies primarily on appropriate imaging and image-guided biopsy. Computed tomography (CT) is the mainstay of hepatic imaging, but magnetic resonance (MR) imaging, ultrasound (US), and nuclear imaging all play a role in the workup.

Evaluation for hepatic metastatic disease is a common indication for imaging the liver in oncology patients. However, cancer does not respect anatomic boundaries, so the hepatic scan is often extended from the thoracic inlet to the pelvic floor (CT of the chest, abdomen, and pelvis).

The sensitivity and specificity of hepatic CT is markedly increased by analyzing the time course of "contrast enhancement" seen in hepatic lesions after a peripheral intravenous bolus injection of contrast medium; "contrast enhancement" is a complex function of perfusion, capillary permeability, and blood volume in a particular lesion. Rapid multidetector scanners and computer analysis allow the radiologist to tailor CT so as to define "enhancement" over time.

MR imaging can be equivalent to—or better than—CT for detection of **hepatic** lesions, but the cost is greater and extension of the examination to the pelvis and chest with similar accuracy is not feasible. US is generally less sensitive than CT or MR for detection of small hepatic lesions.

Although evaluation of the liver for neoplastic disease is the focus of this chapter, the problem of incidentally

18

discovered hepatic masses is relevant, because the liver is very often examined by CT or US for nonmalignant disease, during which solitary or even multiple lesions are identified. Unless these lesions are clearly benign, they must be further characterized by imaging or, in selected cases, biopsy. The radiologist can recommend the most effective method to evaluate such lesions.

Relative Costs: Abdominal CT, enhanced, **$$$**; abdominal MR, unenhanced, **$$$$**; abdominal MR, enhanced, **$$$$**; liver scan with labeled RBCs, SPECT, **$$$**; liver biopsy, CT-guided, **$$$–$$$$**; liver biopsy, US-guided, **$$$**; FDG-PET, **$$$$$**.

PLAN AND RATIONALE

Evaluation of suspected liver mass or suspected metastases when the patient has NO documented contraindication to intravenous contrast medium:

STEP 1: COMPUTED TOMOGRAPHY (CT) WITH INTRAVENOUS CONTRAST MEDIUM (ENHANCED)

When a primary tumor is abdominal—or is extra-abdominal but likely to involve abdominal organs or spaces—abdominal CT is the most appropriate test to search for metastases, adenopathy, and ascites. Enhanced CT can exclude hepatic metastases with a high level of confidence, and when common benign hepatic lesions (especially cysts and hemangiomas) are discovered, they can often be confidently characterized, obviating biopsy.

As contrast medium flows through the liver, the radiologist sets scan parameters that image during specific phases of the circulation. If hepatocellular carcinoma, focal nodular hyperplasia, adenoma, or certain metastases (e.g., from islet cell, carcinoid, or hepatocellular tumors) are suspected, images are best generated during the arterial phase of contrast enhancement, because these metastases may be undetected on routine delayed images. Most other metastases are best seen during the portal venous phase of enhancement when normal liver tissue is maximally enhanced. Suspected hemangiomas can also be imaged in a delayed phase.

Multiple noncystic hepatic masses (especially new masses) are presumed to represent metastatic disease in the proper clinical context. A solitary mass may require biopsy (see **CHAPTER 60**, **Percutaneous Guided Biopsy and Imaging-Guided Therapy**) or another imaging study for clarification.

A normal enhanced CT usually ends the workup.

When intravenous contrast medium is contraindicated, or when the nature of a lesion remains equivocal after enhanced CT but clinical suspicion of hepatic tumor persists:

STEP 2A: MAGNETIC RESONANCE (MR) IMAGING

MR technology has largely overcome problems related to motion artifacts from breathing, bowel peristalsis, and vascular pulsations, and the study does not require the iodinated intravenous contrast medium used for CT. A gadolinium-based contrast medium, which is usually safe even in the presence of renal failure or iodinated contrast-medium allergy, is used. A number of liver-specific MR contrast agents have been developed and may improve lesion detection in selected patients. **Furthermore, MR can often characterize many small liver lesions—as cysts or hemangiomas—that were equivocal on CT, thereby eliminating the need for biopsy or CT follow-up.**

A normal MRI usually ends the workup.

When an equivocal lesion is likely to represent a cyst, when expertise in hepatic MR is unavailable, or in the pediatric oncology population:

STEP 2A: ULTRASOUND (US)

US, although less sensitive for small liver lesions than CT or MR, can often characterize these lesions as cystic or solid, when CT is equivocal. Simple cysts can be ignored whereas solid lesions require further characterization.

US expertise is almost universally available in radiology departments, whereas expertise in hepatic MR is more variable. In the pediatric population, which should avoid unnecessary radiation exposure (from CT) and often cannot tolerate long scanning times (of MR), abdominal US is appropriate to follow patients with known or suspected metastatic disease.

> **When cavernous hemangioma of the liver is suspected after CT or US and MR is contraindicated or nondiagnostic:**

STEP 2A OR 2B: NUCLEAR MEDICINE

Once the mainstay of imaging the liver for metastatic disease, radionuclide scanning of hepatic masses is now relegated almost entirely to a single specific niche—the imaging of "blood pool" in suspected cavernous hemangiomas.

One mL of the patient's blood is drawn and the red blood cells (RBCs) are labeled with a short-lived nuclide, technetium 99m (Tc-99m), after which they are injected intravenously as a bolus. Rapid-sequence images of the liver following the peripheral intravenous injection demonstrate any areas of hyperperfusion, and subsequent static images reveal any areas of local high blood volume, termed "blood pool." Hemangiomas characteristically **do NOT** receive increased blood flow but **do** display a high blood pool.

The study is most sensitive for peripheral lesions 2 cm or more in diameter and when the static images are generated on a single-photon emission computed tomography (SPECT) camera, a device available in virtually all modern nuclear medicine departments.

A definitive nuclear scan for hemangioma ends the workup.

When pathologic characterization is required:

STEP 3: IMAGE-GUIDED PERCUTANEOUS NEEDLE BIOPSY

Most hepatic masses that can be adequately visualized are amenable to percutaneous fine-needle aspiration or core biopsy for pathologic diagnosis. Biopsies are performed using US or CT guidance. MR imaging–compatible needles are also available for the rare lesion seen only by MR. Biopsies are performed on an outpatient basis, using local anesthetic either alone or in combination with conscious sedation (see **CHAPTER 60, Percutaneous Guided Biopsy and Imaging-Guided Therapy**).

SUMMARY AND CONCLUSIONS

1. In adults, contrast-enhanced CT is the appropriate screen for hepatic metastatic disease, unless contrast medium is contraindicated. MR is also highly accurate and can be used when iodinated contrast medium is contraindicated. US is a less sensitive alternative.
2. In follow-up of children with known or suspected metastatic disease, and in screening of certain high-risk adults for hepatocellular carcinoma, US is often the procedure of choice.
3. A normal contrast-enhanced CT or normal MR imaging is sufficient to end the workup.
4. Multiple noncystic hepatic lesions, in the proper context, are considered metastatic.
5. Contrast-enhanced CT can usually characterize common benign hepatic lesions, including cysts and hemangiomas, but if CT is equivocal (generally

in the case of small lesions), MR has greater specificity.

6. When cavernous hemangioma is suspected in lesions 2 cm or larger, and CT and/or MR are equivocal, radionuclide RBC scanning is usually definitive.

7. Percutaneous image-guided needle biopsy, a relatively simple outpatient procedure, can provide tissue if required.

ADDITIONAL COMMENTS

- US is also used to screen some high-risk patients with a history of cirrhosis or hepatitis for hepatocellular carcinoma, because these patients need very frequent monitoring, and repeated CT scans would introduce an unacceptable radiation burden. Finally, **intraoperative** US—in which the sonographer works with a surgeon, placing a high-frequency US probe **directly on the liver surface**—is used to evaluate the liver before partial hepatic resection or ablation; the logic of this procedure is to eliminate the likelihood of metastases in the "good" liver that is to remain after the infiltrated liver is resected or ablated. **This technique is actually the most sensitive imaging modality for detection of small metastases.**

- Recently developed contrast agents can increase the sensitivity and specificity of US for hepatic masses, but these agents are not yet approved in the United States by the Food and Drug Administration.

- A SPECT radionuclide liver scan using Tc-99m-sulfur colloid can sometimes be helpful in diagnosing focal nodular hyperplasia; the radiolabeled colloid particles are phagocytized by reticuloendothelial cells in normal liver and in the lesion, whereas other lesions do not contain such cells and do not accumulate the radiopharmaceutical.

- Fluorodeoxyglucose–positron emission tomography (FDG-PET) is a useful imaging test with a growing number of clinical applications, especially in cancer care (see **CHAPTER 61, PET and PET/CT in Cancer Staging**). PET is not currently approved for hepatic screening, but multiple reports have established that **FDG-PET can detect hepatic metastatic disease when CT findings are normal.**

▐ SUGGESTED READING

Braga L, Guller U, Semelka RC: Modern hepatic imaging. Surg Clin N Am 2004;84:375–400.

Ji H, McTavish JD, Mortele KJ, et al: Hepatic imaging with multidetector CT. Radiographics 2001;21:S71–S80.

Kim CK, Worsley DF: Radionuclide imaging of hepatic tumors. In Ell PJ, Gambhir SS (eds): Nuclear Medicine in Clinical Diagnosis and Treatment, 3rd ed. Philadelphia, Churchill Livingstone, 2004, pp 15–22.

Oliver JH, Baron RL: Helical biphasic contrast-enhanced CT of the liver: technique, indications, interpretation, and pitfalls. Radiology 1996;201:1–14.

Withers CE, Wilson SR: The liver. In Rumack CM, Wilson SR, Charboneau JW (eds): Diagnostic Ultrasound, 2nd ed. St. Louis, Mosby, 1998, pp 87–154.

Bile Leak

INTRODUCTION

Imaging can detect, define, and follow bile leaks that develop after trauma, after open surgery, or as a complication of laparoscopic cholecystectomy. Although computed tomography (CT) and ultrasound (US or sonography) detect abnormal fluid collections in the abdomen, they cannot differentiate bile from other fluids, and they cannot determine whether a leak is ongoing or whether a fluid collection is the result of a **previous leak** that has sealed.

Nuclear biliary tract imaging with technetium 99m (Tc-99m)–hepatobiliary iminodiacetic acid (HIDA) **can detect an active leak at the time of the study.** After intravenous injection, HIDA is rapidly cleared from the circulation, accumulated by the liver, and excreted into the biliary tree. The abdomen is imaged, visualizing the common duct, cystic duct, gallbladder, and duodenum. Imaging can continue until all of the HIDA has been excreted (usually <2 hours, but occasionally 12 to 24 hours).

If the problem is postsurgical **and a T-tube remains in place,** the most direct approach is T-tube cholangiography; contrast medium is injected directly into the T-tube under fluoroscopic control, and the biliary tree is well defined. The procedure is also excellent for detecting stenoses and biliary duct calculi.

Relative Costs: T-tube cholangiogram, **$**; abdominal CT, enhanced, **$$$**; upper abdominal US, **$$**; HIDA, **$$**.

▌ PLAN AND RATIONALE

If the suspected leak is postsurgical and a T-tube remains in place:

STEP 1: T-TUBE CHOLANGIOGRAM

Direct injection of contrast medium under fluoroscopic control, through a T-tube, produces excellent filling and visualization of the extrahepatic biliary tree and much of the intrahepatic tree. Active leaks are almost always defined. If the T-tube cholangiogram is normal, the workup ends, unless there is compelling clinical evidence of an **intermittent** leak.

STEP 2: NUCLEAR HEPATOBILIARY IMINODIACETIC ACID (HIDA) SCAN

In occasional cases a T-tube cholangiogram is normal, yet signs and symptoms suggest an intermittent leak. Because HIDA is excreted over a period of hours, the "window" during which this study can detect an intermittent leak is longer than that of T-tube cholangiogram. Therefore, when an intermittent leak is suspected, a normal T-tube cholangiogram is often followed by HIDA imaging.

Although intraductal lesions and calculi are not well defined by HIDA, the presence of HIDA outside of the normal biliary tree or gut is easily detected. When bile leaks are sought, the T-tube is clamped after intravenous HIDA injection, and often the patient is imaged in the position most likely to elicit pain or leak. Sometimes follow-up images at 24 hours reveal that a slow leak has occurred overnight.

If an active leak appears, the diagnostic workup ends, unless follow-up HIDA studies are required to determine whether the leak has stopped. For purposes of anticipated intervention—either surgical repair/drainage or radiologic "guided" transcutaneous drainage—CT is often required.

Step 3: Computed Tomography (CT)

CT can define the three-dimensional anatomy of a bile collection; without this information transcutaneous drainage is nearly impossible. Furthermore, surgical intervention is greatly expedited by foreknowledge of the extent of a fluid collection.

When no T-tube is in place:

Step 1: Nuclear Hepatobiliary Iminodiacetic Acid (HIDA) Scan

Although intraductal lesions and calculi are not well defined by HIDA imaging, the presence of HIDA outside of the normal biliary tree or gut is easily detected. Often the patient is imaged in the position most likely to elicit pain or leak, and sometimes follow-up images at 24 hours reveal that a slow leak has occurred overnight.

If the HIDA study is normal, the diagnostic workup ends, unless clinical suspicion of an intermittent leak persists. In this very uncommon situation, HIDA can be repeated.

If an active leak appears, the diagnostic workup ends unless follow-up HIDA studies are required to determine whether the leak has stopped. For purposes of anticipated intervention—either surgical repair/drainage or radiologic "guided" transcutaneous drainage—CT is often required.

Step 2: Computed Tomography (CT)

CT defines the three-dimensional anatomy of a bile collection; without this information transcutaneous drainage is nearly impossible. Furthermore, surgical intervention is greatly expedited by foreknowledge of the extent of a fluid collection.

SUMMARY AND CONCLUSIONS

1. When a T-tube is in place, direct injection of contrast medium through the tube—a T-tube cholangiogram—is the first-line procedure for bile leak. Intermittent leaks may remain undetected.
2. When no T-tube is in place or when a T-tube cholangiogram fails to define a suspected intermittent leak, HIDA is appropriate.
3. CT reveals abnormal fluid collections, defines their three-dimensional anatomy, and provides essential information before transcutaneous or surgical drainage; therefore, CT sometimes follows a positive T-tube cholangiogram or HIDA study.

ADDITIONAL COMMENTS

- Patients with suspected bile leak are often postsurgical; dressings, drains, and wounds may inhibit sonography.

5 Pancreatic Mass

INTRODUCTION

Pancreatic adenocarcinoma is the fifth most common cause of cancer-related death in the United States. The prognosis is usually grim, because most pancreatic adenocarcinomas are already unresectable by the time the patient develops symptoms and a mass is discovered. Extension to peripancreatic soft tissues, adjacent organs, and regional lymph nodes is common. Other pancreatic masses include neuroendocrine tumors, a variety of cystic tumors, metastases, focal pancreatitis, and pseudocysts.

Computed tomography (CT), magnetic resonance (MR) imaging, and transabdominal ultrasound (US) can define a pancreatic mass and surrounding abdominal structures. Endoscopic retrograde cholangiopancreatography (ERCP) and endoscopic ultrasound (EUS) can sometimes detect small pancreatic tumors when CT and US findings are normal or equivocal.

ERCP is a somewhat invasive procedure that requires a gastroenterologist with special expertise. The examination is sometimes unsuccessful because of variations in anatomy, regardless of the skill and experience of the endoscopist. Acute pancreatitis can occur as a complication of ERCP in a small percentage of patients.

EUS examines the pancreas using a high-resolution US transducer at the end of an endoscope; it evaluates the pancreatic head in detail but is somewhat less effective in the pancreatic body and tail.

Relative Costs: Abdominal US, **\$\$**; abdominal CT, enhanced, **\$\$\$**; ERCP, **\$\$\$–\$\$\$\$**; endoscopic US, **\$\$\$**; pancreatic biopsy, CT-guided, **\$\$\$–\$\$\$\$**; pancreatic biopsy, US-guided, **\$\$\$–\$\$\$\$**.

▌PLAN AND RATIONALE

For suspected pancreatic carcinoma in the jaundiced patient:

STEP 1: ULTRASOUND (US)

Pancreatic lesions producing jaundice are most likely in the pancreatic head. US defines pancreatic head tumors and often other causes of jaundice, such as a gallstone in the common bile duct or a tumor in the liver or porta hepatis. It also detects bile duct dilation, differentiating obstructive from nonobstructive jaundice (see **CHAPTER 2, Biliary Tract Obstruction/Hepatic Dysfunction**).

If the pancreatic head and bile ducts are normal, and the study is of good quality, the imaging workup for suspected pancreatic cancer ends, and evaluation for nonobstructive jaundice proceeds.

In the presence of jaundice and dilated ducts, CT follows US:

- If US of the pancreas is equivocal or technically limited (e.g., in obese patients or if bowel gas is obscuring the pancreas)
- For staging, when US reveals a pancreatic mass
- If US reveals ductal dilation with no apparent cause (pancreatic head is sonographically normal), to identify a possible extremely subtle obstructing lesion

STEP 2: COMPUTED TOMOGRAPHY (CT)

CT is noninvasive and reliably images the entire pancreas and adjacent structures. A dedicated pancreatic study using multidetector CT with very thin sections through the pancreas during rapid peripheral intravenous infusion of contrast medium is appropriate, followed by delayed (portal venous phase) images to evaluate the remainder of the abdomen.

CT can characterize tumors as unresectable when invasion of soft tissue, encasement of adjacent large blood vessels, or metastatic spread is demonstrated. (Unfortunately, a pancreatic tumor may be unresectable **even without these findings,** because subtle local tumor extension or tiny metastases to the liver or peritoneum may exist, undetected by CT.)

If a pancreatic mass that obstructs biliary drainage is identified, endoscopic or percutaneous biliary stenting is often performed to alleviate jaundice. Before treatment, biopsy is usually appropriate (Step 3, below).

If no pancreatic mass is found, yet clinical suspicion is compelling, or if CT is equivocal, MR, ERCP, or EUS may be definitive.

STEP 3: MAGNETIC RESONANCE (MR) IMAGING, ENDOSCOPIC RETROGRADE CHOLANGIOPANCREATOGRAPHY (ERCP), OR ENDOSCOPIC ULTRASOUND (EUS)

If CT demonstrates a slight abnormality in pancreatic contour or a slight increase in pancreatic size without ductal dilation, a small tumor or anatomic variation may be responsible. Although not recommended as an initial imaging test, unless a patient cannot tolerate the iodinated contrast medium for CT, dedicated MR of the pancreas is often a useful problem-solving technique in these situations. MR cholangiopancreatography (MRCP) can produce images of the biliary and pancreatic ducts that are similar to those of ERCP, though of lower resolution.

Although more invasive, when MR of the pancreas is not readily available, ERCP and/or EUS also play an important role in this situation. Performed by a trained endoscopist, ERCP involves the passage of an endoscope into the duodenum, where the ampulla of Vater is visualized and cannulated. Under fluoroscopy, contrast medium is injected, filling the pancreatic duct and the biliary tree. This study reveals fine anatomic detail of the duct system and can define very small pancreatic and distal common bile duct tumors, as well as ductal stenoses. A biliary stent can also be placed and small tissue samples or brushings can be procured through the endoscope.

Similarly, if CT or US demonstrate biliary or pancreatic duct dilation but an otherwise normal pancreas, a small pancreatic head or ampullary tumor may be responsible, and ERCP and EUS may be helpful.

STEP 3: IMAGING-GUIDED BIOPSY

CT- or US-guided biopsy is appropriate to establish a diagnosis before treatment. Focal pancreatitis can occasionally simulate cancer on CT, and guided biopsy may avoid unnecessary surgery. These procedures are accurate and safe; serious complications are uncommon (see **CHAPTER 60, Percutaneous Guided Biopsy and Imaging-Guided Therapy**).

If CT of the pancreas is normal and the biliary tract is not obstructed, the imaging workup for pancreatic carcinoma in the jaundiced patient ends.

For suspected pancreatic carcinoma in the nonjaundiced patient:

STEP 1: COMPUTED TOMOGRAPHY (CT) (see above)

If a pancreatic mass is defined by CT:

STEP 2: IMAGING-GUIDED BIOPSY (see above)

If no pancreatic mass is defined by CT, yet clinical evidence is compelling:

Step 3: Magnetic Resonance (MR) Imaging, Endoscopic Retrograde Cholangiopancreatography (ERCP), Endoscopic Ultrasound (EUS) (see above)

SUMMARY AND CONCLUSIONS

1. **US is the appropriate first study in jaundiced patients.** It accurately determines whether the biliary system is dilated, may detect non-neoplastic causes of jaundice, effectively reveals many tumors of the pancreatic head, and is less expensive than CT. If a lesion is found in the pancreatic head, CT is appropriate for staging; if US is inconclusive or technically limited, CT is also appropriate.
2. **CT is the initial test of choice for imaging nonjaundiced patients with suspected pancreatic carcinoma,** because the entire pancreas and peripancreatic tissues are defined.
3. Normal findings on CT or US end the workup for pancreatic carcinoma in the jaundiced patient **without** biliary dilation.
4. If CT reveals a suspicious contour abnormality or if pancreatic cancer is suspected despite a normal finding on CT in the nonjaundiced patient, MR, ERCP, EUS, or percutaneous imaging-guided biopsy may help to confirm the presence or absence of tumor.

ADDITIONAL COMMENTS

- Multidetector CT scanners produce extremely thin, high-resolution images during the optimal phase of contrast medium enhancement, without respiratory motion artifact. CT evaluation of peripancreatic vascular invasion has improved sufficiently; **preoperative conventional angiography is no longer necessary.**

- Pancreatic tumor may cause pancreatitis by obstructing the pancreatic duct. **Unexplained pancreatitis that fails to respond to conservative therapy should be studied by ERCP, because ductal obstruction and encasement by a small tumor may be responsible.**

SUGGESTED READING

Brand R: The diagnosis of pancreatic cancer. Cancer J 2001;7:287–297.

Horton KM, Fishman EK: Multidetector CT angiography of pancreatic carcinoma: Part 1, evaluation of arterial involvement. AJR Am J Roentgenol 2002;178:827–831.

Horton KM, Fishman EK: Multidetector CT angiography of pancreatic carcinoma: Part 2, evaluation of venous involvement. AJR Am J Roentgenol 2002;178:833–836.

Kalra MK, Maher MM, Sahani DV, et al: Current status of imaging in pancreatic diseases. J Comput Assist Tomogr 2002;26:661–675.

Reznek RH, Stephens DH: The staging of pancreatic adenocarcinoma. Clin Radiol 1993;47:373–381.

Shin HJC, Lahoti S, Sniege N: Endoscopic ultrasound-guided fine-needle aspiration in 179 cases. Cancer 2001;96:174–180.

Tamm E, Charnsangavej C: Pancreatic cancer: current concepts in imaging for diagnosis and staging. Cancer J 2001;7:298–311.

Pancreatitis

INTRODUCTION

The clinical presentation of acute pancreatitis can vary from mild abdominal discomfort to catastrophic hypovolemia and multi-organ failure. Symptoms include abdominal pain, back pain, nausea, vomiting, anorexia, and fever. Most pancreatitis is related to excessive alcohol intake or underlying gallstones that migrate down the bile ducts and obstruct the pancreatic duct. However, pancreatitis has many potential causes, including medications, congenital abnormalities, abdominal trauma, and metabolic disorders. Most cases (70% to 80%) are mild and self-limiting; however, chronic pancreatitis can develop after repeated episodes of acute inflammation. Although the initial diagnosis and estimation of prognosis are primarily based on clinical history, physical examination, and laboratory tests, imaging plays an important role in management.

Ultrasound (US) is indicated in suspected pancreatitis to evaluate the biliary tract for stones or obstruction. Additional imaging with computed tomography (CT) is appropriate for patients with atypical presentations and those with more severe pancreatitis who may develop complications such as pancreatic hemorrhage or necrosis, pseudocyst, pseudoaneurysm, or abscess.

Overall, CT is the best single imaging test to evaluate the pancreas and surrounding structures. Endoscopic retrograde cholangiopancreatography (ERCP) and endoscopic ultrasound (EUS) can define subtle abnormalities of the biliary and pancreatic ducts and guide interventions to relieve obstruction from stones or strictures;

however, these tests—particularly ERCP—are much more invasive than CT or US.

Relative Costs: US, **$$**; CT, **$$$**; EUS, **$$$**; ERCP, **$$$$**.

PLAN AND RATIONALE

(A) MILD ACUTE PANCREATITIS

STEP 1: ULTRASOUND (US)

Generally, no imaging is required beyond abdominal US to exclude gallstones as a cause and to examine the bile ducts for obstruction (dilation). The patient should fast for at least 4 to 6 hours before US, so that the gallbladder becomes distended with bile. The pancreas itself may appear normal sonographically or show very subtle peri-pancreatic inflammation in mild cases. Whereas the head and body of the pancreas are well seen with US, the pancreatic tail is often incompletely visualized because of overlying bowel gas.

If gallstones are present, elective cholecystectomy is usually warranted, after the acute episode resolves, to prevent future episodes of pancreatitis or cholecystitis.

In the presence of a mild attack, if no calculi or ductal dilation is seen, the workup ends. However, if ongoing biliary obstruction from a common bile duct stone is suspected or if a common duct stone is defined and does not pass spontaneously, then ERCP may be warranted.

STEP 2: ENDOSCOPIC RETROGRADE CHOLANGIOPANCREATOGRAPHY (ERCP)

ERCP is primarily for therapeutic procedures. The procedure involves passage of an endoscope down the esophagus, through the stomach, and into the duo-denum, after which the pancreatic duct is cannulated and contrast medium injected under fluoroscopic guidance. **ERCP generates detailed images of the pancreatic and bile ducts and may define strictures, stones, and congenital abnormalities when other noninvasive studies are negative or equivocal.** During this procedure a papillotomy is feasible, through which a stone can be removed or pass.

ERCP is performed in the radiology department by a skilled gastroenterologist. Unfortunately, injection/manipulation of the pancreas during ERCP can cause iatrogenic pancreatitis.

(B) Severe or Atypical Pancreatitis

Step 1: Computed Tomography (CT)

Overall, the best single imaging test to evaluate the pancreas is CT performed with intravenous contrast medium (contrast enhanced). The scan is timed relative to the peripheral contrast medium infusion so that the pancreas is imaged during maximal pancreatic contrast enhancement; afterward the remainder of the abdomen is scanned. The severity of pancreatitis can be graded and complications—including pancreatic hemorrhage or necrosis, splenic or portal venous thrombosis, pseudoaneurysm, and pseudocyst or abscess formation—can be detected. The bile ducts are also evaluated for obstruction.

Superimposed infectious complications often require intervention. If the patient's condition indicates infection of a necrotic pancreas, surgery is usually required. Infected pseudocysts or abscesses can usually be drained by the radiologist (see **CHAPTER 60, Percutaneous Guided Biopsy and Imaging-Guided Therapy**). Persistent pseudocysts larger than 5 to 7 cm generally are drained percutaneously or surgically marsupialized to the gastrointestinal tract. Unless infection is suspected, marsupialization is not performed for approximately 6 weeks, to allow a mature wall to form around a pseudocyst. **Both CT and US can guide percutaneous aspirations and drainages.**

If CT reveals uncomplicated pancreatitis and gall-stones, the workup ends, **but if CT does not demonstrate stones, US is appropriate.**

STEP 2: ULTRASOUND (US)

Noncalcified gallstones are frequently undetected by CT, so US should be performed to detect them and prevent further attacks. (US is also useful to follow complications such as pancreatic pseudocyst; most pseudo-cysts smaller than 5 cm shrink or remain stable over time and do not require treatment if asymptomatic.)

If US defines calculi in the gallbladder, they should be removed after the acute episode resolves. An obstructing stone in the common duct may require ERCP (see **Mild Acute Pancreatitis,** above).

(C) CHRONIC PANCREATITIS

Chronic pancreatitis is characterized by recurrent episodes of inflammation and pain, leading to varying degrees of glandular fibrosis. **Complications of acute pancreatitis mentioned previously affect these patients as well, but morphologic damage in chronic pancreatitis may also lead to loss of pancreatic exocrine and endocrine function over time.** As the pancreas atrophies, episodes of acute pancreatitis may occur without appreciable elevations of serum amylase and lipase.

STEP 1: ULTRASOUND (US)

US is warranted to exclude cholelithiasis as a cause, but inflammation of the pancreas itself may not be defined. Therefore, if confirmation is required in the presence of normal ultrasound, CT is appropriate.

STEP 2: COMPUTED TOMOGRAPHY (CT)

CT can define acute inflammation as well as chronic changes of pancreatic atrophy, calcification, and ductal dilation. Although CT is less sensitive than ERCP to very early findings of chronic pancreatitis, it is far less invasive and, therefore, comes first.

If confirmation of the diagnosis is necessary in problematic cases, or if an obstructing stone or other abnormality in the pancreatic or bile duct is suspected, ERCP is appropriate.

STEP 3: ENDOSCOPIC RETROGRADE CHOLANGIOPANCREATOGRAPHY (ERCP)

ERCP can show subtle changes in the contour of the pancreatic duct and side branches not visible with CT. ERCP can also demonstrate communication of pseudocysts with the pancreatic ducts and can guide stone removal as well as papillotomy. If the diagnosis remains uncertain even after ERCP, endoscopic ultrasound (EUS) is the remaining option.

STEP 4: ENDOSCOPIC ULTRASOUND (EUS)

EUS, generally performed by a trained gastroenterologist, images the pancreas using a small ultrasound transducer at the end of an endoscope placed in the adjacent stomach and duodenum. It can be used to evaluate both the ducts and pancreatic parenchyma, often allowing a more confident diagnosis of chronic pancreatitis.

SUMMARY AND CONCLUSIONS

1. After a diagnosis of pancreatitis, abdominal US is indicated to rule out gallstones as a cause and to rule out ongoing biliary obstruction, which may

    necessitate endoscopic stone removal or papillotomy.

2. CT is indicated in cases of suspected moderate or severe pancreatitis, which are often associated with complications, or when the clinical presentation is nonspecific. Newer, multidetector CT scanners produce superb images of the pancreas and other abdominal organs, so that the severity of pancreatitis and its various complications can be assessed.

3. ERCP is primarily for therapeutic procedures, although it may be used for diagnosis only, after CT, in problematic cases. **ERCP generates detailed images of the pancreatic ducts and may define strictures, stones, and congenital abnormalities when other noninvasive studies are negative or equivocal.** During this procedure a papillotomy is feasible, through which an obstructing stone can be removed or pass. EUS is used with increasing frequency in the evaluation of **chronic** pancreatitis.

ADDITIONAL COMMENTS

- Occasionally, pancreatic, duodenal, or biliary **malignancies** may obstruct the pancreatic duct and present with an episode of pancreatitis.
- Occasionally, focal, mass-like areas of chronic inflammation may mimic pancreatic carcinoma and cause a diagnostic dilemma (see **CHAPTER 5**, **Pancreatic Mass**). Biopsy of such areas can be guided by CT, transabdominal US, or EUS.
- Magnetic resonance cholangiopancreatography (MRCP) is being used with increased frequency. Carefully performed MRCP can produce images of the biliary and pancreatic ducts similar to, though lower in resolution than, those of ERCP, **thereby avoiding the inherent risk of ERCP-induced pancreatitis. Pancreatic MR imaging can**

substitute for CT in patients unable to tolerate iodinated contrast medium due to renal insufficiency or allergy.

SUGGESTED READING

Ahmad NA, Shah JN, Kochman ML: Endoscopic ultrasonography and endoscopic retrograde cholangiopancreatography imaging for pancreaticobiliary pathology. The gastroenterologist's perspective. Radiol Clin N Am 2002;40:1377–1395.

Balthazar EJ: Staging of acute pancreatitis. Radiol Clin N Am 2002;40:1199–1209.

Maher MM, Lucey BC, Gervais DA, Mueller PR: Acute pancreatitis: the role of imaging and interventional radiology. Cardiovasc Intervent Radiol 2004;27:208–225.

Pitchumoni CS: Pancreatic diseases. In Stein JH (ed): Internal Medicine. St. Louis, Mosby, 1998, pp 2233–2247.

Remer EM, Baker ME: Imaging of chronic pancreatitis. Radiol Clin N Am 2002;40:1229–1242.

Turner MA: The role of US and CT in pancreatitis. Gastrointest Endosc 2002;56(6 Suppl):S241–S245.

7 Acute and Chronic Gastrointestinal Bleeding in the Adult

ACUTE GASTROINTESTINAL BLEEDING

INTRODUCTION

Acute gastrointestinal bleeding, indicated by grossly bloody gastric aspirate, hematemesis, hematochezia, or severe melena, must be differentiated from chronic gastrointestinal bleeding, usually indicated by iron deficiency anemia or stools positive for occult blood. These clinical problems require different imaging approaches.

When endoscopy identifies a bleeding site, emergency diagnostic imaging is unnecessary but when endoscopy is technically unfeasible—or fails because of excessive hemorrhage—emergency imaging plays a key role. Nuclear imaging demonstrates or confirms active bleeding and, if possible, localizes its approximate site, so that **selective** angiography for more precise localization can proceed. **However, massive or life-threatening hemorrhage in a patient not taken directly to the operating room is frequently studied only by angiography.**

Barium in the intestinal lumen hinders subsequent endoscopic, angiographic, and nuclear investigations. Therefore, if any of these studies are contemplated in patients with acute gastrointestinal (GI) bleeding, **an upper GI series or barium enema should be delayed** (see **ADDITIONAL COMMENTS** for the later role of barium studies; **in the acute setting, barium examinations have virtually no role**).

Relative Costs: Tc-99m-RBC bleeding study, **$$$**; visceral abdominal angiogram, superior mesenteric artery (SMA), inferior mesenteric artery (IMA), celiac, **$$$$$.**

PLAN AND RATIONALE

STEP 1: TECHNETIUM 99M–LABELED RED BLOOD CELL (TC-99M-RBC) STUDY

The goal of the nuclear examination is to document active bleeding as a precursor to angiography, which, during an active bleed, is a high-yield procedure.

A few mL of the patient's own red blood cells (RBCs) are removed, labeled with technetium 99m (Tc-99m), and reinjected. The labeled RBCs circulate normally. If bleeding is present, serial images of the abdomen usually reveal focal accumulation of radiolabeled RBCs in the gut lumen. The labeled RBC technique can detect bleeding rates as low as 0.05 to 0.1 mL/minute. Accurate **localization** of the bleeding site, as opposed to **proof that there is on-going bleeding,** requires recognition of specific bowel segments as extravasated radiopharmaceutical along with blood enters the bowel lumen and moves, driven by peristalsis.

Because labeled red cells in the gut lumen are not resorbed, and because pharmaceutical in the circulation persists for hours, bleeding that has occurred **at any time between radiopharmaceutical injection and imaging may be identified. In this respect, the nuclear scan differs markedly from the angiogram, because active bleeding must exist at the time of contrast medium injection for angiographic detection.**

If the nuclear study documents and approximately localizes active bleeding, angiography is appropriate for therapy (embolization) or to better localize the lesion and its vascular anatomy, as a presurgical "road map."

If nuclear imaging documents the presence of active bleeding but does not localize its site,

angiography can often identify the site and even the cause.

If nuclear imaging fails to document active bleeding, most angiographers are reluctant to proceed, because angiography without documentation of an ongoing bleed is a low-yield procedure.

STEP 2: CATHETER ANGIOGRAM

Angiography is usually performed via percutaneous transfemoral arterial puncture. Under fluoroscopic guidance a catheter is threaded cephalad through the aorta and subsequently positioned in the vessel to be studied, usually the superior mesenteric, inferior mesenteric, or celiac artery. (The vessel is selected by the preliminary localization of the bleeding site on a nuclear scan, by clinical signs/symptoms—i.e., upper or lower GI tract—or, if none of these guidelines are available, on statistical grounds.) Then, over several seconds, contrast medium is injected and the abdomen is radiographed repeatedly. Bleeding points are defined as the contrast medium extravasates from the vascular space into the gut lumen; a bleeding rate of at least 0.5 to 1.0 mL/ minute is required at the time of contrast medium injection.

About two thirds of upper GI bleeds originate in the stomach or first portion of the duodenum, and one third result from ruptured esophageal varices. Angiography successfully localizes the source of bleeding in the majority of patients with duodenal and gastric lesions but seldom demonstrates bleeding varices, because the contrast medium is usually very dilute in the late stages of an arteriogram when varices are best visualized. However, if gastric aspirate contains blood and gastroesophageal varices are identified, these varices are usually assumed to represent the bleeding site, even if no contrast medium extravasation during the angiogram is seen. Vascular ectasia (angiodysplasia) of the cecum and ascending colon characteristically presents as small, dilated clusters of arteries and veins on angiography; a specific diagnosis can be made even in the absence of acute bleeding.

SUMMARY AND CONCLUSIONS

1. When endoscopy defines a bleeding source, emergency imaging is usually unnecessary, unless a specific angiographic intervention can treat the hemorrhage.
2. Massive or life-threatening GI hemorrhage not immediately treated surgically should be studied by angiography.
3. When endoscopy fails to find a bleeding source, nuclear imaging is often useful to document (and sometimes approximately localize) active bleeding as a precursor to angiography.
4. Angiography may be invaluable for therapy or more precise localization before surgery, once nuclear imaging has confirmed ongoing hemorrhage. If nuclear imaging reveals no active bleeding, neither will angiography, unless the patient coincidentally rebleeds at the time of the angiogram.
5. Barium studies have no role in the initial evaluation of acute GI bleeding.

ADDITIONAL COMMENTS

- Barium studies do not actually demonstrate bleeding itself, and barium in the GI tract interferes with subsequent angiographic, nuclear, and endoscopic procedures. Therefore **barium exams are best avoided in the initial evaluation of acute bleeding.**
- Meckel's diverticulum may acutely bleed, especially in children. A nuclear study can localize Meckel's diverticulum, regardless of whether bleeding is active. Tc-99m pertechnetate is injected intravenously and the abdomen is imaged. The radiopharmaceutical

concentrates in the ectopic gastric mucosa commonly present in symptomatic Meckel's diverticula.

- **Angiographic treatment of acute GI bleeding is often effective when more conservative therapies have failed.** This method is ideal for high-risk surgical candidates; in other patients, it is an important temporizing measure, permitting surgery at the most opportune time, rather than as an emergency. The angiographic technique most commonly used is selective intra-arterial embolization, most commonly with a temporary agent, such as Gelfoam slurry or pledgets, which is resorbed days to weeks later, allowing the vessel to heal. Vessel selection must be precise to control the bleed but preserve collateral flow in the GI tract. Supers selectivity may not be an option for postsurgical patients whose native blood supply has been disrupted; thus, they are at an increased risk of bowel ischemia/infarction.

  When sufficiently selective catheterization is impossible, or the site lacks collateral flow to supply adjacent bowel, intra-arterial infusion of vasopressin may be initiated. Vasopressin infusion requires an indwelling arterial catheter and careful monitoring for 24 to 48 hours, usually in an intensive care unit. Its effectiveness is probably due to smooth muscle contraction of both the GI tract wall and the vascular tree, reducing blood flow and promoting thrombosis. The complications of vasopressin therapy are usually minor and easily managed. Bowel infarction is very unusual if excessive vasospasm is avoided.

- A variation in angiographic diagnosis involves the infusion of agents such as heparin, streptokinase, or urokinase that **provoke or prolong** bleeding. This technique, diagnostic pharmacoangiography, is sometimes useful when bleeding has stopped by the time of diagnostic angiography. The short-term resumption of bleeding permits precise localization. This procedure, however, introduces the risk of uncontrollable bleeding and is performed with **extreme** trepidation.

CHRONIC GASTROINTESTINAL BLEEDING

▌ INTRODUCTION

Chronic gastrointestinal (GI) bleeding usually presents with iron deficiency anemia or stools positive for occult blood.

Colonoscopy and upper intestinal tract endoscopy have largely replaced venerable barium exams in the evaluation of chronic bleeding. "Virtual colonoscopy," a computed tomography (CT)-based imaging examination of the colon, has recently been developed, but its indications are highly specific (see **ADDITIONAL COMMENTS**), and it is not considered a first-line test in the workup of chronic GI bleeding.

Relative Costs: Small bowel barium study, **$**; enteroclysis, **$**; visceral abdominal angiogram, IMA, SMA, celiac, **$$$$$**; Meckel's diverticulum nuclear scan, **$$**; virtual colonoscopy, **$$$**.

▌ PLAN AND RATIONALE

STEPS 1 AND 2: CALL THE GASTROENTEROLOGIST, NOT THE RADIOLOGIST!

When the entire gut is to be surveyed for a chronic bleeding site, upper and lower GI endoscopy should precede any imaging studies.

However, if no bleeding site is found, the small bowel must be studied by imaging.

STEP 2: SMALL BOWEL SERIES AND, IF AVAILABLE, ENTEROCLYSIS

The standard small bowel series, which is simply a series of abdominal X-rays after oral ingestion of barium, is notorious for missing small lesions. Although meticulous technique may improve the sensitivity of standard exams, some institutions use "enteroclysis" as their primary small bowel study in patients with a high likelihood of disease.

For enteroclysis, a nasoduodenal tube is inserted and positioned with its tip near the ligament of Treitz, and a small balloon is inflated to maintain this position. Barium is introduced at about 100 mL/minute. The distal progression of barium is followed fluoroscopically. Air, water, or even methylcellulose may be added through the tube after barium for better mucosal coating.

Enteroclysis is available in only a limited number of centers. Because the examination is lengthy and requires a nasoduodenal tube, it is somewhat uncomfortable, although without major risk.

If findings from upper and lower endoscopy and a small bowel series (preferably enteroclysis) are negative, angiography is the next option.

STEP 3: ANGIOGRAPHY

Angiography can occasionally identify lesions that cause chronic blood loss.

After percutaneous transfemoral introduction, a catheter is advanced into the aorta. The major feeding vessels of the GI tract are catheterized and contrast medium injected, defining the vascular pattern of the gut and any lesions. In cases of **chronic**—as opposed to **acute**—bleeding, extravasation of contrast material into the bowel lumen is typically **not** seen, because the rate of bleeding is too slow and usually intermittent (below 1.0 mL/minute). However, the vascular pattern of some lesions that cause chronic bleeding can be identified, particularly arteriovenous malformations, including angiodysplasia of the colon, especially in the elderly; they are assumed to represent the bleeding source when other abnormalities are not defined. Occasionally, small neoplasms undetected by endoscopy and even entero-clysis are discovered.

If angiography fails to define a lesion that could slowly bleed, Meckel's diverticulum is rarely responsible.

STEP 4: RADIONUCLIDE MECKEL'S DIVERTICULUM SCAN

Meckel's diverticulum may rarely produce chronic GI bleeding, even in adults. The lesion can sometimes be identified, because its ectopic gastric mucosa concentrates a radiopharmaceutical, Tc-99m pertechnetate, within 2 hours of intravenous injection. Sensitivity of the pertechnetate scan is approximately 75% when ectopic gastric mucosa is present.

SUMMARY AND CONCLUSIONS

1. Endoscopy identifies the majority of lesions responsible for chronic bleeding.
2. Enteroclysis is a barium study of the small intestine. Some centers perform enteroclysis as their usual small intestinal series, whereas others perform a routine small bowel study first.
3. Endoscopy and small bowel studies usually precede angiography.
4. In chronic bleeding, angiography does not define the active bleeding site but locates abnormal vascular patterns, such as angiodysplasia, arteriovenous malformation, and neoplasm, which may produce chronic blood loss.
5. Meckel's diverticulum scans are sometimes useful, especially in children.

ADDITIONAL COMMENTS

- Nuclear medicine techniques for evaluation of acute gastrointestinal bleeding are not useful in chronic bleeding, because the rate of blood loss in chronic bleeding is too low.
- In adults, a Meckel's diverticulum scan usually follows endoscopy and an angiogram, but in children it is earlier in the workup, because the lesion is a more common cause of chronic bleeding in the pediatric population, and endoscopy is much more traumatic for children.

- The venerable barium enema and upper GI series, once the principal diagnostic imaging studies in chronic GI bleeding, are now afterthoughts. However, in cases of chronic bleeding, after all else has failed, an upper GI series is a worthwhile study, because endoscopy is highly operator dependent and there may be endoscopic blind spots in the stomach, sometimes dependent upon gastric anatomy. The examination is simple to perform, safe, and rapid; there is no downside.

- "Virtual colonoscopy" is a CT examination of the abdomen. Preparation for the study is the same as for actual colonoscopy, but less sedation is required during the examination. Nonetheless, a rectal (not colonic) tube is required, and the colon must be distended with air before imaging. The CT data are computer-manipulated so that the colon can be viewed in conventional "slice" mode or displayed so that the colon is seen from the inside, as if visualized through a conventional colonoscope, called the "fly through" mode. The accuracy of virtual colonoscopy compared with that of conventional colonoscopy is now under study; early data indicate that they are roughly equivalent. However, conventional examinations allow a biopsy of a lesion when it is identified, whereas the "virtual" examination identifies lesions that must **later** be biopsied through a standard scope.

  Some advocates recommend that "virtual colonoscopy" replace the conventional "garden hose" examination for chronic GI bleeding and colon cancer screening. This conclusion is premature and problematic, because (1) many who have undergone conventional colonoscopy report that the most demanding part of the procedure is the prep **before** the procedure, and this prep **is the same for both examinations** (both require an empty, clean colon); (2) although less sedation is required for the "virtual" examination, "less" is not necessarily an advantage for the general population, because the sedation reduces discomfort, and the air insufflation for the "virtual" examination is universally reported as uncomfortable; and (3) a lesion identified on the "virtual" examination must then be biopsied through a conventional scope.

Therefore, we suggest that current indications for "virtual colonoscopy" be limited to (1) patients with sufficient anxiety to prevent conventional colonoscopy; (2) patients with comorbid conditions severe enough to contraindicate full conscious sedation; and (3) patients with a known, partially occluding colonic lesion that will not permit passage of a scope but will permit passage of air. The surgeon needs to know "what is on the other side," and virtual colonoscopy is ideal for this purpose.

Acknowledgment. The authors gratefully acknowledge the critical help of Garin Tomaszewski, MD, Assistant Professor of Radiology, State University of New York School of Medicine and Biomedical Sciences at Buffalo, NY, and Director, Section of Angio/Interventional Radiology, The Roswell Park Cancer Institute, Buffalo, NY.

8 Acute and Chronic Mesenteric Ischemia

INTRODUCTION

Mesenteric ischemia is an increasingly common problem in our aging population. Both chronic and acute ischemia represent a diagnostic challenge for clinicians and radiologists; both need to maintain a high index of suspicion when faced with abdominal pain in the appropriate clinical context.

Acute mesenteric ischemia most frequently results from acute insult(s), such as hypotension or embolus, often superimposed upon pre-existent atherosclerosis of the mesenteric arterial circulation. In a minority of patients, the acute event is a thrombosis in the mesenteric venous system. Alternatively, ischemia may follow bowel obstruction.

In acute small bowel mesenteric ischemia, patients present with pain and elevation of both the white cell count and serum lactic acid, sometimes with diarrhea and/or vomiting. **Unfortunately, symptoms, especially in the nonocclusive forms of acute mesenteric ischemia, are often nonspecific.**

Acute small bowel ischemia is an emergency with a high mortality rate and usually requires immediate surgery (resection of infarcted bowel, if the patient is a surgical candidate, often with a vascular arterial bypass), **whereas most patients with acute colonic ischemia (i.e., ischemic colitis) are managed conservatively. Prognosis is directly related to the duration of the ischemic event and the extent of bowel infarction.**

Chronic mesenteric ischemia most often affects older adults with high-grade atherosclerotic

52

stenoses (or occlusions) of at least two of the three mesenteric arteries (celiac, superior mesenteric, and inferior mesenteric). The classic history is postprandial pain (abdominal angina) out of proportion to physical findings, along with weight loss and anorexia.

For two generations, the diagnostic imaging study for mesenteric ischemia was conventional catheter angiography. Recently, computed tomography (CT) and magnetic resonance (MR) imaging, especially when applied as CT angiography (CTA) and MR angiography (MRA), have supplanted catheter angiography for the diagnosis of both acute and chronic mesenteric ischemia, because CT/CTA and MR/MRA **can evaluate both the bowel itself and its associated mesenteric vascular system.**

Relative Costs: CT/CTA, **$$$**; MR/MRA, **$$$$**.

PLAN AND RATIONALE

(A) Acute Mesenteric Ischemia

Step 1: Computed Tomography/Computed Tomographic Angiography (CT/CTA) or Magnetic Resonance Imaging/Magnetic Resonance Angiography (MR/MRA)

For patients with suspected acute mesenteric ischemia, the test of choice is CT/CTA.

A typical protocol includes the rapid peripheral administration of intravenous contrast medium (with or without oral contrast medium), usually along with a "neutral" oral contrast agent (water), **followed by imaging as the intravenously injected contrast medium passes through the arteries of the mesentery and as it later fills the portal veins, creating images of both the arterial and venous circulation.**

The condition of the bowel itself—especially of the small bowel—is evaluated. Bowel wall thickening and/or dilation, abnormal perfusion, and findings of bowel compromise, including gas in the wall and mesenteric venous system, can be identified. The "arterial phase" images can be reconstructed to demonstrate the central arterials in multiple planes and with three-dimensional imaging to reveal stenoses, occlusions, and central emboli, and the "venous phase" images identify mesenteric venous thrombosis. The latest scanners can define smaller, more peripheral vascular lesions as well.

MR/MRA is an alternative for patients who cannot tolerate iodinated contrast medium (see **INTRODUCTION** to this book for a discussion of this topic). However, for patients who can tolerate iodinated contrast medium, CT/CTA is preferable, because of its much shorter scanning times, lower cost, and compatibility with virtually all life support systems, and because the status of the bowel and complications of ischemia (such as air in the bowel wall) are more readily identified.

(B) CHRONIC MESENTERIC ISCHEMIA

Where advanced MR techniques and MR expertise are available:

STEP 1: ADVANCED MAGNETIC RESONANCE/MAGNETIC RESONANCE ANGIOGRAPHY (MR/MRA)

Advanced MR/MRA can estimate blood flow to the bowel, both before and after a meal "challenge," but even without this special technique, MRA can estimate the patency of the central mesenteric arteries.

We emphasize that advanced MRA (where available) provides the dual advantages of a safer gadolinium-based contrast medium and the information provided by a postprandial meal "challenge."

Where advanced MR techniques are unavailable:

STEP 1: COMPUTED TOMOGRAPHY/COMPUTED TOMOGRAPHIC ANGIOGRAPHY (CT/CTA)

CT/CTA is capable of demonstrating stenoses in the major mesenteric arteries and is an acceptable alternative where a postprandial meal "challenge" with MR/MRA is not available.

STEP 2: INTERVENTIONAL RADIOLOGY: CONVENTIONAL CATHETER ANGIOGRAPHY

Conventional catheter angiography remains the best test for demonstrating the smaller arteries of the mesenteric circulation as well as collaterals, and catheter angiography remains a mainstay of therapy.

The interventional radiologist can treat a minority of acute mesenteric ischemia patients with direct infusion of a vasodilator into the mesenteric arterial circulation, in cases of nonocclusive ischemia—if bowel infarction has not yet occurred. Alternatively, catheter techniques may be appropriate for treatment of some patients with acute embolic or thrombotic occlusions. Selection of such patients is an emergent matter to be discussed between the surgeon and interventional radiologist.

Some patients with chronic mesenteric ischemia can be treated with angioplasty/stent placement.

SUMMARY AND CONCLUSIONS

1. **CTA is the test of choice for suspected acute mesenteric ischemia.** The condition of the bowel itself can be defined (normal versus ischemic/infarcted), along with the presence or absence of vascular disease: mesenteric arterial stenosis, occlusion or emboli, and mesenteric venous patency. The bowel findings on CTA, however, are often not specific for ischemia, especially earlier in the disease course, and careful

correlation with the status of the vasculature and the patient's status is needed.

2. For suspected chronic mesenteric ischemia, either CTA or MRA can evaluate the central mesenteric arteries. Advanced MRA can study blood flow after a meal challenge (i.e., postprandial ischemia).

3. Catheter angiography remains superior to CTA and MRA for showing the entire arterial and venous mesenteric circulation, although it is no longer the primary test for evaluation of either acute or chronic mesenteric ischemia. A variety of angiographic techniques can treat mesenteric ischemia, although many patients require definitive surgery.

ADDITIONAL COMMENTS

- Careful correlation of the imaging findings and clinical information is essential in patients with suspected chronic mesenteric ischemia, **because the presence and severity of stenoses do not necessarily correlate with the clinical diagnosis.** Similarly, CT/CTA in acute mesenteric ischemia may be nonspecific, and correlation with the history, physical, and laboratory findings is key.

- Ischemic colitis usually presents with nonspecific colonic thickening on CT; however, the typical distribution of left colonic involvement, extending from the splenic flexure caudad, should suggest the diagnosis in the correct clinical setting. Other portions of the colon may also be affected.

- The esophagus, stomach, and duodenum are only rarely sites of mesenteric ischemia.

- Plain x-rays may suggest or even diagnose acute mesenteric ischemia in some patients (e.g., thickened bowel loops; air in the bowel wall, portal/mesenteric veins, or under the diaphragm), **but their sensitivity and specificity are grossly inferior**

to CT/CTA, and plain films should not be a primary test when the diagnosis is suspected.

- Stenoses of the celiac and superior mesenteric arteries can be identified on ultrasound (US, or sonography), using a variety of techniques (e.g., before and after eating); **however, we do not advocate US for the workup of patients with suspected mesenteric ischemia—particularly in acute ischemia—because of limited visualization of the aortic branches in larger adults and limited visualization of the small bowel.**

- Diffuse spasm related to nonocclusive acute mesenteric ischemia is best demonstrated on conventional angiography—and then can be treated with intra-arterial vasodilators if appropriate—but is potentially also defined by CT angiography.

- The differential diagnosis of mesenteric ischemia is lengthy and includes hypercoagulable states, iatrogenic etiologies, vasculitis, radiation therapy, drugs, and invasive tumors.

▌ SUGGESTED READING

Chang JB, Stein TA: Mesenteric ischemia: acute and chronic. Ann Vasc Surg 2003;17:323–328.

Chow LC, Chan FP, Li KC: A comprehensive approach to MR imaging of mesenteric ischemia. Abdom Imaging 2002;27:507–516.

Cognet F, Ben Salem D, Dranssart M, et al: Chronic mesenteric ischemia: imaging and percutaneous treatment. Radiographics 2002;22:863–880.

Horton KM, Fishman EK: Multi-detector row CT of mesenteric ischemia: can it be done? Radiographics 2001;21:1463–1473.

Kirkpatrick ID, Kroeker MA, Greenberg HM: Biphasic CT with mesenteric CT angiography in the evaluation of acute mesenteric ischemia: initial experience. Radiology 2003;229:91–98.

Martinez JP, Hogan GJ: Mesenteric ischemia. Emerg Med Clin N Am 2004;22:909–928.

Oldenburg WA, Lau LL, Rodenberg TJ, et al: Acute mesenteric ischemia: a clinical review. Arch Intern Med 2004;164:1054–1062.

Wiesner W, Khurana B, Ji H, Ros PR: CT of acute bowel ischemia. Radiology 2003;226:635–650.

Small Bowel Obstruction

INTRODUCTION

Small bowel obstruction (SBO) is common. Eighty percent or more of all intestinal obstructions occur in the small bowel, and 80% of these result from adhesions or hernias. Another cause is metastatic cancer; abdominal or pelvic infection/inflammation (e.g., perforated diverticulitis, perforated appendicitis, inflammatory bowel disease) is less frequent, and primary small bowel tumor is relatively rare. Small bowel dilation may also result from "downstream" large bowel obstruction.

Sometimes the diagnosis of SBO is straightforward, but it can be difficult. SBO also must be differentiated from adynamic ileus, which may follow any abdominal insult or result from a wide variety of extra-abdominal or systemic diseases.

The hallmark of SBO is a "transition zone" at the junction of normal and obstructed bowel, unless the site of obstruction is at the ileocecal valve, in which case the entire small bowel is dilated, mimicking adynamic ileus.

Adynamic ileus usually responds to conservative therapy—nasogastric tube drainage and medical treatment of the underlying disorder—whereas many patients with SBO require surgery.

Relative Costs: Plain films, **$**; CT, **$$$**.

▌PLAN AND RATIONALE

STEP 1: PLAIN RADIOGRAPHS (PLAIN FILMS): SUPINE, UPRIGHT, AND DECUBITUS (PATIENT LIES ON HIS/HER SIDE)

Although plain films are severely limited compared with computed tomography (CT), they can be useful when (1) an immediate approximate answer is requested **and the patient cannot go to CT, or CT is not immediately available;** (2) the index of suspicion for SBO is very high, surgery is planned, and the specific localizing information potentially provided by CT is not going to change patient management; and (3) the clinical index of suspicion is relatively low, and negative plain films would end the workup.

Establishing the presence or absence of free intraperitoneal air is key, because in the setting of SBO, free air almost always indicates bowel perforation. Air rises in the abdomen, so that **upright** films can be used to diagnose or exclude free air seen under the diaphragm. If the patient is too ill for erect films, decubitus films may reveal air **along the upright flank. An upright chest film is strongly recommended, because free air under the diaphragms is usually better seen on a chest film than on an abdominal film.**

The plain film (and CT) diagnosis of small bowel obstruction rests on the fact that proximal to an obstruction the bowel distends, usually with fluid and swallowed air, whereas distal to an obstruction it empties of both, forming a "transition zone" between dilated and collapsed small bowel. The transition zone represents the site of obstruction (e.g., adhesion, hernia, tumor). **Thus, typical findings in "high-grade" SBO include multiple dilated small bowel loops, with decreased or absent colonic gas (Fig. 9-1).** Air-fluid levels of unequal heights in each dilated bowel loop may appear on upright or decubitus radiographs, because active

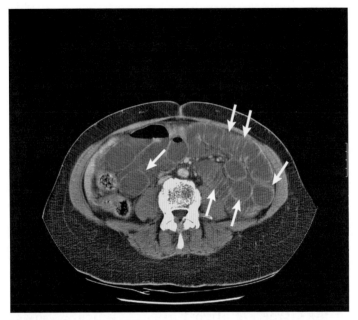

Figure 9-1. Abdominal CT in a 54-year-old woman with high-grade distal small bowel obstruction secondary to adhesions related to previous hysterectomy. CT with intravenous contrast medium demonstrates multiple dilated small bowel loops (*arrows*). The right colon is collapsed.

peristalsis continues proximal to an obstruction, and at the instant of film exposure it is likely that air is at different heights in the proximal and distal loops of any given actively contracting bowel segment.

Although the diagnosis is clear in some patients, **the diagnosis of SBO on plain films is often tenuous:** adynamic ileus may resemble a "lower grade" SBO, dilated small bowel loops filled with fluid (but not air) may be radiographically invisible or difficult to identify, and air-fluid levels of unequal heights on a given segment may result from other conditions. Moreover, a very proximal SBO may present with few dilated bowel loops, and the bowel proximal to the obstruction may be empty of air as a result of repeated vomiting; further-more, in early obstruction, colonic gas may remain (the bowel distal to the obstruction has not yet had time to empty). Finally, even if the diagnosis of SBO can be established, the site of obstruction may not be evident, nor the cause, and the status of the small bowel (and surrounding structures) may not be well defined. **Therefore, plain films are significantly less accurate than CT for the diagnosis of SBO.**

Step 2: Computed Tomography (CT)

CT is the definitive test of choice for suspected SBO.

CT is much more accurate than plain films, because it frequently demonstrates the transition zone (**or, if SBO is absent, may reveal an alternate diagnosis**) and may define **the cause of the obstruction. CT is sufficiently accurate that adhesions, the most common cause of SBO, can be confidently inferred in the postsurgical patient, when CT fails to define another cause.**

Many radiologists avoid oral contrast medium when SBO is suspected, especially if the obstruction may be high grade, because (1) if SBO **is** present, oral contrast medium further distends the proximal bowel; (2) oral contrast medium delays the scan (abdominal CT is usually performed about an hour after contrast medium ingestion, so that the contrast medium satisfactorily opacifies distal bowel loops, and although this protocol is ideal when the goal is to differentiate bowel loops from masses, in the case of high-grade SBO **a delay is undesirable**); (3) intragastric contrast medium may be vomited and aspirated by a severely obstructed patient; (4) oral contrast medium is unlikely to reach the point of obstruction; and (5) during SBO, water in dilated small bowel loops serves as an intrinsic contrast medium.

Oral contrast medium may be used in select cases, however, at the discretion of the radiologist.

Secondary bowel ischemia may be more readily identified after intravenous contrast medium, so this medium is appropriate in suspected **high-grade** SBO, but intravenous contrast medium is not needed simply to establish or exclude SBO.

CT also can demonstrate "closed-loop" obstruction (a characteristic 180-degree semi-circular orientation of dilated bowel loops around the mesentery); in this event, **immediate surgery is required. (Closed-loop obstruction occurs from blockage at two separate points—two sites of adhesion, an internal hernia, or small bowel volvulus—which can lead to bowel strangulation, decreased blood supply, and bowel infarction.)**

STEP 3: FOLLOW-UP PLAIN RADIOGRAPHS, FOLLOW-UP COMPUTED TOMOGRAPHY (CT), OR ADDITIONAL SMALL BOWEL STUDIES (SMALL BOWEL FOLLOW-THROUGH, ENTEROCLYSIS, AND CT ENTEROCLYSIS)

Imaging follow-up depends on the patient's clinical status. After surgery or during conservative management, no additional imaging may be necessary, although as-needed plain radiographs can be used to confirm the absence of recurrent SBO or adynamic ileus.

Whether to use conventional fluoroscopic imaging studies or special variations of these studies for patients immediately following or during conservative management of SBO is controversial. **Such studies, including enteroclysis and CT enteroclysis, are contraindicated in high-grade SBO, but they can be performed when the obstruction is resolving, low grade, or intermittent.** In problematic cases, these examinations can sometimes determine whether an obstruction persists and can sometimes define the cause.

The conventional small bowel examination or "small bowel follow-through" involves oral administration of barium and sequential fluoroscopic and radiographic study of the barium column as it progresses distally. The specific cause of obstruction may be difficult to identify, **because the barium column is progressively diluted by intraluminal fluid as it progresses, reducing its visibility.**

Particularly if the workup has been inconclusive, enteroclysis can be more precise and can detect subtle lesions, including adhesions and tumors. However, the procedure is demanding for the patient and requires special radiologic expertise. Under fluoroscopic control, the end of a long trans-nasal tube is placed into the proximal jejunum. Barium, followed by a solution of methylcellulose, is infused (either by hand injection or by mechanical pump) directly into the jejunum. The barium-methylcellulose column is followed as it progresses to the site of obstruction. The study is preferable to a basic small bowel follow-through, because it is usually faster and delivers a contrast medium bolus directly into the small bowel **without significant dilution** of the barium. Serial radiographs define the obstruction. The study may be modified into CT enteroclysis; rather than serial radiographs, a CT immediately follows luminal contrast medium administration, and intravenous contrast may also be administered. **CT enteroclysis combines the optimal luminal distention and contrast enhancement of enteroclysis with the cross-sectional advantages of CT.**

SUMMARY AND CONCLUSIONS

1. Plain films have significant limitations for the diagnosis or exclusion of SBO but can be performed initially in several circumstances: if the patient cannot immediately go to CT and a high-grade obstruction is suspected, when the surgeon wants only confirmation prior to surgery, or if the clinical index of suspicion is relatively low and a negative plain film study would end the workup.
2. Ideally, supine, upright, and decubitus radiographs should be included.
3. Free intraperitoneal air in a patient with an SBO almost always indicates bowel perforation. The best plain radiograph to show free intraperitoneal gas is an **upright chest film.**

4. **CT is the test of choice for suspected SBO.** The technique we prefer is **with intravenous but without oral contrast medium.**

5. The hallmark of SBO on CT is the identification of a transition zone, unless the site of obstruction is at the ileocecal valve. CT may also reveal the cause of the SBO.

6. **Findings of closed-loop obstruction on CT should prompt immediate surgery, as irreversible small bowel necrosis may occur or may have already occurred.**

7. Follow-up imaging studies, especially if the patient is initially managed conservatively, include repeat plain films, repeat CT, or additional testing—small bowel follow-through, enteroclysis, or CT enteroclysis.

ADDITIONAL COMMENTS

- Closed-loop obstruction may be difficult to diagnose on plain films, because there is insufficient gas trapped in the closed loop to produce characteristic air-fluid levels. The fluid-filled bowel loops may produce a "pseudotumor," but this appearance is not specific. Plain film findings in closed-loop obstruction can even be normal.

- With current CT technology, the imaging data set can be easily manipulated (into various reconstructions), which may assist in identification of a transition zone or an internal hernia.

- Other etiologies of SBO that may be identified or suggested on CT include Crohn's disease, intussusception, luminal foreign body, and a gallstone (in "gallstone ileus").

- Ultrasound has a limited role in the evaluation of SBO. Hyperperistaltic, dilated, and fluid-filled small bowel loops are directly visualized, but the presence, absence, and site of a transition zone usually cannot be established.

- "Capsule endoscopy" (the patient swallows a pill containing a tiny camera that transmits pictures of the gut to a receiver) has become a major factor in the workup of small bowel disease. However, **in the setting of SBO, capsule endoscopy is contraindicated, because the pill may become lodged proximal to the obstruction.**

SUGGESTED READING

Balthazar EJ, Birnbaum BA, Megibow AJ, et al: Closed-loop and strangulating intestinal obstruction: CT signs. Radiology 1992;185:769–775.

Boudiaf M, Soyer P, Terem C, et al: CT evaluation of small bowel obstruction. Radiographics 2001;21:613–624.

Furukawa A, Yamasaki M, Takahasi M, et al: CT diagnosis of small bowel obstruction: scanning technique, interpretation, and role in diagnosis. Semin US CT MRI 2003;24:336–352.

Harlow CL, Stears RL, Zeligman BE, Archer PG: Diagnosis of bowel obstruction on plain abdominal radiographs: significance of air-fluid levels at different heights in the same loop of bowel. Am J Roentgenol 1993;161:291–295.

Maglinte DD, Kelvin FM, Rowe MG, et al: Small-bowel obstruction: optimizing radiologic investigation and nonsurgical management. Radiology 2001;218:39–46.

Megibow AJ, Balthazar EJ, Cho KC, et al: Bowel obstruction: evaluation with CT. Radiology 1991;180:313–318.

Sandrasegaran K, Maglinte DD, Howard TJ, et al: The multifaceted role of radiology in small bowel obstruction. Semin US CT MRI 2003;29:319–335.

Appendicitis/ Diverticulitis

SUSPECTED APPENDICITIS

INTRODUCTION

Appendicitis is the most common indication for emergency abdominal surgery in the western world. Although it can occur at any age, appendicitis is most common during the second decade of life; its lifetime risk is about 7%. Although the clinical diagnosis is straightforward in some patients, in others—especially the elderly, young children, and women of childbearing age—it is often challenging. Elderly patients often manifest few (or nonspecific) clinical signs and symptoms; infants and young children give no history and are prone to appendiceal perforation; and gynecologic disease (rupture of an ovarian cyst, pelvic inflammatory disease, and ovarian torsion) in women of childbearing age commonly mimics appendicitis. In these patients, computed tomography (CT) may be extremely helpful. Moreover, even in young adult males, **CT is more accurate than clinical findings and can suggest or establish alternative diagnoses, demonstrate complications such as perforation or abscess, and serve as a preoperative "road map."**

CT reduces the rate of negative exploratory surgery and is therefore particularly cost-effective. Its accuracy in appendicitis is 95% to 98%, it is more accurate than sonography, and it is also superior for defining other processes

in the abdomen and pelvis that may mimic appendicitis.

Relative Costs: US, **$**; CT, **$$$**.

PLAN AND RATIONALE

For all patients (except for pregnant women or women of childbearing age in whom the likelihood of gynecologic disease is high):

STEP 1: COMPUTED TOMOGRAPHY (CT)

The entire abdomen and pelvis are imaged. Most radiologists administer both oral and intravenous contrast medium to best prove that the appendix is normal or abnormal and optimally demonstrate alternative conditions.

If either a normal or clearly abnormal appendix (Fig. 10-1) is identified or if the appendix is not identified but the examination findings are otherwise negative, the imaging workup almost always ends.

Occasionally, when the initial CT is equivocal for appendicitis, or when the patient's complaints worsen after initially negative or equivocal CT findings, short-interval repeat CT (e.g., in 12 to 24 hours) is appropriate. Normal findings on repeat CT end the workup, but if an alternative diagnosis is established or suggested, the imaging workup proceeds, depending on the specific findings.

CT also defines complications of appendiceal perforation, such as abscess, and can be a road map for surgery; for example, it is helpful for the surgeon to know preoperatively if the appendix is atypical in location (retrocecal or in the right mid- or upper abdomen).

For pregnant women or women of childbearing age in whom the probability of gynecologic disease is high:

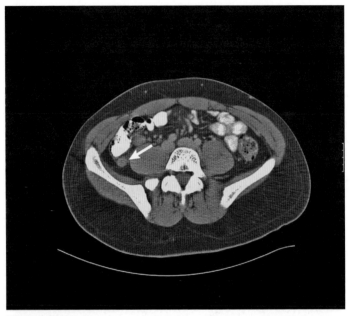

Figure 10-1. Abdominal CT in a 23-year-old man with right lower quadrant pain. CT shows an enlarged (12 mm in diameter) fluid-filled retrocecal appendix (*arrow*) in cross-section, with an enhancing wall and mild surrounding inflammatory changes. Appendicitis was confirmed at surgery.

STEP 1: ULTRASOUND (US, OR SONOGRAPHY)

Multiple investigations have proven the superiority of CT over US for suspected appendicitis, in both adults and children, even when US is performed by an expert, and thus the role of sonography in suspected appendicitis has diminished. However, when radiation is to be avoided (e.g., in pregnant women or women of childbearing age), or when gynecologic disease is likely and the pretest probability of appendicitis is low, US is a reasonable first option.

A "graded compression" technique is used. A linear (i.e., rectangular) transducer is placed over the point of maximal tenderness. The underlying bowel is slowly and gently compressed and displaced. The normal appendix, although often difficult to identify, is a tubular, compressible structure, with a transverse diameter of 6 mm or less. A noncompressible appendix with a transverse diameter of more than 6 mm (in adults or children) is highly suggestive of appendicitis. Periappendiceal abscess or collections may also be identified. Color Doppler sonography (see the **INTRODUCTION** to this book for a brief discussion of Doppler ultrasound) augments the examination and may reveal increased blood flow in the wall of an inflamed appendix. If the appendix is not identified, the remainder of the pelvis and abdomen is examined to seek other possible causes of symptoms. **Unlike CT, US is operator dependent and may fail when the appendix is obscured by bowel gas or when the patient is obese or very tender and cannot tolerate the examination.**

Transvaginal sonography is complementary to transcutaneous US.

If the appendix is not identified and there is no clear alternative diagnosis, then CT is appropriate in the face of significant symptoms.

SUMMARY AND CONCLUSIONS

1. CT is the best imaging examination for almost all patients with suspected appendicitis. Radiologists generally administer both oral and IV contrast medium.

2. The traditional approach of blind surgical exploration of the acute abdomen is obsolete unless the diagnosis is completely straightforward.

3. Although its role has diminished, US may be useful, when performed by an expert radiologist/ sonographer, in selected patients: pregnant women (avoiding radiation is key) or a woman of childbearing age when gynecologic disease is likely. However, CT may ultimately be necessary in many of these patients.

■ ADDITIONAL COMMENTS

- Some hospitals with strong pediatric radiology groups prefer US as the initial test in young children with suspected appendicitis, but in the absence of an experienced pediatric radiologist, or in a general rather than pediatric hospital, we prefer CT.
- CT findings of appendicitis include a distended, fluid-filled appendix with an "enhancing" wall, which may be associated with inflammatory changes in the adjacent fat (see **INTRODUCTION** to this book for a discussion of the enhancement phenomenon).
- Appendicoliths (hard, sometimes calcified debris in the appendix) can be discovered on CT or other imaging tests (e.g., on plain films or on US), but if the appendix is otherwise normal, an isolated appendicolith does not indicate appendicitis.
- Magnetic resonance (MR) imaging without contrast medium (nonenhanced) is an emerging test that appears to be better than US in pregnant patients with suspected appendicitis. Radiation is avoided, appendicitis can be diagnosed or excluded with higher accuracy than with US, and alternative diagnoses are often possible. (MR is believed to be safe in pregnancy, particularly in the second and third trimesters.)

DIVERTICULITIS

■ INTRODUCTION

Diverticulitis is the most common cause of left lower quadrant pain in adult males and is also relatively common in women. Diverticular disease has been associated with a western lifestyle and an aging population. Onset may be acute or subacute, associated with change in bowel habits, fever, and an elevated white cell count. The clinical findings are often nonspecific and may be simulated by a variety of alternative diagnoses; therefore, routine imaging of all patients with suspected diverticulitis has been advocated. Although much more commonly affecting the sigmoid and/or descending colon, right-sided and even transverse diverticulitis may also occur. Attacks commonly recur. The appropriate management of diverticulitis remains controversial (i.e., which patients should undergo resection—at the time of the first attack or after multiple recurrences), but the test of choice for suspected diverticulitis is clearly CT.

▌ PLAN AND RATIONALE

STEP 1: COMPUTED TOMOGRAPHY (CT)

CT is appropriate for all patients with suspected diverticulitis, particularly when complications are suspected. For this purpose the venerable barium enema (BE) is now obsolete. Although a BE will show diverticu**losis** and complications of diverticulitis (such as fistulas and communicating pericolonic pus collections/abscesses), **it cannot reveal the inflammatory changes in the adjacent fat, the associated mesenteric and fascial thickening, or the small noncommunicating pericolonic fluid collections that are the hallmarks of the disease.**

Regardless of whether it is truly cost-effective for patients with a suspected first episode of diverticulitis to undergo CT or whether CT should be reserved for patients who do not respond to conservative management, the reality of current practice is that **most patients do initially undergo CT**—to confirm the clinical diagnosis, to search for complications, to establish a baseline, and to exclude alternative diagnoses.

Several CT protocols are effective for patients with suspected diverticulitis, and each has advantages and disadvantages; most radiologists use both oral and intravenous contrast medium. This protocol optimally defines pericolonic pus collections and alternative diagnoses (such as pyelonephritis or gynecologic disease). Other protocols involve only rectal contrast medium (usually water soluble), which unlike oral contrast medium reaches the descending colon almost

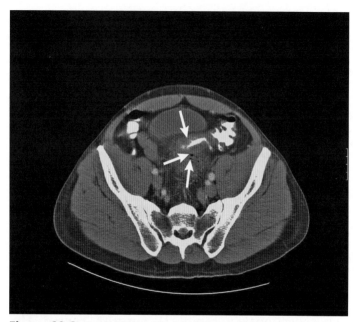

Figure 10-2. Pelvic CT in a 38-year-old man with fever and left lower quadrant abdominal pain, due to sigmoid diverticulitis. CT shows thickening of the sigmoid colonic wall (*top arrow*) in association with diverticulosis, inflammation in the adjacent fat, and an extraluminal gas collection (*lower arrows*), representing a localized sigmoid perforation.

instantly, speeding up the examination. Alternatively, CT without **any** contrast medium permits immediate imaging; this protocol is most useful in patients with ample fat around the colon, so that the presence or absence of inflammatory changes within fat adjacent to the colon can be identified.

CT also defines localized "microperforations" (i.e., small collections of extraluminal gas) (Fig. 10-2) as well as abscesses and secondary small bowel obstruction, and the technique is effective for optimal patient management, guiding drainages of pericolonic fluid collections/abscesses, and following up progress of the disease.

SUMMARY AND CONCLUSIONS

1. CT is appropriate for all patients with suspected diverticulitis, and it is ideal for defining suspected complications. The best protocol, however, remains unproven; we prefer both oral and intravenous contrast medium.
2. As in cases of suspected appendicitis, CT is very useful for revealing alternative diagnoses.

ADDITIONAL COMMENTS

- **US** is inferior to CT for diverticulitis, but for a woman of childbearing age, when gynecologic disease is likely on clinical grounds, sonography is a reasonable first option.
- Very mild cases of diverticulitis can be subtle, **even on CT.** Findings may include colonic wall thickening, which could simply represent chronic wall hypertrophy related to diverticul**osis.**
- In a small percentage of patients presenting with what initially appears to be diverticulitis, there may be an underlying neoplasm, usually perforated colonic adenocarcinoma. Underlying colon cancer should be kept in mind in the senior age group, especially if the patient has undergone no previous colon cancer screening.

SUGGESTED READING (Suspected Appendicitis)

Terasawa T, Blackmore CC, Bent S, Kohlwes RJ: Systematic review: computed tomography and ultrasonography to detect acute appendicitis in adults and adolescents. Ann Intern Med 2004;141:537–546.

Urban BA, Fishman EK: Targeted helical CT of the acute abdomen: appendicitis, diverticulitis, and small bowel obstruction. Semin US CT MRI 2000;21:20–39.

Wijetunga R, Doust B, Bigg-Wither G: The CT diagnosis of acute appendicitis. Semin US CT MRI 2003;24:101–106.

Wilson EB: Surgical evaluation of appendicitis in the new era of radiographic imaging. Semin US CT MRI 2003;24:65–68.

■ SUGGESTED READING (Diverticulitis)

Ambrosetti P, Jenny A, Becker C, et al: Acute left colonic diverticulitis—compared performance of computed tomography and water-soluble contrast enema: prospective evaluation of 420 patients. Dis Colon Rectum 2000;43:1363–1367.

Kaiser AM, Jiang JK, Lake JP, et al: The management of complicated diverticulitis and the role of computed tomography. Am J Gastroenterol 2005;100:910–917.

Kircher MF, Rhea JT, Kihiczak D, Novelline RA: Frequency, sensitivity, and specificity of individual signs of diverticulitis on thin-section helical CT with colonic contrast material: experience with 312 cases. Am J Roentgenol 2002;178:1313–1318.

Urban BA, Fishman EK: Targeted helical CT of the acute abdomen: appendicitis, diverticulitis, and small bowel obstruction. Semin US CT MRI 2000;21:20–39.

Part II

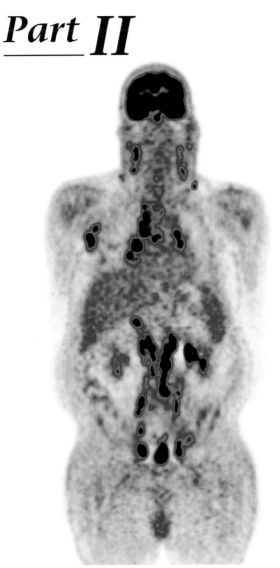

Genitourinary

11 Renal Colic/Unilateral Upper Urinary Tract Obstruction

INTRODUCTION

Unilateral upper urinary tract obstruction is defined as obstruction of a single kidney and/or its corresponding ureter.

Renal "colic" is the pain caused by an obstructing ureteral stone—the most common cause of unilateral urinary tract obstruction and a very common reason for imaging in emergency departments. The lifetime incidence is up to 12%, and the correct clinical diagnosis is often unclear, although patients usually present with flank pain that may radiate to the back or the groin, with or without hematuria. Most ureteral stones are believed to arise from initially asymptomatic calculi that develop in the renal medullary pyramids, enter the urinary tract, and migrate into the ureter, where they cause acute obstruction and pain—sometimes extremely severe.

Over the past decade, **computed tomography (CT) performed without oral or intravenous contrast medium ("unenhanced" or "nonenhanced") has become the imaging test of choice to establish or exclude an obstructing ureteral stone. For a variety of reasons—speed, accuracy, better sizing of stones and determination of "stone burden," and, particularly, for establishing alternative diagnoses—CT has completely replaced the venerable intravenous urogram or pyelogram (IVU or IVP).** CT is also better than ultrasound (US, or sonography), because most **ureteral** calculi are extremely difficult to identify on sonography.

Other much less common causes of unilateral obstruction include blood clot, stricture, and tumor;

these have a variety of clinical presentations—acute, subacute, or chronic, with or without hematuria (see **CHAPTER 12, Hematuria**). Imaging is appropriate in the setting of flank (i.e., probably renal) pain, when a stone or other etiology is suspected. Regardless of the cause of unilateral urinary tract obstruction (unless there is a solitary kidney or pre-existing renal insufficiency), blood urea nitrogen (BUN) and creatinine remain normal.

Relative Costs: CT, unenhanced, **$$$**; CT, enhanced, **$$$**; US, **$$**; MR, **$$$$**.

▌PLAN AND RATIONALE

(A) Suspected Renal Colic

Step 1: Computed Tomography (CT) without Contrast Medium ("Unenhanced" or "Nonenhanced" or "Noncontrast" CT)

CT without contrast medium was first introduced as a test for suspected obstructing ureteral stone in 1995. The examination is rapid (no patient preparation required). Accuracy is extremely high, because almost **all urinary tract stones are sufficiently dense to be seen by CT.** Also, almost all patients with obstruction develop some degree of unilateral secondary findings such as hydronephrosis, hydroureter, edema of fat around the kidney and/or ureter, or swelling of the kidney. **The severity of findings correlates with the duration and degree of obstruction.** Because renal colic is rarely bilateral, the opposite side serves as an intrinsic control. CT can also reveal concurrent calculi in the kidneys, which indicate that the patient may be at future risk of subsequent renal colic and/or have a metabolic abnormality that predisposes to stone formation.

Findings on CT are very useful for planning patient management. For example, a 2-mm stone at the ureterovesical junction (the junction

between the distal ureter and bladder) is extremely likely to pass with only conservative management (pain medication, intravenous hydration), whereas an 8-mm stone at the ureteropelvic junction (junction of the ureter and renal pelvis) is likely to need urologic intervention.

CT is invaluable for demonstrating alternative causes of pain that can simulate renal colic. Pyelonephritis (appearing on CT as a swollen kidney with surrounding edema, but usually without significant hydronephrosis or hydroureter), appendicitis, diverticulitis, colitis, ovarian cysts, pancreatitis, and even ruptured abdominal aortic aneurysm can sometimes be diagnosed by nonenhanced CT.

In a minority of patients, the ureteral stone may have passed by the time of CT; pain may decrease or persist due to residual ureteral spasm. In such cases, a calculus is either absent or seen in the bladder. **The vast majority of these patients are managed conservatively, without further imaging. However, if the radiologist suspects an alternative urinary tract process causing obstruction, or if the patient's pain does not resolve, additional testing may be indicated** (see **Unilateral Upper Urinary Tract Obstruction, below**).

If CT is diagnostic of an obstructing ureteral stone or is completely negative without concern for a significant alternative abdominal diagnosis (e.g., the patient is believed to have spinal/vertebral pain and will be followed up appropriately), or if CT conclusively demonstrates an alternative diagnosis or is consistent with a recently passed stone, the imaging workup ends.

If suspicion of abdominal disease persists, despite negative findings on CT, or to clarify a CT that is equivocal for an alternative diagnosis:

STEP 2: REPEAT "ENHANCED" CT (WITH INTRAVENOUS AND SOMETIMES ORAL CONTRAST MEDIUM)

A normal "enhanced" CT ends the workup.

Alternative diagnoses made on enhanced CT are dealt with individually.

(B) UNILATERAL UPPER URINARY TRACT OBSTRUCTION PROBABLY UNRELATED TO STONE DISEASE

Many conditions besides calculi may cause upper urinary tract obstruction—ureteral stricture (postinflammatory, postsurgical, or congenital), retroperitoneal fibrosis, ureteral tumor (usually transitional cell cancer), metastatic disease to the ureter, extrinsic obstruction by posterior abdominal masses, and even intraureteral endometriosis.

If ureteral obstruction is acute (e.g., from a blood clot secondary to an underlying bleeding renal mass), patients may present with suspected renal colic and initially undergo a nonenhanced CT (see **Suspected Renal Colic, Step 1,** above).

For suspected unilateral upper urinary tract obstruction **probably unrelated to stone disease,** US is an appropriate initial examination.

STEP 1: ULTRASOUND (US, OR SONOGRAPHY)

Sonography is a good test for determining whether subacute or chronic unilateral upper urinary tract obstruction is present. However, **sonography usually does not reveal the cause or the level of the obstruction.**

If sonography findings are completely normal, the *upper tract* workup ends, but the workup continues if disease in the more distal urinary tract (ureter or bladder) is suspected clinically (e.g., hematuria; see **CHAPTER 12, Hematuria**).

Patients with extremely acute urinary tract obstruction often have no or minimal/subtle

hydronephrosis on sonography, because the collecting systems may not yet have had time to dilate; in such cases, short-interval repeat sonography in 12 to 24 hours is an inexpensive and effective option.

If sonography reveals any significant dilation, CT or magnetic resonance (MR) imaging is appropriate to establish the cause.

STEP 2: COMPUTED TOMOGRAPHY (CT) OR MAGNETIC RESONANCE (MR) IMAGING

CT is the imaging test of choice for evaluating suspected or probable unilateral upper urinary tract obstruction, once sonography has confirmed that some dilation is present. In contrast to US, the retroperitoneum is readily visualized on CT, and intrinsic ureteral lesions such as tumor and/or stricture, as well as extrinsic processes (secondary ureteral invasion/compression by an adjacent mass), are very well shown. In general, intravenous contrast medium (with or without oral contrast medium) is the key to demonstrating normal and abnormal anatomy, and to confirm that if there is unilateral dilation of the renal collecting system and ureter, there is **obstruction as well as dilation,** because **obstruction affects the excretion rate of contrast medium in addition to producing physical enlargement of the collecting system. In other words, a rough evaluation of renal function, as an indication of obstruction, is possible with contrast medium** (see **ADDITIONAL COMMENTS** for the role of nuclear studies in this regard).

MR is equally effective. One advantage of MR imaging is that heavily T2-weighted images (or so-called "MR urography") may help in evaluation of the exact site of obstruction; for example, a "filling defect" (caused by an intraureteral blood clot and/or tumor) may be shown at the transition zone from dilated ureter to collapsed ureter. (See **INTRODUCTION** to this book for a discussion of MR technology and image weighting.)

Once the cause of the obstruction has been defined, the diagnostic workup ends, but imaging is key to the next step in therapy: **decompression.**

STEP 3: DECOMPRESSION OF THE OBSTRUCTED URINARY TRACT: RETROGRADE PYELOGRAM OR ANTEGRADE PYELOGRAM

A unilateral upper urinary tract obstruction may be decompressed from below: a urologist passes a cystoscope through the urethra and bladder into the ureter and attempts to visualize the obstruction. Diagnostic and therapeutic choices include biopsy, stent placement, and even (at selected centers) endoscopic ultrasound (EUS); during the procedure contrast medium may be instilled under fluoroscopy, producing a "retrograde pyelogram," which may show subtle **ureteral** abnormalities undetectable by other modalities. Alternatively, if there is obstruction at the uteropelvic junction or high in the ureter, an interventional radiologist may puncture the collecting system percutaneously, using US guidance, and place a nephrostomy tube. Introduction of contrast medium followed by fluoroscopy produces an "antegrade pyelogram" that can provide some additional diagnostic detail (see **CHAPTER 60**, **Percutaneous Guided Biopsy and Imaging-Guided Therapy**).

SUMMARY AND CONCLUSIONS

1. CT without oral or intravenous contrast medium is the imaging test of choice for patients with suspected renal colic. The examination is extremely accurate for the diagnosis or exclusion of an obstructing ureteral stone, permits precise stone sizing and localization, determines the overall "stone burden," shows secondary findings of obstruction in almost all patients with an

obstructing ureteral stone, and reveals significant alternative or additional diagnoses.

2. In patients with a negative nonenhanced CT, in the face of continued strong clinical suspicion of a significant alternative diagnosis, or in patients with equivocal nonenhanced CT, the study should be repeated with intravenous and sometimes oral contrast medium.

3. The workup of known or strongly suspected **unilateral upper urinary tract obstruction unrelated to stone disease is similar to that of bilateral obstruction and includes sonography, CT, and/or MR;** more invasive testing/procedures include retrograde or antegrade studies, with the prime therapeutic goal of decompression.

ADDITIONAL COMMENTS

• Plain radiographs, although previously the diagnostic mainstay of renal colic, are substantially inferior to CT for demonstrating urinary tract calcifications, particularly within the ureter. For calculi dense enough and large enough to be clearly visible, however, plain films may be used **to follow up** patients with urinary tract calcifications. In some patients, for whom the evolution of findings would make a major difference in management, CT may be serially repeated to determine if the stone is still present and where. Caution is appropriate in following young stone formers, so that their radiation burden from serial CT examinations is not excessive.

• US is appropriate as an alternative to CT for suspected renal colic when radiation dose is a concern in children and pregnant women. However, the yield is disappointingly low, and the authors favor either a special lower-dose CT or, when available, **MR urography;** the latter requires no contrast medium. To date, large series showing the accuracy and utility of MR urography in both children and pregnant women have not been published to our knowledge.

- The classic IVP and IVU (intravenous pyelogram or intravenous urogram—terms synonyms for the same examination) have been completely eliminated by CT in almost all situations, particularly for acute renal colic and hematuria (see **CHAPTER 12, Hematuria**).

- Sometimes sonography and/or CT reveals a collecting system that is significantly dilated without evidence of obstruction in any part of the urinary tract. This pattern represents a diagnostic conundrum. Such a system may represent the residual "stretching" of previous-but-now-relieved obstruction, usually on the basis of stones that formed previously and then passed. A Lasix diuretic renogram can provide a definitive diagnosis. The Lasix renogram, performed in all nuclear medicine departments, is based upon the fact that an intravenous Lasix infusion augments urine flow and empties a dilated but not obstructed system rapidly, whereas a truly obstructed system does not drain rapidly under the pressure of augmented urine output. Because a radionuclide that is excreted by the kidney is used to image the kidney, the radioactivity in the kidney can easily be quantified and its passage through the kidney plotted as a function of time and compared to normal values as well as the contralateral "control."

▌ SUGGESTED READING

Abramson S, Walders N, Applegate KE, et al: Impact in the emergency department of unenhanced CT on diagnostic confidence and therapeutic efficiency in patients with suspected renal colic: a prospective study. AJR Am J Roentgenol 2000;175:1689–1695.

Katz DS, Scheer M, Lumerman JH, et al: Alternative or additional diagnoses on unenhanced helical computed tomography for suspected renal colic: experience with 1000 consecutive examinations. Urology 2000;56:53–57.

Manthey DE, Teichman J: Nephrolithiasis. Emerg Med Clin North Am 2001;19:633-652.

Rucker CM, Menias CO, Bhalla S: Mimics of renal colic: alternative diagnoses at unenhanced helical CT. Radiographics 2004;24:S11–S33.

Sudah M, Vanninen RL, Partanen K, et al: Patients with acute flank pain: comparison of MR urography with unenhanced helical CT. Radiology 2002;223:98–105.

Tamm EP, Silverman PM, Shuman WP: Evaluation of the patient with flank pain and possible ureteral calculus. Radiology 2003;228:319–329.

Teichman JM: Acute renal colic from ureteral calculus. N Engl J Med 2004;350:684–693.

12 Hematuria

INTRODUCTION

Hematuria—especially microscopic hematuria—is a common problem, and most patients **do not** have an underlying lesion, such as a renal mass, that can be identified by imaging. Although gross hematuria usually prompts a urologic workup and imaging studies, the diagnosis, etiology, and management of asymptomatic microscopic hematuria are controversial. Up to 15% of normal individuals may have occasional hematuria; therefore, the American Urological Association has strictly defined microscopic hematuria as three or more red blood cells per microscopic high-power field on at least two of three urinalyses obtained from specimens midstream "clean-catch."

The causes are legion (urinary tract obstruction, infection, tumor, obstructing ureteral stone) and the presentation variable (painless or painful). In select patients, especially those with gross or painful hematuria and middle-aged to older patients with recurrent hematuria—clinical or occult—imaging may be indicated.

Invariably, computed tomography (CT) is the test of choice.

Relative Costs: CT, enhanced, **\$\$\$**; US, **\$\$**; MR, **\$\$\$\$**.

PLAN AND RATIONALE

(A) PAINLESS RECURRENT HEMATURIA

(See also **CHAPTER 13, Renal Mass.**)

STEP 1: COMPUTED TOMOGRAPHIC UROGRAPHY (CT UROGRAPHY)

The consensus among radiologists is that CT urography, a multiphasic contrast-enhanced abdominal CT, is the test of choice for the evaluation of painless, recurrent hematuria. This exam has replaced the venerable intravenous urogram (IVU), also sometimes called an intravenous pyelogram (IVP).

CT images are generated before, during, and shortly after a peripheral intravenous contrast medium infusion. CT's sensitivity and specificity for depicting and assisting the radiologist in characterizing renal lesions are superior to those of IVU, and CT images can be computer manipulated, reformatted, and adjusted in a variety of ways (e.g., to create images in multiple planes and to see through contrast medium that might obscure ureteral and bladder lesions).

Initial noncontrast-medium–enhanced images of the abdomen (and sometimes pelvis) are obtained, followed by contrast-enhanced imaging of the kidneys, followed by thin-section images of the kidneys, ureters, and bladder during the "excretory" phase of contrast medium (starting several minutes after contrast medium administration).

The bladder may be filled by having the patient drink a large glass of water before the scan, and an abdominal "compression device" may be placed over the lower abdomen to distend the ureters. A radiologist reviews the images, looking for an "enhancing" renal mass (see **INTRODUCTION** to this book for a discussion of the "enhancement" phenomenon), a ureteral or bladder mass, an obstructing stone, or other causes of the hematuria.

After CT urography, the imaging workup usually ends.

STEP 2: CYSTOSCOPY

Even state-of-the-art multidetector CT cannot reveal small bladder or ureteral masses, and if hematuria persists, cystoscopy, performed by a urologist, is indicated.

(B) HEMATURIA ASSOCIATED WITH ACUTE PAIN

STEP 1: CT OF THE ABDOMEN AND PELVIS WITHOUT ORAL OR IV CONTRAST MEDIUM, FOR A SUSPECTED URETERAL STONE

(See also **CHAPTER 11, Renal Colic.**) **The imaging test of choice for patients with suspected renal colic (i.e., due to an obstructing ureteral stone) is CT of the abdomen and pelvis, without oral or intravenous contrast medium.**

For urinary tract stones, the sensitivity and specificity of CT are very high, the exact size and location of stones can be determined, findings of associated obstruction are identified, **and alternative diagnoses—many in the differential diagnosis of hematuria associated with pain (e.g., pyelonephritis, appendicitis, diverticulitis)—can be suggested or defined.**

In selected cases, the examination can be repeated while the patient is still on the CT table or soon after, with intravenous and/or oral contrast medium, to clarify the initial CT findings. Nonenhanced CT (supplemented by enhanced CT as needed) can identify less common genitourinary tract causes of hematuria associated with acute pain, such as renal tumor. Generally, the workup ends with CT.

SUMMARY AND CONCLUSIONS

1. CT urography is the test of choice for imaging patients with recurrent painless hematuria and has replaced intravenous urography.
2. A negative result on CT urogram, in the face of continuing hematuria, is followed by cystoscopy to exclude a small bladder or ureteral mass or similar lesion.

3. In patients with hematuria associated with acute pain, the initial imaging examination is usually CT of the abdomen and pelvis **without oral or intravenous contrast medium.** In selected cases, the examination can be repeated while the patient remains on the CT table, with intravenous contrast medium.

ADDITIONAL COMMENTS

- A variety of tests is used in the evaluation of patients with hematuria **following significant abdominal and pelvic trauma,** including contrast-enhanced CT of the abdomen and pelvis, CT cystography, and retrograde fluoroscopic studies (e.g., retrograde urethrography, cystography). Generally, a routine abdominal and pelvic CT is performed first, with supplemental CT cystography performed as needed (especially if there are pelvic fractures, there is gross hematuria, and there is free pelvic fluid on initial CT). If a Foley catheter cannot be easily placed into the bladder, then retrograde contrast studies under fluoroscopy are indicated, if the patient's clinical condition is stable.
- Ultrasound **(US) is an appropriate imaging study for hematuria in children but is more limited in adults.** Although it may be used as an initial examination in adults to look for a renal or bladder mass, its sensitivity for tumors and other conditions (such as pyelonephritis) is lower than that of CT.
- CT urography can show urinary tract abnormalities such as papillary necrosis and some small transitional cell carcinomas.
- In lieu of multiphasic CT, especially when imaging younger patients to eliminate the radiation dose, or when imaging patients with a contraindication to iodinated contrast medium, **we suggest magnetic resonance (MR) imaging of the abdomen. A**

variety of sequences can be used, including MR urography (heavily T2-weighted sequences) and contrast-enhanced sequences with gadolinium.

▌SUGGESTED READING

Caoili EM, Cohan RH, Korobkin M, et al: Urinary tract abnormalities: initial experience with multi-detector row CT urography. Radiology 2002;222:353–360.

Caoili EM, Inampudi P, Cohan RH, Ellis JH: Optimization of multi-detector row CT urography: effect of compression, saline administration, and prolongation of acquisition delay. Radiology 2005;235:116–123.

Chow LC, Sommer FG: Multidetector CT urography with abdominal compression and three-dimensional reconstruction. Am J Roentgenol 2001;177:849–855.

Joffe SA, Servaes S, Okon S, Horowitz M: Multi-detector row CT urography in the evaluation of hematuria. Radiographics 2003;23:1441–1456.

Kawashima A, Glockner JF, King BF Jr: CT urography and MR urography. Radiol Clin North Am 2003;41:945–961.

Kawashima A, Vrtiska TJ, LeRoy AJ, et al: CT urography. Radiographics 2004;24:S35–S58.

Lang EK, Macchia RJ, Thomas R, et al: Improved detection of renal pathologic features on multiphasic helical CT compared with IVU in patients presenting with microscopic hematuria. Urology 2003;61:528–532.

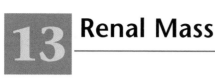

13 Renal Mass

INTRODUCTION

Although renal masses in adults are often discovered during the workup of urinary tract problems, they are also detected incidentally during abdominal imaging for other reasons.

The vast majority of renal masses can be characterized by ultrasound (US) or contrast-enhanced computed tomography (CT). **Nuclear imaging and angiography have no primary role in the study of renal masses.** Magnetic resonance (MR) imaging is used only as a problem-solving tool in select cases (e.g., in patients with renal insufficiency or intolerance to iodinated contrast medium).

A major goal of imaging is to characterize renal lesions as either simple cysts or complex (partly cystic/partly solid) masses; this differentiation is key, **because simple renal cysts are very common benign lesions (present in 50% of the population older than 50 years of age) and require no treatment.** Although solid or complex masses have many etiologies—benign and malignant—**solid masses are considered malignant until proven otherwise. Renal cell carcinoma and transitional cell carcinoma constitute the majority of these renal malignancies.**

Relative Costs: Abdominal US, **$$**; abdominal CT, enhanced, **$$$**; renal biopsy, CT-guided, **$$$$**; renal biopsy, US-guided, **$$$–$$$$**.

▌PLAN AND RATIONALE

STEP 1: ULTRASOUND (US, OR SONOGRAPHY)

US is usually the preferred initial test, because it is inexpensive, readily available, uses no ionizing radiation or contrast medium, and can accurately differentiate simple cysts from solid or complex lesions. Also, US can exclude urinary tract obstruction or stones.

If sonography proves that a lesion is a simple cyst, the workup ends.

If sonography reveals that a lesion is solid, or that a cystic lesion is "indeterminate" (i.e., does not meet all criteria for benignity), CT is the next step.

When the patient can tolerate intravenous contrast medium:

STEP 2: COMPUTED TOMOGRAPHY (CT)

Properly performed CT is currently the best imaging test to evaluate suspicious renal masses.

The radiologist must be notified in advance that evaluation of a suspicious renal mass is requested, so that a dedicated renal CT protocol can be selected. First, a scan without contrast medium (unenhanced) demonstrates calcifications or hemorrhage and defines the lesion's baseline density. This is followed by a study during intravenous contrast medium infusion to define the lesion's "enhancement." (Enhancement is a complex function of vascularity, capillary permeability, and blood volume.) Finally, delayed images display the anatomy of the collecting systems.

If a renal mass has typical benign cystic features, or can be characterized as a specific benign solid lesion such as an angiomyolipoma, the workup ends.

If CT reveals a solid mass or a complex cystic mass with certain features (contrast enhancement, solid components, calcifications, or thick septations), the mass is considered malignant until proven otherwise (Fig. 13-1). Biopsy can provide confirmation (see **CHAPTER 60, Percutaneous Guided Biopsy and Imaging-Guided Therapy**), but such patients almost always proceed directly to surgery. (In this context, note that CT also provides important pretreatment staging information—i.e., evidence of vascular invasion, direct extension to adjacent organs, lymphadenopathy, or metastases).

CT almost always ends the presurgical workup, but in patients (1) who are **not** candidates for surgical resection; (2) with a known or suspected underlying malignancy where **a metastasis to the kidney is likely;** (3) with a suspected **nonmalignant lesion** (infection, hemorrhagic cyst) that **cannot** be fully characterized by CT; and (4) who are undergoing **non-surgical management** such as radiofrequency ablation, **image-guided biopsy is often appropriate to establish a histologic diagnosis.**

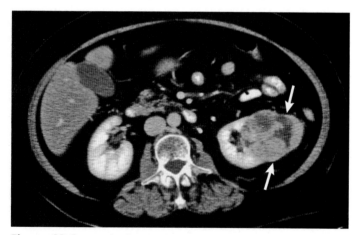

Figure 13-1. Renal cell carcinoma. CT shows a solid enhancing mass in the lateral aspect of the left kidney (*arrows*). The right kidney is normal.

When the patient cannot tolerate intravenous contrast medium:

STEP 2: MAGNETIC RESONANCE (MR) IMAGING

MR is appropriate for patients who, because of allergy or renal insufficiency, cannot tolerate the intravenous contrast medium used for CT. MR uses a gadolinium-based contrast agent, which is generally well tolerated in this population. Carefully performed renal MR, though insensitive to calcification, is equivalent to CT for detection and characterization of renal lesions.

STEP 3: PERCUTANEOUS IMAGING-GUIDED NEEDLE ASPIRATION/BIOPSY/DRAINAGE

Renal biopsies are performed under CT or US guidance on an outpatient basis (see **CHAPTER 60, Percutaneous Guided Biopsy and Imaging-Guided Therapy**). Fine-needle aspiration or core biopsies provide tissue for cytology/histology. If infection is suspected, a fine-needle aspiration can confirm the diagnosis and obtain material for culture. If indicated, catheter drainage of renal or perirenal abscesses is possible.

SUMMARY AND CONCLUSIONS

1. Renal cysts are extremely common and rarely cause symptoms. US is an accurate and inexpensive initial test that can characterize a lesion as cystic (ignore) or solid (likely malignant). If a mass is not a simple cyst on sonography, CT is next.
2. Most solid and mixed cystic and solid (complex) masses on US or CT are considered malignant until proven otherwise, **unless they have specific benign characteristics like fat that indicate an angiomyolipoma.**

3. If a patient cannot tolerate iodinated contrast medium because of allergy or renal insufficiency, MR can accurately evaluate renal masses.
4. Because of the high pretest probability that a solid renal mass represents a renal cell carcinoma, percutaneous biopsy is rarely indicated and should be reserved for the evaluation of renal masses in patients who are poor surgical risks or when there is a strong reason to believe that the mass represents a nonsurgical process such as a metastasis, lymphoma, abscess, or benign lesion.

ADDITIONAL COMMENTS

- Discovery of "incidental" renal masses has increased with the growth of cross-sectional imaging in medicine. In many cases (i.e., elderly and infirm patients) it is reasonable to take a conservative approach to such lesions. Many are benign (e.g., angiomyolipoma, oncocytoma), and even if malignant, many grow extremely slowly. Follow-up imaging with US or CT over time may allow the physician to document stability or very slow growth and estimate the risk that a lesion poses to the patient in relation to other health concerns.
- Angiography is usually reserved for evaluation and treatment of suspected vascular masses such as arteriovenous malformations. Some surgeons request angiographic embolization of hypervascular masses before surgery to reduce operative blood loss or to palliate patients with inoperable masses. Assessment of tumor invasion of the renal veins and/or inferior vena cava can usually be accurately made during renal CT, Doppler US, or MR, and no longer requires angiography.
- For two generations, the standard radiographic examination of the urinary tract was the intravenous pyelogram (IVP), also known as the intravenous urogram (IVU). This study is simply a series of plain

films of the abdomen after a peripheral intravenous injection of contrast medium, which is excreted by the kidneys, thereby opacifying and visualizing the urinary tract. The study is simple and inexpensive, and therefore naively appealing, **but although an IVP may initially demonstrate a mass, it cannot differentiate a cyst from a solid mass and has no value in the workup beyond initial mass detection. Note also that an IVP is not an appropriate screen after hematuria, because a normal IVP does not exclude a renal mass.**

█ SUGGESTED READING

Bosniak MA: The use of the Bosniak classification system for renal cysts and cystic tumors. J Urol 1997;157:1852–1853.

Hartman DS, Choyke PL, Hartman MS: A practical approach to the cystic renal mass. Radiographics 2004;24:S101–S115.

Lockhart ME, Smith JK: Technical considerations in renal CT. Radiol Clin North Amer 2003;41:863–875.

Sheth S, Scatarige JC, Horton KM, et al: Current concepts in the diagnosis and management of renal cell carcinoma: role of multidetector CT and three-dimensional CT. Radiographics 2001;21:S237–S254.

Thurston W, Wilson SR: The urinary tract. In Rumack CM, Wilson SR, Charboneau JW (eds): Diagnostic Ultrasound, 2nd ed. St. Louis, Mosby, 1998, pp 329–397.

Volpe A, Panzarella T, Rendon RA, et al: The natural history of incidentally detected small renal masses. Cancer 2004;100:738–745.

Wehle MJ, Thiel DD, Petrou SP, et al: Conservative management of incidental contrast-enhancing renal masses as safe alternative to invasive therapy. Urology 2004;64:49–52.

Zhang J, Pedrosa I, Rofsky NM: MR techniques for renal imaging. Radiol Clin North Amer 2003;41:877–907.

Renal Failure/ Obstructive Uropathy

▌INTRODUCTION

The initial imaging evaluation of renal failure, acute or chronic, requires a determination of renal size and **exclusion of urinary tract obstruction.** Ultrasound (US) is the initial test for this evaluation. Computed tomography (CT) and magnetic resonance (MR) imaging are useful for further assessment of patients with newly diagnosed hydronephrosis/hydroureter.

Relative Costs: US, **$$**; CT, **$$$**; MR, **$$$$**.

▌PLAN AND RATIONALE

STEP 1: RENAL SONOGRAM OR ULTRASOUND (US)

US is the primary and initial imaging examination in the evaluation of renal failure.

US is quick, easily performed (unless the patient is very obese), noninvasive, and inexpensive. Renal size is measured, parenchymal thickness estimated, the pelvicalyceal systems and proximal ureters evaluated for dilation, and morphologic lesions, including calculi, cysts, and masses, are shown.

Normal-size or enlarged kidneys are common in **acute** renal failure, whereas small, irregularly contoured (i.e., scarred) kidneys indicate **chronic** disease. Moreover, the parenchymal reflection of ultrasound (echotexture) may be increased in renal failure, especially when chronic; this finding is nonspecific and indicates "medical renal disease." Using color and power Doppler techniques, blood flow to the kidneys can also be defined (see the

INTRODUCTION to this book for a brief discussion of Doppler ultrasound).

Less than 5% to 10% of renal failure is due to bilateral urinary tract obstruction. However, **obstruction is the most easily correctable cause of renal failure, so excluding bilateral obstruction is key.** Causes of **bilateral** urinary tract obstruction include pelvic masses and prostatic hypertrophy that blocks the bladder outlet. **Dilation of the renal collecting systems and ureters is the hallmark of obstruction; therefore, a normal sonogram effectively excludes obstruction, ending the workup.**

When obstruction is excluded, an enormous variety of medical conditions, including hypertensive or diabetic nephropathy, collagen vascular disease, drug toxicity, and glomerulonephritis, may be responsible for the renal failure. The role of imaging is then limited to determining the partition of renal function between each kidney, if clinically required (see **ADDITIONAL COMMENTS**), and guiding renal biopsy. Sonography is the best guidance method.

When US demonstrates bilateral hydronephrosis, the bladder should be sonographically evaluated immediately **after** the patient voids. If the bladder remains full after voiding, **the kidneys should be reevaluated after the bladder is emptied via Foley catheter,** because an overdistended bladder may cause collecting system dilation by exerting back pressure on the distal ureters, producing the spurious appearance of obstruction by an organic lesion.

In the presence of an empty bladder and persistent bilateral hydronephrosis/hydroureter, the lower abdomen and pelvis are sonographically examined for masses, which can cause bilateral ureteral obstruction. **However, sonography often fails to define the cause and level of the obstruction, because overlying bowel gas often obscures much of the retroperitoneal region between the bladder and the renal pelves.**

If examination of the lower abdomen and pelvis is unrevealing, equivocal, or suboptimal

in the presence of bilateral hydronephrosis (with or without evidence of hydroureter), the retroperitoneum and pelvis require further study with other cross-sectional imaging (i.e., MR or CT).

> **Thus, if bilateral hydroureter/hydro-nephrosis is present without a clear etiology demonstrated by sonography:**

STEP 2: COMPUTED TOMOGRAPHY (CT) OR MAGNETIC RESONANCE (MR) IMAGING

CT or MR can be used to evaluate the retroperitoneum and pelvis between the kidneys and the bladder when there is bilateral hydronephrosis/hydroureter. The advantage of MR compared with CT is that the intravenous contrast medium used for MR is gadolinium based and is not contraindicated in the presence of renal failure, whereas even the safest iodinated contrast media for CT are somewhat nephrotoxic. In fact, even without contrast medium the ureters are well demonstrated on MR, due to the high signal intensity of urine within dilated ureters.

On CT and MR both the level of the obstruction and the underlying lesion (e.g., a uterine carcinoma) are better seen than on US. **However, in the presence of bilateral hydronephrosis/hydroureter no underlying lesion may be identified, in which case the differential diagnosis includes bladder outlet obstruction and bilateral ureteral stricture.**

After bladder outlet obstruction has been excluded, urinary tract decompression is usually next.

STEP 3: URINARY TRACT DECOMPRESSION

Patients with bilateral hydroureter/nephrosis and renal failure usually undergo cystoscopy (performed by a urologist) and placement of stents in both ureters.

Contrast medium, under fluoroscopic guidance (usually in an operating room setting), may be injected retrograde, to visualize the ureters and guide stent placement.

An antegrade approach may substitute when retrograde stent placement is not possible. Under fluoroscopic or US guidance, each dilated renal pelvis is punctured percutaneously with a fine needle, and a nephrostomy catheter is then placed to decompress the upper urinary tract (or in some patients, a combination nephrostomy tube/ureteral stent may be placed, if the site of obstruction can be crossed). Antegrade studies and nephrostomy tubes are usually the realm of the interventional radiologist.

SUMMARY AND CONCLUSIONS

1. Sonography is the imaging test of choice for the evaluation of renal failure, because it is rapid, noninvasive, usually easily performed, and inexpensive. Renal size and the status of the renal collecting systems and ureters are accurately determined.
2. Bilateral urinary tract obstruction, a relatively uncommon cause of renal failure, is excluded with a very high degree of accuracy. If no obstruction exists, imaging is limited to guiding a biopsy, or, in select patients, determining renal function with radionuclide techniques (see **ADDITIONAL COMMENTS**).
3. If bilateral hydronephrosis/hydroureteronephrosis is present without a clear etiology on sonography, CT or MR may be indicated to search for under-lying distal lesions.
4. Imaging can guide antegrade and retrograde procedures that decompress the urinary tract.

ADDITIONAL COMMENTS

- In patients whose kidneys are not well seen by US (e.g., obese patients), CT or MR may be required to visualize the kidneys and evaluate them for hydronephrosis. **The safer contrast medium of MR is a distinct advantage in this regard.**

- US is easily repeated to follow patients with renal failure, to serially evaluate renal size, and to exclude interval development of obstruction.

- A nuclear renal scan can measure the total and individual function of each kidney (i.e., "split renal function"). This measurement is sometimes considered to be more useful than blood urea nitrogen or serum creatinine, because it partitions function of the kidneys individually.

- Although plain films may show urinary tract calcifications and skeletal changes in patients with chronic renal failure, as well as vascular calcifications in patients with underlying diabetes or abnormalities related to the renal failure itself, plain films of the abdomen and pelvis do not have a diagnostic role in the workup of most patients with renal failure.

- **Although imaging findings in renal failure may be nonspecific, in select instances they may be highly specific or at least greatly narrow the differential diagnosis. For example, renal cortical calcification suggests prior renal cortical necrosis or oxalosis, and enlargement of both kidneys by numerous cysts is characteristic of polycystic renal disease.**

- Rarely, in extremely **acute** bilateral obstruction, the pelvicalyceal systems are **NOT** dilated, **because the sonogram has been performed before the systems have had time to dilate.** These cases represent a diagnostic conundrum. **A repeat sonogram is effective in 1 to 2 days, but the problem is determining which patients require a repeat study. The best guide is to repeat the sonogram when in doubt, because the test is inexpensive, readily available, and noninvasive.**

- Renal arterial occlusion is an uncommon cause of renal failure. In renal artery occlusion by emboli (or due to other arterial causes such as aortic dissection), color and power Doppler sonography are useful, supplemented as needed by MR with contrast medium (enhanced), to document the presence or absence of perfusion to one or both kidneys. These techniques have largely supplanted nuclear scans for **acute** renal arterial occlusion.

- When **urethral** obstruction is suspected, voiding cystourethrography is helpful for defining lesions such as post-traumatic or postinflammatory strictures in adults. Under fluoroscopy the bladder is catheterized and filled with contrast medium, and the patient then voids following catheter removal. Reflux of contrast medium from the bladder into the ureters is also identified.

- Sometimes US and/or CT reveals a collecting system that is **significantly dilated with no evidence of obstruction in any part of the urinary tract.** Such a system may represent the residual "stretching" from previous but now relieved obstruction. **A Lasix diuretic renogram can provide a definitive diagnosis.** The Lasix renogram, performed in all nuclear medicine departments, is based upon the fact that an intravenous Lasix infusion augments urine flow and empties a dilated but not obstructed system rapidly, whereas a truly obstructed system does not drain as rapidly under the pressure of augmented urine output. Because a radionuclide that is excreted by the kidney is used to image the kidney, the radioactivity in the kidney can easily be quantified and its passage through the kidney plotted as a function of time and compared to normal values as well as the contralateral "control."

SUGGESTED READING

O'Neill WC: Sonographic evaluation of renal failure. Am J Kid Dis 2000;35:1021–1038.

15 Renovascular Hypertension

INTRODUCTION

Hypertension is a major health problem that affects nearly 60 million Americans. However, the vast majority have primary or "essential hypertension"; renovascular disease accounts for only 1% to 4%.

Clinical signs of renovascular hypertension include (1) uncontrolled blood pressure despite optimal antihypertensive therapy with three to four drugs, (2) malignant hypertension with evidence of encephalopathy or retinopathy, (3) onset of hypertension in persons younger than 30 years or older than 50 years of age, (4) abrupt onset of hypertension, (5) rapid worsening of preexisting hypertension, (6) decreased renal function after treatment with angiotension-converting enzyme (ACE) inhibitors, (7) a flank or abdominal bruit, and (8) unilateral small kidney in a hypertensive patient.

Most renovascular lesions are atherosclerotic. However, in young women fibromuscular dysplasia is more common. Rare causes of high-renin hypertension **without** an **intrinsic** renovascular lesion include renal cysts, renal neoplasms, polycystic renal disease, Page kidney, and even calyceal dilation secondary to obstruction. **In all of these conditions reduced blood flow through a renal artery (intrinsic narrowing or extrinsic pressure) results in renal ischemia, to which the affected kidney responds by releasing renin, a potent hypertensive agent; the ensuing elevation in blood pressure increases perfusion pressure to the affected kidney, maintaining renal function over the short term**

but adversely affecting the contralateral kidney and multiple other systems.

For many years, a noninvasive physiologic test was first recommended to establish that there was in fact a high-renin state produced by a poorly perfused kidney. (Classical thinking was that no purpose is served by initially ordering invasive imaging exams to show the renal arteries and define areas of narrowing, unless there is a proven high-renin state, because many incidental stenoses occur without producing hypertension, and repair of such stenoses would be ineffective, not to mention risky and expensive.) The recent development of **noninvasive arterial imaging** has changed the algorithm in many medical centers. These noninvasive arterial imaging tests, CTA (computed tomographic angiography) and MRA (magnetic resonance angiography), are rapid, safe, and nearly 100% sensitive for stenoses. After CTA or MRA defines a stenosis, a physiologic study to prove high renin is almost always appropriate before repair.

Relative Costs: ACE-inhibitor nuclear renal scan, **$$$**; CTA, **$$$**; MRA, **$$$$**; catheter renal arteriogram with angioplasty and stent placement, **$$$$$–$$$$$$**.

▌ PLAN AND RATIONALE

> **If renal function is not severely compromised, there is no acute or chronic obstruction, and there is no contra-indication to iodinated contrast medium:**

STEP 1: COMPUTED TOMOGRAPHIC ANGIOGRAPHY (CTA)

Multidetector CT scanners have changed radiology's entire approach to diagnostic angiography. Traditional catheter angiography required a vascular puncture and passage of a catheter into the blood vessel of interest, followed by injection of contrast medium, during which radiographs were taken, revealing the vessel in exquisite detail. Such studies are invasive, expensive, and **inappropriate as a screening tool. Incredibly, equivalent vascular visualization can now be routinely achieved by a rapid, peripheral intravenous (e.g., antecubital) injection of contrast medium, followed by a well-timed CT scan, as the contrast medium passes through the body's central blood vessels.** Moreover, other renal lesions, including tumors, cysts, and parenchymal scarring, are clearly defined.

If CTA is normal, the workup ends; there is no stenosis to repair, and other rare nonvascular lesions are excluded.

If CTA reveals vessel narrowing, a physiologic study to establish that there is high-renin secretion by the affected kidney is appropriate.

STEP 2: ACE-INHIBITOR RADIONUCLIDE RENAL SCAN (SCINTIGRAPHY)

In patients with good or only moderately compromised renal function, the ACE-inhibitor renal scan effectively establishes whether there is high-renin secretion by the underperfused kidney. (In some protocols, ACE-inhibitor therapy is discontinued before the test, so contact with the nuclear medicine physician is essential before scheduling in order to achieve optimum sensitivity.) The examination uses radiopharmaceuticals that are excreted by glomerular filtration, such as technetium 99m–diethylenetriamine pentaacetic acid (Tc-99m-DTPA), or by tubular secretion, such as technetium 99m–mercaptoacetyltriglycine (Tc-99m-MAG-3).

In some protocols the test involves two phases: **(1)** An initial intravenous injection of Tc-99m-DTPA or Tc-99m-MAG-3 is followed by rapid-sequence "flow" images and later "static" images. The uptake of radiopharmaceutical by each kidney is quantitated, providing an indicator of renal function (glomerular filtration rate [GFR] if Tc-99m-DTPA is used or effective renal plasma flow [ERPF] if Tc-99m-MAG-3 is used). The GFR or ERPF for each kidney is calculated **individually.** Alternatively, individual pharmaceutical uptake curves are generated. **(2)** Subsequently, an ACE inhibitor is administered, and a second dose of radiopharmaceutical is injected; the patient is re-imaged, and the renal function or uptake curves for each kidney are recalculated. Other protocols use only a one-phase test, with the patient on ACE-inhibitor treatment before the study.

A stenotic renal artery decreases blood flow to the **afferent** arterioles of the glomeruli of the affected kidney. In response to this ischemia, the kidney attempts to preserve glomerular filtration pressure by constricting its **efferent** arterioles and by increasing renal arterial blood flow. The mechanism through which these adaptations occur is the angiotensin-renin axis; the ischemic kidney releases renin, a powerful hypertensive agent that also constricts the efferent arterioles. **ACE inhibitors block the effect of renin,** so that blood pressure falls and the compensatory vasoconstriction of the efferent arterioles abates. Because the arterioles of the ischemic kidney are "normally" in a state of maximal constriction to maintain filtration pressure, arteriolar relaxation causes a precipitous fall in filtration pressure, **dropping that kidney's GFR and ERPF,** and adversely affecting its pharmaceutical uptake curves. **Thus, the kidney whose function falls is the high-renin secretor.** A negative study usually ends the workup.

A positive study result is followed by conventional catheter renal arteriography and repair.

STEP 3: CONVENTIONAL CATHETER RENAL ARTERIOGRAM, ANGIOPLASTY, AND STENT

The common femoral artery is punctured percutaneously, and a catheter is advanced craniad through the aorta; contrast medium is injected as films are exposed. Aortography is performed first to look for accessory renal arteries; then, the renal arteries are individually catheterized and visualized, along with the renal parenchyma. The arteriogram therefore guides the following angioplastic repair, during the same procedure.

A balloon at the end of the catheter is inflated at the site of the stenosis, widening the artery. A repeat arteriogram is performed to evaluate the degree of dilation and serve as a post–percutaneous transluminal angioplasty (PTA) baseline. A sleeve of mesh-like material (a "stent") is almost always placed at the site of ostial lesions to maintain arterial patency.

Long- and short-term outcomes of lesions repaired with angioplasty are quite favorable; fibromuscular dysplasia responds especially well. The procedure is safe and well tolerated in most cases. However, rare complications, such as renal arterial rupture or uncontrolled renal arterial dissection, can occur.

If renal function is severely compromised or there is another contraindication to iodinated contrast medium:

STEP 1: MAGNETIC RESONANCE ANGIOGRAPHY (MRA)

Severely failing kidneys should not be exposed to the high doses of iodinated contrast medium required for CTA; therefore, MRA is appropriate.

MRA, like CTA, requires only a peripheral intravenous injection of contrast medium, but the technique uses gadolinium–diethylenetriamine pentaacetic acid (Gd-DTPA) or a similar gadolinium chelate. This contrast medium is safe in patients with a contraindication to the iodinated contrast medium used for CTA.

Renal MRA is more complex than CTA, more time-consuming, more expensive, and less available. Whereas CTA is available in virtually all hospitals and in many freestanding imaging centers, MRA of the kidneys is performed only in larger centers.

If no stenosis is defined, the workup ends.

However, the demonstration of a stenosis by MRA does not necessarily indicate that the lesion is responsible for hypertension.

If MRA was selected as the screen because of a contraindication to iodinated contrast medium but renal function is not severely compromised, an ACE-inhibitor nuclear scan is appropriate (see Step 2, above). Repair proceeds if the ACE-inhibitor scan is abnormal.

However, in cases in which MRA was selected as the screen because of advanced renal failure, an ACE-inhibitor nuclear scan often is inaccurate, because renal function is too poor for accurate quantitation. In these cases a positive MRA can be problematic (see **ADDITIONAL COMMENTS,** below).

SUMMARY AND CONCLUSIONS

1. CTA is becoming the primary study for imaging the renal arteries for diagnostic purposes, especially in departments with a strong CT section. A normal CTA finding has an extremely high negative predictive value, excluding renal artery stenosis.

2. In radiology departments that use ACE-inhibitor renal scan as the screen, **contact with the nuclear physician before the study is essential, so that antihypertensive therapy can be discontinued, if that is called for by the particular protocol involved.**

3. When there is renal failure or another strong contraindication to iodinated radiographic contrast medium, MRA is effective (in fact, as the speed and availability of MRA improve, MRA could well replace CTA as the primary screen).

4. In the absence of renal failure, **a stenosis demonstrated by CTA or MRA should be followed by an ACE-inhibitor renal scan to confirm that the kidney distal to the stenosis is in fact a high renin secretor.** In advanced renal failure, the renal scan is unreliable.

5. In renal failure, the demonstration of a severe stenosis will sometimes lead to repair even with-

out proof that the stenosis has produced a high-renin state, in the hope that better perfusion will improve renal function. The issue is controversial (see **ADDITIONAL COMMENTS,** below).

6. Most renovascular lesions are amenable to PTA and stenting.

ADDITIONAL COMMENTS

- Ultrasound (US) has been advocated as a primary screen for renal artery stenosis, because it is completely noninvasive and inexpensive. However, the technique is extremely operator dependent; in excellent hands it is highly sensitive, but elsewhere it is fraught with false negatives (accuracy of US is believed to be approximately 70%, as opposed to more than 90% for CTA or MRA). Therefore, in a general algorithm for the renovascular hypertension workup, we prefer CTA and MRA, which are standardized and more readily available.

- In patients with renal failure who must be screened with MRA, the issue of whether to repair a stenosis is unresolved. Some internists and nephrologists steadfastly refuse to authorize repair in the absence of functional proof that the lesion has caused a high-renin state, and, in these cases, renal vein renin sampling can be considered. For this procedure a femoral vein is punctured and a catheter is passed craniad through the inferior vena cava to the renal veins, which are catheterized individually and sampled for a renin assay, sometimes before and after ACE-inhibitor administration. **The procedure has had variable results and is totally unsuitable as a screen;** it is mentioned here only in the context of those very uncommon patients whose renal failure contraindicates ACE-inhibitor scintigraphy. Moreover, a strong argument can be made for simply ablating a kidney with only 10% to 15% of residual function, because it contributes little and is basically a "renin factory." Thus, whether stenosis repair and using a stent are worthwhile in such a case is usually a decision jointly made by a nephrologist and an interventional radiologist.

- Very recent work has shown that the gadolinium-based contrast media **for MR imaging** can also be used **for CTA.** Thus, patients with a contraindication to iodinated radiographic contrast medium (currently used for CTA) **could undergo CTA with the gadolinium-based compounds.** At the time of this writing, such use would be "off label" and prohibitively expensive, but it may well be approved in the future; if so, MRA may lose its place in the workup.

Acknowledgment. The authors gratefully acknowledge the help and suggestions of Charles Ray, MD, Chief, Interventional Radiology, Denver Health Medical Center, Denver, Colorado.

▌SUGGESTED READING

Soulez G, Oliva VL, Turpin S, et al: Imaging of renovascular hypertension: respective values of renal scintigraphy, renal Doppler US, and MR angiography. Radiographics 2000;20:1355–1368.

16 Scrotal Pain/Mass

INTRODUCTION

Scrotal disease in adults generally presents as new onset of pain or a palpable mass. The differential diagnosis of acute scrotal pain includes ischemia (from torsion of the spermatic cord), epididymitis/orchitis, trauma, and tumor. The differential diagnosis of a scrotal mass includes malignant or benign neoplasm, hydrocele, varicocele, epididymal or testicular cyst, scrotal hernia, and acute or chronic epididymitis. **Some of these processes require immediate surgical intervention; in acute ischemia, for example, viability of the testicle declines sharply after only 6 hours.**

Scrotal imaging plays a key role in the evaluation. The clinical differentiation between causes of an acutely painful scrotum is difficult, and a palpable mass must be characterized as **intratesticular** or **extratesticular. Solid intratesticular masses are considered malignant until proven otherwise, whereas extratesticular masses are almost always benign.**

Applicable techniques include ultrasound and nuclear imaging, **but ultrasound (US, sonography) is generally the first and only examination required for a mass. However, for the acutely painful scrotum, when torsion is a consideration, the chosen examination often depends on which is available on an emergency basis.**

Relative Costs: Scrotal US, **$$**; nuclear scrotal scan, **$$**.

▌PLAN AND RATIONALE

Acutely painful scrotum, without previous trauma:

STEP 1: COLOR DOPPLER ULTRASOUND (US, SONOGRAPHY)

After acoustical gel is applied to the skin, the transducer is placed on the scrotum, and high-resolution images of the testes and other scrotal contents are produced. The inguinal canal and abdomen can also be examined. Conventional US supplies strictly anatomic information, but **color Doppler US also provides an excellent assessment of blood flow to the testes.** Acute ischemia of the testis, caused by torsion of the spermatic cord (called "testicular torsion," usually occurring in children and adolescents), can be identified, and any underlying morphologic lesions are also revealed. Epididymo-orchitis, a common cause of pain in the adult population, can be accurately diagnosed. The workup of acute scrotal pain almost invariably ends with color Doppler US. US delivers no ionizing radiation.

Prior to the refinement of color Doppler US, nuclear imaging was the examination of choice for evaluation of the acute scrotum. It is very accurate for excluding the diagnosis of testicular torsion. **Therefore, although color Doppler US has generally replaced nuclear imaging as the initial study of choice in the setting of suspected testicular torsion, nuclear imaging remains a viable choice if US is not immediately available.**

If color Doppler sonography is unavailable on an emergency basis:

STEP 1: NUCLEAR SCAN

Nuclear scrotal scanning is available virtually everywhere; the equipment and technique are highly standardized. A bolus of technetium 99m–pertechnetate is injected intravenously, and serial images of the scrotum are rapidly generated. **This sequence reveals perfusion of the testes as the bolus of radioactivity passes through the scrotal vessels—a "radionuclide angiogram." "Static" images, which reflect the presence or absence of hyperemia, are then obtained. The contralateral asymptomatic testis serves as a control.**

Acute ischemia of the testis, caused by torsion of the spermatic cord, appears as **decreased perfusion** on the nuclear scan. In striking contrast, inflammatory lesions such as epididymo-orchitis produce **increased perfusion.** The findings are less clear-cut in testicular abscess or in torsion more than 1 day old (missed torsion). Also, an unsuspected testicular tumor occasionally presents as acute, painful swelling, caused by tumor hemorrhage or accompanying epididymo-orchitis; in such unusual cases the nuclear findings may be confusing.

When the nuclear scan is definitive, as it usually is in acute torsion or epididymitis-orchitis, the imaging workup ends. When the nuclear scan is equivocal, US may be helpful (see **Step 1,** above).

Acute painful swelling, after trauma:

STEP 1: ULTRASOUND (US, SONOGRAPHY)

Sonography is the best initial imaging study after acute scrotal trauma. Intrascrotal injuries, including hematoma (intra- or extratesticular), hematocele, and epididymal injury, are readily demonstrated. The testicle is also evaluated for ischemia and for fracture or capsular rupture, which require surgical repair. Follow-up US of intratesticular abnormalities detected after trauma is important, because testicular malignancies occasionally present with pain that is incorrectly attributed to minor trauma.

Scrotal mass:

STEP 1: ULTRASOUND (US, SONOGRAPHY)

The primary diagnostic consideration in a patient with a palpable mass or a painless, swollen scrotum is tumor. Sonography can clearly show whether a scrotal mass is intra- or extratesticular. **A solid intratesticular lesion is presumed to be malignant until proven otherwise.** Scrotal lesions with a fluid component, such as complicated and uncomplicated hydroceles and epididymal or testicular cysts, can be evaluated and followed. Other conditions causing a mass, including hernias, chronic epididymitis, and abscess, can usually be characterized. **The nuclear scan is generally not helpful in the evaluation of a scrotal mass.**

SUMMARY AND CONCLUSIONS

1. Suspected testicular torsion is a diagnostic emergency, because surgery within 6 hours of torsion can save an ischemic testis.
2. Both color Doppler US and the nuclear scan are sensitive and specific for establishing or excluding acute testicular torsion. US is preferred, because it delivers no ionizing radiation, shows the anatomy and pathology with better spatial resolution, and also evaluates the scrotal contents for other abnormalities.
3. US is appropriate for testicular pain and swelling that is clearly post-traumatic. Color Doppler US analysis should always be included, because ischemia sometimes follows testicular trauma.
4. US is appropriate for evaluation of a suspected scrotal mass. Characterization and localization of a lesion are important because solid intratesticular masses are considered malignant until proven otherwise.

ADDITIONAL COMMENTS

- US is the best method for screening the clinically normal scrotum for occult disease, for example, in the search for a primary testicular tumor in the patient with metastatic disease or as a harbor for metastasis in patients with hematologic neoplasms or lymphoma.
- Scrotal magnetic resonance (MR) imaging sometimes serves a useful problem-solving role for further characterization of a testicular or paratesticular mass in selected patients.

SUGGESTED READING

Dambro TJ, Stewart RR, Carroll BA: The scrotum. In Rumack CM, Wilson SR, Charboneau JW (eds): Diagnostic Ultrasound, 2nd ed. St. Louis, Mosby, 1998, pp 791–821.

Dogra V, Bhatt S: Acute painful scrotum. Radiol Clin North Am 2004;42:349–363.

Dogra VS, Gottlieb RH, Oka M, Rubens DJ: Sonography of the scrotum. Radiology 2003;227:18–36.

Nussbaum-Blask AR, Bulas D, Shalaby-Rana E, et al: Color Doppler sonography and scintigraphy of the testis: a prospective, comparative analysis in children with acute scrotal pain. Pediatr Emerg Care 2002;18:67–71.

Zuckier LS: The genital tract. In Ell PJ, Gambhir SS (eds). Nuclear Medicine in Clinical Diagnosis and Treatment, 3rd ed. Philadelphia, Churchill Livingstone, 2004, pp 1657–1684.

Adnexal Mass/Pelvic Pain

INTRODUCTION

An adnexal mass may be detected on physical examination, may be noted as an incidental finding on imaging studies, or may be suspect in patients with pelvic discomfort/vaginal bleeding. The differential diagnosis is quite extensive and differs for pre- and postmenopausal women. In the former, a serum beta–human chorionic gonadotropin (bHCG) should be determined; if bHCG is positive, ectopic pregnancy must be excluded (see **CHAPTER 18, Ectopic Pregnancy**).

Causes of adnexal mass include ovarian cyst, para-ovarian cyst, teratoma (dermoid), endometrioma, tubo-ovarian abscess, hydrosalpinx, exophytic uterine fibroid, ovarian torsion, and benign or malignant ovarian tumor. Most adnexal masses in premenopausal women are transient and reflect benign changes, usually simple or hemorrhagic functional ovarian cysts. **The likelihood of an ovarian mass representing a malignant neoplasm increases with age, especially after menopause. Unfortunately, most malignant ovarian tumors are incurable at the time of diagnosis, because they often do not cause symptoms until the disease has spread beyond the ovary.**

Ultrasound (US) is the initial procedure of choice when an adnexal mass is suspected. It can establish the presence or absence of a mass and determine its relationship to the uterus and ovaries. The sonographic appearance of a lesion, in combination with the clinical presentation, allows a confident diagnosis to be made in most cases, and, if the appearance of the lesion is indeterminate, a short-term follow-up establishes whether it should be excised. Magnetic resonance (MR) imaging and computed tomography (CT) are appropriate in select cases to further characterize indeterminate masses.

Although pelvic pain in women is commonly related to ovarian/adnexal lesions, gastrointestinal and urologic causes must also be considered. If clinical findings do not indicate gynecologic disease, other imaging modalities, particularly CT, may be more useful.

Relative Costs: Pelvic US, **$$**; abdominal US, **$$**; transvaginal US, **$$**; pelvic MR, **$$$$**; pelvic CT, **$$$**.

▌ PLAN AND RATIONALE

If an adnexal mass is suspected and the bHCG is positive (in women of childbearing age), ectopic pregnancy must be excluded (see CHAPTER 18, Ectopic Pregnancy).

If an adnexal mass is suspected in a postmenopausal woman or a premenopausal woman with a negative bHCG, or if pelvic pain of gynecologic origin is likely:

STEP 1: PELVIC ULTRASOUND (SONOGRAPHY, US), TRANSVAGINAL

Transvaginal ultrasound (TVUS) is the initial examination of choice to evaluate the uterus, ovaries, and adnexa.

A probe with a small high-resolution transducer at its end is placed within the vagina, close to the uterus and adnexa. The bladder should be emptied before this examination. **In recent years, TVUS has largely replaced conventional transabdominal US as the initial examination of choice, because it depicts the uterus and adnexa with a higher degree of resolution and avoids the discomfort of the full-bladder transabdominal examination.**

(Transabdominal sonography is used selectively to examine large masses or lesions in the upper pelvis that may lie beyond the imaging range of the transvaginal probe. The bladder is filled to displace bowel loops, which normally obscure the uterus and ovaries, so the pelvic structures can be imaged through the fluid in the bladder.)

Most ovarian masses can be fully characterized sonographically. Simple functional ovarian cysts or follicles contain only fluid, have a thin wall, and are unilocular. Sonographic follow-up is indicated only if a cyst is large or symptomatic. Postmenopausal ovarian cysts can develop, and most are benign; simple cysts less than 5 cm in size can be safely followed sonographically.

In premenopausal women, a sonographically complex collection representing a hemorrhagic corpus luteal cyst is frequently seen after ovulation and can be a cause of significant pelvic pain. The pain is generally transient, and short-term follow-up US during a different phase of the menstrual cycle (usually in 6 weeks) typically shows complete resolution.

A dermoid is usually asymptomatic and detected as an incidental finding. The sonographic appearance is very suggestive, but pelvic CT may be requested by the radiologist for confirmation.

Uterine fibroids are easily seen and can be followed sonographically. Exophytic uterine fibroids may cause a palpable adnexal mass, and this diagnosis can usually be made by showing contiguity of the mass with the uterus. If not, pelvic MR can usually differentiate fibroids from ovarian masses.

Hydrosalpinx is easily defined sonographically. Endometriomas, tubo-ovarian abscesses, and ovarian torsion present with pelvic pain and can usually be diagnosed by their sonographic appearance in combination with the appropriate clinical presentation.

Ovarian neoplasms generally appear sonographically as solid or complex (cystic and solid) masses. In the postmenopausal woman, any suspicious solid or complex adnexal mass, or, in the premenopausal woman, any solid or complex

adnexal mass that does not resolve with short-term follow-up, should be considered suspicious for tumor, and laparoscopic surgical evaluation is appropriate.

If ultrasound of the adnexa is inconclusive or suboptimal:

STEP 2: MAGNETIC RESONANCE (MR) IMAGING OR COMPUTED TOMOGRAPHY (CT)

After suboptimal or inconclusive US, the uterus and adnexa, as well as local lymph nodes, can be visualized well with MR. In the case of a sonographically inde-terminate adnexal mass, MR can sometimes characterize a lesion as benign, obviating surgery for diagnostic purposes. MR is particularly useful in the diagnosis of dermoids, uterine leiomyomas, endometriomas, and simple cysts. **However, in the absence of clear evidence of tumor extension or metastases, MR cannot differentiate benign from malignant epithelial ovarian tumors.** MR staging of suspected ovarian malignancy is not as accurate as laparoscopy, which visualizes smaller peritoneal implants. CT is useful for characterizing suspected dermoids when fat and calcification are seen within the lesion.

If nongynecologic disease is suspected as a cause of pelvic pain:

STEP 3: COMPUTED TOMOGRAPHY (CT)

Acute pelvic pain can also reflect **underlying gastro-intestinal or urologic disease.** Clinical and/or laboratory findings can pinpoint common problems such as gastroenteritis or urinary tract infection; pelvic CT is especially useful in patients with **atypical** symptoms and when US results of the uterus and ovaries are negative but clinical symptoms persist. For example, in patients with pain in the right or left pelvis and signs of infection, appendicitis or diverticulitis must be considered (see **CHAPTER 10, Appendicitis/ Diverticulitis**).

When pelvic pain persists after imaging is normal, laparoscopy is warranted.

SUMMARY AND CONCLUSIONS

1. US is the initial study for a suspected adnexal mass and for pelvic pain likely related to the uterus and adnexa. TVUS optimally defines the uterus and ovaries; US is inexpensive, accurate, readily available, and delivers no ionizing radiation. Pelvic US can easily be repeated to re-evaluate adnexal lesions that are likely benign.
2. If TVUS is equivocal, or if visualization of the adnexa is limited, MR can define and help to characterize a number of benign adnexal masses, including leiomyomas, endometriomas, and dermoids. CT can also be useful in problematic cases, especially when nongynecologic disease such as appendicitis or diverticulitis is suspected and in the diagnosis of a suspected dermoid.

ADDITIONAL COMMENTS

- Some past studies using TVUS and Doppler waveforms demonstrated low-resistance blood flow in malignant ovarian masses, which may contain abnormal tumor vasculature (see **INTRODUCTION** to this book for a brief discussion of Doppler US). However, additional studies have shown that a number of benign lesions may have similar blood flow patterns, especially in premenopausal women, and that the morphologic features of a mass (appearance and growth) are the most important indicators of the need for surgery.

- Screening US for asymptomatic patients with an increased risk of ovarian cancer (i.e., strong family history of ovarian carcinoma or breast carcinoma and certain inherited gene mutations) has been advocated, but its value continues to be controversial. US screening is currently under investigation.
- As the number of cross-sectional imaging examinations has increased, more ovarian cysts are discovered as incidental findings. If a cyst is large or shows suspicious features, US is indicated for further characterization.

SUGGESTED READING

Benacerraf BR, Shipp TD, Bromley B: Is a full bladder still necessary for pelvic sonography? J Ultrasound Med 2000;19:237–241.

Cannistra SA: Cancer of the ovary. N Engl J Med 2004;351:2519–2529.

Filly RA: Ovarian masses . . . what to look for . . . what to do. In Callen PW (ed): Ultrasonography in Obstetrics and Gynecology, 3rd ed. Philadelphia, WB Saunders, 1994, pp 625–640.

Jeoug YY, Outwater EK, Kanf HK: Imaging evaluation of ovarian masses. Radiographics 2000;20:1445–1470.

Levine D, Gosink BB, Wolf SI, et al: Simple adnexal cysts: the natural history in postmenopausal women. Radiology 1992;184:653–659.

Salem S, Wilson SR: Gynecologic ultrasound. In Rumack CM, Wilson SR, Charboneau JW (eds): Diagnostic Ultrasound, 3rd ed. St. Louis, Elsevier-Mosby, 2005, pp 527–587.

Webb EM, Green GE, Scoutt LM: Adnexal mass with pelvic pain. Radiol Clin North Am 2004;42:329–348.

Ectopic Pregnancy

INTRODUCTION

Ectopic pregnancy (EP) is a potentially life-threatening first trimester complication. A substantial rise in the incidence of EP has been documented over the last several decades, primarily attributed to an increase in pelvic inflammatory disease. Other risk factors include prior EP, tubal surgery, endometriosis, and in vitro fertilization. Although these factors increase the risk of EP, the condition can occur in any woman of child-bearing age.

The presentation of EP is often relatively nonspecific. Most patients present with pelvic pain and abnormal vaginal bleeding. If the history and physical examination and a positive pregnancy test suggest EP, and the patient is hemodynamically stable, pelvic ultrasound (US) is indicated to evaluate the uterus and adnexa. US is also key to following patients managed with nonsurgical methods and following stable patients with a positive serum beta–human chorionic gonadotropin (bHCG) level but no definite evidence of intrauterine or ectopic pregnancy.

Relative Costs: Transvaginal ultrasound (TVUS), **$$**; transabdominal ultrasound or transabdominal sonography (TAS), **$$**.

PLAN AND RATIONALE

If a patient presenting with suspected ectopic pregnancy is hypotensive and unstable, emergency surgical exploration is indicated; such an urgent presentation is uncommon, and almost always time permits determination of the bHCG level. bHCG is crucial, because **a negative serum bHCG effectively excludes pregnancy (ectopic or intrauterine).**

If bHCG is positive:

STEP 1: TRANSVAGINAL ULTRASOUND (TVUS)

TVUS is the imaging test of choice for evaluating women with possible EP.

The resolution of TVUS is superior to that of transabdominal sonography (TAS), and it detects intrauterine pregnancies and adnexal abnormalities earlier and more accurately. To perform the test, the bladder is emptied and a probe with a small, high-resolution ultrasound transducer at its end is advanced into the vagina, close to the uterus and adnexa.

Sonographic detection of an **intrauterine** pregnancy is crucial, **because intrauterine gestation virtually excludes EP; only 1 in 7000 EPs coexist with intrauterine pregnancy.**

Detection of an intrauterine pregnancy depends upon the stage of fetal development as indicated by the serum quantitative bHCG. **When bHCG is more than 1000 IU/L** (second international standard), **a normal intrauterine pregnancy, if present, should be conclusively demonstrated by TVUS.** If an intrauterine pregnancy is **not** found, indirect findings of EP (adnexal hematoma or free pelvic blood) may suggest the diagnosis of EP. However, an extrauterine embryo and/or a fetal heartbeat are the only direct findings of EP, and these are seen in only 17% to 28% of cases.

When the serum quantitative **bHCG is less than 1000 IU/L,** an intrauterine pregnancy **may not be reliably demonstrated,** even with TVUS. If the patient's condition is clinically stable, no intrauterine pregnancy is seen, and no other abnormalities are found in the pelvis, one of three scenarios is possible: (1) there is a viable intrauterine pregnancy that is too early to be seen; (2) there is a nonviable pregnancy that is aborting; or (3) there is an early ectopic pregnancy that cannot be identified. **Careful clinical follow-up and serial quantitative serum bHCG are indicated.**

In a normal first trimester pregnancy, the serum bHCG usually doubles about every 2 days. If the fetus is aborting, the bHCG level decreases, whereas in an EP the bHCG level increases, but at a slower rate than in a normal pregnancy. **Once the bHCG level approaches 1000, TVUS should be repeated. However, the timing of the repeat examination(s) must be tailored to the individual patient; occasional EPs occur in which the bHCG level does not increase or increases at the rate of a normal pregnancy.**

In recent years, medical management of EP has grown in importance. The use of methotrexate, administered intramuscularly or by direct injection, can decrease patient morbidity and help preserve patient fertility. Methotrexate is generally reserved for stable patients with a small, nonruptured EP, a bHCG less than 5000 to 10,000, and no significant comorbidities.

SUMMARY AND CONCLUSIONS

1. TVUS is the test of choice for evaluating women with suspected EP. If the patient is clinically stable, a quantitative serum bHCG level followed by TVUS is appropriate. **A negative serum bHCG effectively excludes a viable ectopic or intrauterine pregnancy.**
2. **Detection of an intrauterine pregnancy virtually excludes EP** (see **ADDITIONAL COMMENTS** regarding rare heterotopic pregnancies, below).
3. When the serum bHCG is more than 1000, a normal intrauterine pregnancy should be seen with TVUS. If an intrauterine pregnancy is not seen, the likelihood of EP rises, although an early or incomplete abortion is also possible. The only definitive sonographic sign of EP is visualization of an extrauterine embryo or fetal heartbeat.

4. If the serum bHCG is less than 1000, and no intrauterine pregnancy or evidence of ectopic pregnancy is found, stable patients require careful clinical follow-up with serial bHCG measurements. If the bHCG reaches 1000, TVUS should be repeated to look for an intrauterine or ectopic pregnancy. **A negative sonogram never excludes EP if the bHCG is positive.**

▌ADDITIONAL COMMENTS

- If TVUS is not desired (as in many teenage patients), and the bHCG is more than 1800, an acceptable alternative to initial TVUS is transabdominal sonography (TAS), with the uterus and adnexa visualized through a filled bladder. An intrauterine pregnancy, if present, should be visible at this bHCG level. However, if no intrauterine pregnancy is identified, TVUS is appropriate.
- If the serum bHCG is less than 1000, TVUS is nonetheless appropriate. Although the study is often normal and the results inconclusive, EP may be discovered on TVUS, despite the low bHCG.
- If an intrauterine gestation is identified by sonography, the likelihood of an EP coexisting with the intrauterine gestation (a heterotopic pregnancy) is very low (incidence approximately 1:7000). However, the incidence of heterotopic pregnancy is increasing. **Caution should be used if a patient has known risk factors for EP and especially if she is undergoing in vitro fertilization, which places her at a much higher risk for heterotopic pregnancy.**
- An uncommon cause of markedly elevated bHCG is molar pregnancy, which is usually readily diagnosed by TVUS.
- Rarely, ectopic pregnancy can present after the first trimester as an intra-abdominal mass.

▓ SUGGESTED READING

Filly RA: Ectopic pregnancy. In Callen PW (ed): Ultrasonography in Obstetrics and Gynecology. Philadelphia, Saunders, 1994, pp 641–658.

Fleischer A, Pennell RG, McKee MS, et al: Ectopic pregnancy: features at transvaginal sonography. Radiology 1990;174:375–378.

Lazarus E: What's new in first trimester ultrasound. Radiol Clin North Am 2003;41:663–679.

Lyons EA, Levi CS: The first trimester. In Rumack CM, Wilson SR, Charboneau JW (eds): Diagnostic Ultrasound, 3rd ed. St. Louis, Elsevier-Mosby, 2005, pp 1069–1125.

Webb EM, Green GE, Scoutt LM: Adnexal mass with pelvic pain. Radiol Clin North Am 2004;42:329–348.

Abnormal Uterine Bleeding

INTRODUCTION

The differential diagnosis of abnormal uterine bleeding (AUB) is extensive but heavily age dependent. AUB in premenopausal women is often related to hormonal imbalance and in middle-aged women may signal the onset of menopause. Changes in menstruation during childbearing age may indicate pregnancy. During pregnancy early worrisome complications, including ectopic pregnancy and miscarriage, must be considered (see **CHAPTER 18, Ectopic Pregnancy**). Post-menopausal bleeding is always a cause for concern, because up to 10% of these patients have an underlying malignancy.

Other causes of AUB include uterine fibroids, adenomyosis, endometrial hyperplasia, polyps, infection, cervical/endometrial cancer, underlying coagulopathy, many medications including some herbal supplements, and thyroid or pituitary disease.

Imaging, particularly pelvic ultrasound (US), frequently plays an important role in the diagnostic evaluation by defining a specific cause or by excluding significant uterine lesions.

Relative Costs: Transvaginal US (TVUS), **$$**; pelvic MR, **$$$$**.

PLAN AND RATIONALE

STEP 1: PELVIC ULTRASOUND (US), TRANSVAGINAL (TVUS)

In young women **with a normal pelvic examination** and a **negative pregnancy test,** most bleeding is related to hormonal variation and is managed expectantly or treated with oral contraceptives. **Pelvic US is reserved for patients with persistent or unexplained symptoms, an abnormal pelvic exam, a limited physical exam (obesity), accompanying pelvic pain, or postmenopausal bleeding.**

Transvaginal ultrasound (TVUS) is the initial imaging examination to evaluate the uterus, ovaries, and adnexa. TVUS has largely replaced the conventional transabdominal examination, because it depicts the uterus and adnexa with a higher degree of resolution and avoids the discomfort of a full-bladder transabdominal US study.

With the bladder emptied, a small, high-resolution transducer is placed within the vagina, close to the uterus and adnexa. (Transabdominal sonography [TAS], performed with the bladder filled—to displace bowel loops that could obscure pelvic organs—is selectively used (1) to examine large masses; (2) in very young patients— younger than 18 years of age; and (3) for patients unable to tolerate TVUS. Also, many sonographers still prefer to study **all** patients **initially** with transabdominal US and then proceed to TVUS).

The uterine wall (myometrium) is examined carefully during TVUS. Uterine fibroids, a common cause of menorrhagia, are easily seen, and their size, number, and location defined. (Fibroids can be serially followed sonographically, if necessary.) Adenomyosis, in which endometrial tissue grows into the myometrium, can frequently be suggested sonographically (by uterine enlargement and heterogeneity) but is often difficult to differentiate from fibroids.

The thickness of the endometrial lining is also evaluated. Abnormal thickening may be due to **hyperplasia, polyps, submucosal fibroids, or endometrial cancer.** The most accurate time to evaluate the endometrium in premenopausal patients is during the first week after menstruation, before normal physiologic changes cause thickening. Fortunately, this is also the optimal time for ovarian sonographic evaluation.

Magnetic resonance (MR) imaging is frequently useful in the evaluation of suspected adenomyosis and in patients with bulky or complex fibroids (see **Step 2, Magnetic Resonance Imaging,** below).

If the cause of uterine bleeding remains obscure and nongynecologic conditions (coagulopathy, endocrine abnormalities, medication-related bleeding) have been excluded, endometrial biopsy, sonohysterography, or direct endoscopic hysterography usually follow (see **Step 2, Sonohysterography/Endoscopic Hysterography,** below).

STEP 2: SONOHYSTEROGRAPHY/ENDOSCOPIC HYSTEROGRAPHY

OR

STEP 2: MAGNETIC RESONANCE (MR) IMAGING

Sonohysterography

Sonohysterography, a more invasive US study used to evaluate a suspected endometrial abnormality, entails injecting 5 to 10 mL of sterile water into the endometrial canal through a thin plastic catheter. The water creates a gap between the normally juxtaposed linings of the endometrial canal, so that they can be seen in detail; focal endometrial abnormalities (polyps, hyperplasia, submucosal fibroids) can be differentiated from diffuse endometrial thickening (Fig. 19-1). Localized endometrial lesions can be biopsied under hysteroscopic visualization.

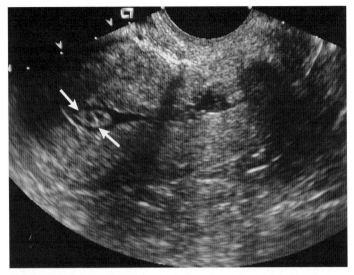

Figure 19-1. Sonohysterogram showing an endometrial polyp in a patient with abnormal uterine bleeding. Sterile saline had been injected into the endometrial cavity and outlines the polyp (*arrow*). The polyp was subsequently excised under hysteroscopic guidance.

Endoscopic Hysteroscopy

A trained gynecologist inserts a small endoscope with biopsy instruments directly into the endometrial cavity; direct hysteroscopy is more accurate for focal lesions than nondirected "blind" endometrial sampling and traditional dilation/curettage.

MR

MR is more accurate than TVUS for the diagnosis of adenomyosis and in gauging the depth of penetration of endometrial carcinoma. Bulky or complex fibroids can be difficult to fully assess sonographically; MR is therefore often performed for preoperative planning or prior to fibroid therapy by uterine fibroid embolization (UFE).

SUMMARY AND CONCLUSIONS

1. AUB has many causes, largely dependent on patient age and presentation. When uterine **lesions**—such as fibroids, adenomyosis, or endometrial pathology, as opposed to endocrine abnormalities—are suspected or must be excluded, TVUS is the examination of choice.

   TVUS is a quick, cost-effective, and accurate evaluator of the uterus and adnexa.
2. Sonohysterography provides a more detailed examination of the endometrium and can characterize endometrial abnormalities as a diffuse or focal process. For focal abnormalities, direct hysteroscopic biopsy by the gynecologist is more accurate than traditional "blind" procedures.
3. MR is appropriate for some uterine lesions, particularly adenomyosis or complex fibroids, and is commonly used for evaluation prior to therapeutic UFE.

ADDITIONAL COMMENTS

- Cervical carcinoma as a cause of AUB is generally diagnosed by direct physical examination and biopsy. Cross-sectional imaging (CT and MR) is usually reserved for subsequent disease staging or follow-up.
- The age-old therapy for troublesome uterine fibroids has been hysterectomy. The past 5 years, however, have seen the rise of an alternative therapy, uterine fibroid embolization (UFE). Because UFE involves at most a one-night hospital stay (and in some centers is an entirely outpatient procedure), and because it is associated with a myriad of other advantages (no abdominal/pelvic scar, lower risk of infection, lower cost, less pain, and less overall morbidity), the procedure is gaining ground.

UFE is performed by an interventional radiologist, who catheterizes the artery or arteries that feed the fibroids and injects microembolic particles, which deprive the lesions of their blood supply. After this, they rapidly involute. The procedure is performed via percutaneous transfemoral arterial puncture under conscious sedation. Preoperative MR is frequently recommended to evaluate the uterus, because some fibroids are not amenable to embolic therapy.

SUGGESTED READING

Mihm LM, Quick VA, Brumfield JA, et al: The accuracy of endometrial biopsy and saline sonohysterography in the determination of the cause of abnormal uterine bleeding. Am J Obstet Gynecol 2002;186:858–860.

Salem S, Wilson SR: Gynecologic ultrasound. In Rumack CM, Wilson SR, Charboneau JW (eds): Diagnostic Ultrasound, 3rd ed. St. Louis, Elsevier-Mosby, 2005, pp 527–587.

Shwayder JM: Pathophysiology of abnormal uterine bleeding. Obstet Gynecol Clin North Am 2000;27:219–234.

Smith-Bindman R, Kerlikowski K, Feldstein VA, et al: Endovaginal ultrasound to exclude endometrial cancer and other endometrial abnormalities. JAMA 1998;280:1510–1517.

20 Adrenal Mass

INTRODUCTION

Adrenal masses incidentally found on cross-sectional imaging (usually computed tomography [CT]) for non-adrenal problems or in patients with a known primary tumor and undergoing a workup for metastatic disease represent a significant problem for both referring clinicians and radiologists. Most of these adrenal lesions, **even in patients with a known malignancy elsewhere, are benign**—usually adenomas but sometimes hyperplasia, myelolipomas, cysts, or hemorrhage. Autopsy series have revealed grossly visible non-functioning adenomas in 2% to 9% of adults (the higher numbers probably include macronodular hyperplasia as well as nonfunctioning adenomas). These lesions normally are less than 3 cm in diameter, but nonfunctioning adenomas occasionally may be larger. Much less commonly, the imaging workup specifically targets the adrenals because of a clinical adrenal syndrome: Cushing's syndrome, primary aldosteronism, or pheochromocytoma.

The mainstay of initial cross-sectional imaging for a suspected adrenal mass is CT, and likewise, the overwhelming majority of incidentally detected adrenal masses, or adrenal masses discovered during the workup for malignancy, are found on CT. Magnetic resonance (MR) imaging also has a role in the workup, and fluorodeoxyglucose–positron emission tomography (FDG-PET) is increasingly important in the adrenal evaluation **of cancer patients** (see **CHAPTER 61, PET and PET/CT in Cancer Staging**). Ultimately, however, CT-guided biopsy may be required, **partic-**

ularly when the presence or absence of adrenal metastases would greatly impact the care plan.

In a few patients with suspected **functioning adrenal tumors,** additional nuclear medicine techniques and adrenal venous sampling apply.

Relative Costs: CT, unenhanced, **$$**; CT, enhanced, **$$$**; MR, **$$$$**; FDG-PET, **$$$$$**; adrenal venous sampling, **$$$$$$**; CT-guided biopsy, **$$$$**.

PLAN AND RATIONALE

(A) THE ENDOCRINOLOGICALLY SILENT ADRENAL MASS/THE INCIDENTAL ADRENAL LESION ON AN INITIAL ABDOMINAL CT

In patients without a known extra-adrenal malignancy and an adrenal mass initially discovered on an abdominal CT:

STEP 1: COMPUTED TOMOGRAPHY (CT) DENSITY MEASUREMENTS/ADDITIONAL CT IMAGES

Abdominal CT is almost invariably performed after a peripheral intravenous infusion of contrast medium; the iodine-based contrast medium "enhances" (increases the radiographic density of) almost all tissues. ("Enhancement" is a complex function of a tissue's blood flow, blood volume, and capillary permeability.) **Thus, when an adrenal mass is incidentally discovered on an abdominal CT, the patient has usually already had contrast medium infused; understanding this fact is key to understanding the subsequent sequence of the workup.**

The interpreting radiologist first compares the current study to previous studies (if any) to determine whether the lesion has been stable in size; he or she then measures the lesion's density.

If the lesion's density is equal to or lower than that of water, the lesion is almost certainly benign.

If the mass is significantly **denser** than water, it is nonetheless likely an adenoma, because primary adrenal cortical carcinoma is rare, and the lesion is not likely to be a metastasis in the absence of a known primary malignancy (although some adrenal masses cannot be clearly characterized as benign or malignant on the initial analysis). For these lesions, additional CT images are helpful; the "enhancement" of benign lesions decreases rapidly over time (contrast medium "washout"), whereas the washout kinetics of malignant adrenal lesions are much, much slower.

The initial density analysis, with a subsequent washout analysis, almost always ends the workup, but in a few cases a repeat CT or MR is appropriate.

STEP 2: ADDITIONAL IMAGING WITH COMPUTED TOMOGRAPHY (CT) OR MAGNETIC RESONANCE (MR)

Because this discussion involves the incidentally discovered adrenal mass found on a CT, and because CT is usually contrast enhanced, it is not possible in this scenario to measure the density of the adrenal lesion on the initial CT **without** circulating contrast medium. **The contrast medium has already been administered.** Thus, for lesions whose nature is ambivalent after **Step 1** above, the logical approach is to return the patient to the radiology department **for an additional nonenhanced CT at a later time** (and, if needed, additional enhanced and delayed images); density measurements according to this protocol usually end the workup.

Alternatively, MR can substitute for CT. MR includes what is referred to as "in-phase" and "out-of-phase" sequences; if the adrenal mass becomes darker on the out-of-phase images compared with the in-phase images, the finding is consistent with an adenoma and the workup ends.

Most experts on adrenal imaging prefer follow-up CT to MR for the majority of adrenal lesions that are indeterminate on initial contrast-enhanced CT, because nonenhanced CT combined (when needed) with additional contrast-enhanced CT and delayed washout analysis can accurately characterize almost all adrenal lesions, whereas some adrenal adenomas (so-called "lipid poor" adenomas) mimic the appearance of metastases on in-phase and out-of-phase MR sequences. **The choice of MR versus CT, however, simply is not "cut and dried," and whether to use MR should be a joint decision of the clinician and the radiologist, tailored to the individual patient.**

If **Steps 1** and **2** do not confirm that the lesion is an adenoma, follow-up imaging (CT or MR) is performed in several months, or, in some circumstances, biopsy is appropriate.

STEP 3: COMPUTED TOMOGRAPHY (CT)-GUIDED BIOPSY

When an adrenal lesion is large and/or heterogeneous (i.e., consists of various types of nonfatty tissue) or if an extra-adrenal malignancy is discovered, biopsy should be considered (see **Step 3, Adrenal Biopsy,** later; see also **CHAPTER 60, Percutaneous Guided Biopsy and Imaging-Guided Therapy**).

In patients with a known extra-adrenal malignancy and an adrenal mass initially discovered on an abdominal CT:

STEP 1: COMPUTED TOMOGRAPHY (CT) OR MAGNETIC RESONANCE (MR) IMAGING

The initial evaluation of patients with a **known** extra-adrenal malignancy and an adrenal mass found on an abdominal CT—usually in the course of the staging or restaging of the primary tumor—follows **Steps 1** and **2**, earlier. However, **in these patients the analysis should be relentlessly pursued to certainty or**

virtual certainty, even to biopsy, especially if an adrenal metastasis would alter patient management. (This scenario commonly applies to potentially resectable non–small-cell lung cancer that presents with an adrenal mass [or masses]; even these patients are more likely to have an adenoma than an adrenal metastasis, but **certainty in diagnosis is the goal, rather than high probability,** so rapid definitive diagnosis should apply, rather than follow-up.)

If available, FDG-PET is often extremely helpful.

STEP 2: FLUORODEOXYGLUCOSE–POSITRON EMISSION TOMOGRAPHY (FDG-PET)

Many cancer patients now undergo FDG-PET as part of their initial tumor staging (see **CHAPTER 61, PET and PET/CT in Cancer Staging**), and the procedure is very useful in the analysis of adrenal masses in the presence of a primary tumor elsewhere, when CT has been equivocal. FDG-PET produces images that reflect the uptake of radiolabeled glucose in various tissues, including tumors. Almost invariably, malignant tumors use more glucose than benign tumors or adjacent tissue, so with a few exceptions the test is a sensitive indicator of malignancy. Uptake of glucose is referred to as "metabolic activity."

FDG-PET has a very high negative predictive value in adrenal malignancies. A normal result on adrenal FDG-PET is a virtual guarantee of benignity.

FDG-PET's **specificity** is not as good, because **some benign adenomas are metabolically active.**

Overall, when the patient has a known primary tumor, and FDG-PET is available, a normal FDG-PET of the adrenals ends the workup.

However, **metabolically active masses should be considered malignant until proven otherwise.** Lesions that are equivocal should proceed to biopsy.

STEP 3: ADRENAL BIOPSY

In patients for whom an adrenal metastasis would alter patient management, biopsy is appropriate to prove that a metabolically active adrenal mass is indeed a metastasis (particularly in patients with otherwise-resectable non–small-cell lung cancer). Biopsy may be performed by a radiologist using imaging guidance, typically CT (see **CHAPTER 60, Percutaneous Guided Biopsy and Imaging-Guided Therapy**).

(B) THE SUSPECTED ENDOCRINOLOGICALLY ACTIVE ADRENAL MASS

Cushing's syndrome

STEP 1: COMPUTED TOMOGRAPHY (CT) WITHOUT INTRAVENOUS OR ORAL CONTRAST MEDIUM

In the majority of cases, Cushing's syndrome develops from adrenal cortical hyperplasia related to pituitary stimulation, but in the minority of cases it is related to an adrenal adenoma or, less commonly, adrenal carcinoma. In hyperplasia, both adrenal glands are usually symmetrically enlarged and are visualized as such on CT. Cortisol-producing tumors are usually large, and almost all are detected using CT. Typically, CT is performed without oral or intravenous contrast medium.

CT of the adrenals is rarely falsely positive or negative. Therefore, if CT finding is normal, the workup for a functioning adrenal cortisol–producing tumor usually ends.

STEP 2: ADRENAL VENOUS SAMPLING

In the relatively rare circumstance of a negative or equivocal CT finding (e.g., it is unclear whether there is an actual **focal** adrenal mass in a patient with mild bilateral adrenal enlargement, or in a patient with bilateral focal adrenal masses), adrenal venous sampling, described many years ago, remains an appropriate procedure before possible surgical intervention.

This study involves percutaneous femoral vein puncture and placement of catheters by an interventional radiologist into the right and left adrenal veins. Gentle injection of contrast medium visualizes the veins, and blood samples are drawn from each, and from the inferior vena cava, sometimes after pharmacologic stimulation. This technically demanding examination is effective for localizing functioning lesions but is invasive, and its availability is limited.

Primary aldosteronism

STEP 1: COMPUTED TOMOGRAPHY (CT) WITHOUT INTRAVENOUS OR ORAL CONTRAST MEDIUM

Adenomas cause about 80% of primary aldosteronism; most are less than 2 cm in diameter. CT without oral or intravenous contrast medium can detect most adenomas. However, because small nonfunctioning adrenal adenomas are common, and because these cannot be differentiated from a functioning adenoma by CT alone, some investigators advocate adrenal venous sampling.

STEP 2: ADRENAL VENOUS SAMPLING

(See **Cushing's syndrome, Step 2**.) Adrenal venous sampling may be appropriate before surgery to increase diagnostic confidence regarding the appropriate adrenal gland for surgery; certainty in terms of lateralization is particularly important for suspected aldosterone-producing adrenal tumors, because the CT findings in these tumors are more often equivocal or nondiagnostic.

Pheochromocytoma

About 90% of pheochromocytomas are located in the adrenals (10% bilateral), but 10% are extra-adrenal, involving para-aortic or paracaval sympathetic nervous tissue. Unusual locations include the chest and the urinary bladder. Malignant pheochromocytomas are rare but can metastasize.

Pheochromocytoma may be suspected when patients have labile, severe, or uncontrolled hypertension and/or spells manifested by headache, palpitations, sweating, or abdominal pain; have elevated basal plasma nor-epinephrine and/or persistently elevated urinary excretion rates for catecholamines; and have historical, clinical, or laboratory evidence for syndromes in which pheochromocytomas occur with increased frequency (multiple endocrine neoplasia [MEN] 2A or B, neuro-fibromatosis, and von Hippel-Lindau disease). However, there may be only minor symptoms or borderline intermittent laboratory abnormalities, and occasionally pheochromocytoma may be completely asymptomatic.

In our experience, the vast majority of patients referred for imaging with suspected pheochromocytoma **do not** have this diagnosis.

STEP 1: COMPUTED TOMOGRAPHY (CT) OR MAGNETIC RESONANCE (MR) OF THE ABDOMEN AND PELVIS

CT of the abdomen and pelvis is the initial imaging study for suspected pheochromocytoma, because most intra-adrenal pheochromocytomas are relatively large and easily identified. Although there was initial concern regarding the administration of intravenous contrast medium to patients with pheochromocytoma (and although intra-arterial contrast medium should not be administered, especially when performing invasive abdominal angiography), **there is no convincing evidence that intravenous contrast medium is unsafe in such patients.**

Alternatively, MR may be the initial examination of the adrenals and abdomen/pelvis in patients with a suspected pheochromocytoma. MR requires no contrast medium, and pheochromocytomas have a typical appearance on MR—quite bright on T2-weighted imaging.

STEP 2: NUCLEAR META-IODOBENZYLGUANIDINE (MIBG) SCAN

In cases in which CT and/or MR findings are equivocal or negative, yet there is compelling clinical and/or laboratory evidence of a pheochromocytoma, MIBG scintigraphy is the appropriate next imaging test. Tagged with iodine-131, MIBG is injected intravenously, and the patient is imaged over the course of several days. (MIBG is a chemical precursor of catecholamines, and, as such, is accumulated by catecholamine-producing tissue.) The technique is safe and noninvasive but provides relatively limited anatomic information compared with CT or MR.

MIBG is highly effective for demonstrating extra-adrenal metastases and recurrent or malignant lesions; however, it should not be an initial screening examination for pheochromocytoma.

SUMMARY AND CONCLUSIONS

1. Almost all incidental adrenal masses discovered on abdominal CT in patients **without a known primary extra-adrenal tumor** are benign. Repeat CT **without** (and if needed **with**) intravenous contrast medium, MR, and sequential follow-up can be performed if the initial examination is not diagnostic of a benign process (particularly an adenoma). Further imaging and follow-up should be considered on a patient-by-patient basis.

2. For patients **with a known extra-adrenal malignancy** and an adrenal mass incidentally discovered on CT, a similar approach applies, especially if an adrenal metastasis would alter

patient management. However, in these patients expeditious **diagnostic certainty** is the goal, pursued to biopsy if necessary.

3. FDG-PET plays an increasing role in the workup of patients with various malignancies. **If an adrenal mass is not metabolically active, it is very likely benign;** however, the converse is not true, as some adrenal adenomas are metabolically active.

4. Adrenal biopsies have declined in recent years because of the increased accuracy of CT and MR and the development of FDG-PET.

5. CT is also the mainstay for the initial diagnosis of adrenal lesions in patients with suspected cortisol-producing or aldosterone-producing tumors. CT or MR should be performed as the initial imaging test for suspected pheochromocytoma. Additional workup of these patients, when necessary, can be performed with adrenal venous sampling or MIBG tagged with iodine-131.

ADDITIONAL COMMENTS

- Adrenal hyperplasia is a relatively common finding on cross-sectional imaging, particularly in elderly patients with chronic cardiac disease. The adrenal glands are symmetrically and diffusely enlarged, and there is usually no focal mass. Such findings require no specific imaging or clinical follow-up.

- Benign adrenal lesions (adenomas and myelolipomas) are occasionally bilateral.

- Adrenal cortical carcinoma is a rare malignancy with a poor prognosis, that typically presents as a large, heterogeneous mass. Lymphadenopathy, venous invasion, and metastases may be present at diagnosis or occur shortly after initial diagnosis.

- Adrenal hemorrhage in adults may occur bilaterally, for example in a patient with sepsis who is on anticoagulation therapy, or unilaterally following trauma. The affected adrenal(s) are enlarged and hyperdense (most evident on nonenhanced images) with ill-defined margins. Management is conservative.

- Adrenal myelolipomas are benign lesions that have a characteristic appearance on cross-sectional imaging studies, due to their macroscopic fat content. **Unless large and/or symptomatic, they should not be resected (or biopsied).** Rarely, myelolipomas may occur in the abdomen and pelvis outside the adrenal glands.

- Rare causes of adrenal masses include adrenal cysts and "collision" tumors (metastasis intermingling with an adenoma). The former are usually benign, and the latter should be considered when a heterogenous adrenal lesion is encountered on cross-sectional imaging in the correct clinical setting. **In general, when an adrenal lesion has a heterogeneous appearance (and the heterogeneity is not due to the presence of fat), caution is advised, because it may represent a necrotic metastasis or adrenal cortical carcinoma.**

- Ultrasound is not an appropriate adrenal imaging modality in adults, because it is inferior to CT and MR.

Part III

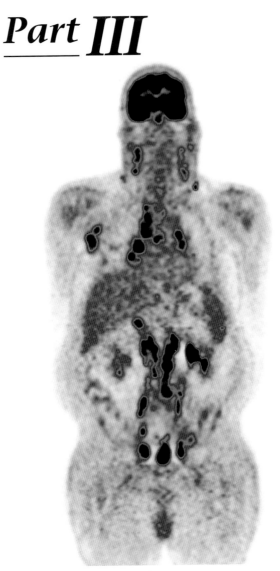

Chest

Solitary Pulmonary Nodule

▌INTRODUCTION

For two generations the solitary pulmonary nodule (SPN) was defined as a round or ovoid lung lesion less than 3 cm in diameter, usually identified first on a chest radiograph. In recent years, however, many much smaller SPNs have been identified on computed tomography (CT) of the chest, often as incidental findings. Although some SPNs are malignant, in most age groups the majority are benign—commonly, granulomas, intrapulmonary lymph nodes, or hamartomas, or, less commonly, benign bronchial adenomas. Moreover, a host of other lesions, ranging from rheumatoid nodules to sarcoid lesions, can appear as SPNs. **The goal of imaging is to differentiate benign from possibly malignant SPNs, without a biopsy when possible.** This differentiation depends primarily upon three factors: calcification, growth rate, and metabolic state (i.e., the accumulation of fluorodeoxyglucose [FDG] on positron emission tomography [PET]).

This chapter concerns the evaluation of a **solitary** lung lesion with no obvious central (hilar or mediastinal) mass on the initial chest radiograph **or** the finding of a **solitary** lung lesion on CT. (Noncalcified adenopathy, multiple noncalcified lung lesions, or a central mass suggests malignancy and the subsequent workup focuses on establishing a tissue diagnosis and the extent of disease by CT, PET, and biopsy, but that workup differs completely from the analysis of a SPN.) This chapter assumes that other indicators of malignancy, such as positive sputum cytology, are absent.

Patient age and history (particularly **cigarette smoking**) influence the decision-making process, and these must be provided to the radiologist.

Relative Costs: Posteroanterior (PA) and lateral chest radiography (films), **$**; PA, lateral, and oblique chest films, **$**; chest CT, with contrast medium, **$$$**; chest CT, without contrast medium, **$$**; chest lesion biopsy, CT-guided, **$$$$**; FDG-PET, **$$$$$**.

PLAN AND RATIONALE

When the initial SPN is detected on a chest film:

STEP 1: ADDITIONAL CHEST RADIOGRAPHS

After nodule detection with standard PA and lateral films, supplementary oblique or apical lordotic films may be required to prove that the nodule is truly intra-pulmonary. Sometimes, at the discretion of the radiologist, additional films are exposed with lead markers on skin lesions or the nipples to prove that these confusing "pseudonodules" are extrapulmonary. Obviously, if the "nodule" is proven to be an extraneous extrapulmonary density, the workup ends.

Certain characteristic patterns of calcification virtually assure benignity, and such calcifications may be obvious on chest films. When calcifications characteristic of benignity are identified, the workup ends, but when calcifications are absent or ambiguous, **every attempt must be made to obtain previous films to establish whether the lesion has grown.** In recent years a number of classic patterns previously considered to establish malignancy or benignity reliably (e.g., smooth versus speculated margins) have been discarded as unreliable, **but ABSENCE OF GROWTH has endured as an indication of benignity.** The criterion for benignity is generally considered to be 2 years of size stability for lesions discovered on a chest film.

If old chest films establish that the lesion has been stable for 2 years, the workup ends.

If old films are not available, or if previous films establish that the lesion is enlarging, CT is appropriate.

STEP 2: COMPUTED TOMOGRAPHY (CT)

CT confirms the presence of the nodule, maps its exact location, and often reveals additional unsuspected findings (other nodules or disease in the hila, mediastinum, or pleura). The additional findings frequently suggest alternative diagnoses, such as metastatic disease, and therefore shift the diagnostic focus away from SPN.

Although morphologic criteria like margins and shape are suggestive, they are in fact unreliable, even on CT, but the presence or absence of certain calcification patterns is characteristic of benignity. Sometimes benign calcification can be defined by CT, even when calcifications were **not** defined by chest films.

If the calcification pattern of a SPN is typically benign, the workup ends.

If no calcifications characteristic of benignity are defined by CT, the lesion is indeterminate, and further imaging depends upon the lesion's size and the patient's smoking history.

When the lesion is at least 1 cm in diameter, FDG-PET is appropriate.

When the lesion is less than 1 cm in diameter, serial follow-ups by CT are appropriate.

When the initial SPN is detected by CT:

See **Step 2: Computed Tomography** (above). The workup then proceeds according to CT findings and the lesion's size.

STEP 3A: FLUORODEOXYGLUCOSE–POSITRON EMISSION TOMOGRAPHY (FDG-PET), FOR LESIONS AT LEAST 1 CM IN DIAMETER

PET in combination with FDG has revolutionized the workup of the SPN, because the uptake of FDG in the nodule is **a reflection of its glucose avidity and, thus, of its metabolism.** Because tumors almost always aggressively accumulate glucose to support their rapid growth, an FDG-avid lesion is always a worrisome finding. Glucose avidity on PET is expressed as the "standardized uptake value" (awkwardly abbreviated SUV).

Although high FDG avidity is worrisome, it is **NOT** specific, because a large number of non-neoplastic inflammatory conditions, from compact pneumonias to sarcoid, can generate high SUVs. **Thus, a positive finding on a FDG-PET study for SPN does NOT indicate malignancy; rather, it indicates a worrisome lesion that requires a tissue diagnosis.** However, the predictive value of a negative finding on a FDG-PET study is very, very high, because only a very few ominous neoplasms fail to aggressively accumulate FDG, including bronchoalveolar carcinoma (BAC), carcinoid, and, occasionally, very, very low-grade adenocarcinoma.

Thus:

Nodules that accumulate FDG need a tissue diagnosis.

Nodules that do not accumulate FDG should be followed radiographically for 2 years; because these nodules are at least 1 cm in diameter, chest films, which are less expensive than CT, can be used, unless the nodule is superimposed over the hila, mediastinum, or major blood vessels. These superimposed structures interfere with accurate measurement. A radiologist should decide whether serial CT scans or chest films are appropriate.

Stability for 2 years ends the workup.

STEP 3B: SERIAL FOLLOW-UPS FOR LESIONS LESS THAN 1 CM IN DIAMETER

For purely technical reasons, PET is unable to reliably determine the FDG uptake of lesions less than 1 cm in diameter. (This inability does **NOT** imply that glucose uptake per unit volume of tumor is less in smaller lesions than in larger ones; rather, it derives from the physics of the PET scanner itself.) Thus, in such small lesions the criterion that determines whether to biopsy is **rate of growth,** and **the rate of growth of small lesions is best determined by CT.** Furthermore, we emphasize that measuring such small lesions on CT assumes that the scanner is helical and that thin sections are used; **archaic "stop and shoot" scanners, or helical scanners with thick sections, are completely inadequate to this purpose.**

THUS: Although most lesions at least 1 cm in diameter that are not overlapped by the hila, mediastinum, or heart may be followed by chest films, smaller lesions are appropriately followed by CT.

Follow-up intervals for CT are controversial, but in adults with a smoking history close follow-up is prudent: 3, 6, and 12 months followed by 2 and 3 years is reasonable. Any documented growth mandates biopsy.

Stability for 3 years ends the workup.

Nonsmokers should also be followed for 3 years with CT, but the follow-up intervals are controversial and many thoracic physicians advocate longer intervals between examinations.

STEP 4: IMAGING-GUIDED BIOPSY OR THORACOSCOPIC WEDGE RESECTION

When a tissue diagnosis is mandatory (FDG-avidity and/or lesion growth), consultation with a thoracic surgeon is often appropriate, because some lesions can be resected by video-assisted thoracoscopic wedge resection, a minimally invasive thoracic surgical technique that permits concurrent diagnosis and treatment.

Most SPNs larger than 1 cm in diameter are amenable to CT-guided percutaneous, transthoracic needle biopsy. The procedure is usually performed under a medication regimen called "conscious sedation," which provides good pain control without major risks of respiratory depression or hypotension. The likelihood of obtaining adequate tissue for a pathologic diagnosis is very high, particularly when the radiologist works with a pathologist on site, in the radiology department, who examines the specimen immediately to determine its adequacy.

The procedure takes from 30 minutes to 1 hour, depending upon the size and position of the lesion. The most common complication is pneumothorax, almost always small, requiring only observation; if larger, pneumothorax is usually treated by a small-bore chest tube, without the need for a thoracic surgeon.

A benign biopsy ends the workup, whereas a malignant biopsy is followed by appropriate further therapy.

SUMMARY AND CONCLUSIONS

1. Standard frontal and lateral chest films are sometimes supplemented with additional views to confirm the intrathoracic location of an apparent nodule and to identify calcification. If calcification characteristic of benignity is identified, the workup ends.

2. If no characteristic calcifications are seen, previous chest films must be sought to establish the SPN's growth rate. **A nodule that has not changed in size for at least 2 years on serial chest films is considered benign. Growth of any nodule is worrisome for malignancy, despite its configuration.**

3. CT can establish whether the nodule is truly solitary and whether there is unsuspected disease elsewhere—other nodules in the mediastinum, hila, or pleura. CT can often characterize nodules as **almost certainly benign** or **indeterminate.**

4. Indeterminate nodules are studied differently, according to their size. SPNs at least 1 cm in diameter are examined by FDG-PET. **High FDG accumulation is worrisome and mandates tissue diagnosis by CT-guided biopsy or video-assisted thoracoscopic surgery.**

5. Low FDG accumulation on PET is reassuring, but follow-up is indicated.

6. For PET-negative (non–FDG-avid) nodules 1 cm or larger, chest films are acceptable for follow-up, and 2 years of stability ends the workup.

7. CT is best for follow-up of lesions less than 1 cm in size, and for these small lesions 3 years of follow-up is prudent, for smokers and nonsmokers alike. More frequent follow-up intervals, however, are usually advocated for smokers.

ADDITIONAL COMMENTS

- When sputum cytology is positive and the chest film is normal, chest CT and bronchoscopy are appropriate, but a thorough ear, nose, and throat examination and esophagoscopy should accompany these studies, because the abnormal cytology may originate from malignant lesions of the nose, oropharynx, nasopharynx, mouth, trachea, or upper esophagus. FDG-PET studies of the chest have to date not been helpful in this matter.

- Positive sputum cytology establishes the presence of malignancy but does not localize a lesion itself. Cytology is more likely negative when the lesion is an isolated, malignant, peripheral nodule.

- Although bronchoscopy is an established and pivotal tool for evaluating chest malignancy, it is often fruitless in the evaluation of a peripheral nodule with no central mass/adenopathy.

- Magnetic resonance (MR) imaging and CT have been used to define the perfusion of a nodule after peripheral intravenous injection of contrast medium. Malignant nodules usually exhibit greater perfusion than benign nodules, but this analysis is less reliable than FDG-PET for larger SPNs and is unreliable in very small SPNs.

  For many years CT was used to quantitate the calcium content of a SPN by comparing the lesion to a calcium-containing target called a "phantom." This technology has been superseded by PET-FDG for nodules at least 1 cm in diameter, and for smaller lesions it has been superseded by serial CT scans to assess growth.

- The alert reader will have noted that we suggest 3 years of CT follow-up for small lesions yet only 2 years of chest films follow-up for larger lesions. This discrepancy relates to the inherent difficulties in established growth rates in small versus larger lesions; by definition, lesions seen on a chest film must be **at least** 5 to 7 mm in diameter. The problem is that very tiny lesions cannot be defined sufficiently, even by CT, to be **sure** that no significant growth has occurred from year to year, and a very small change **in diameter** indicates a large change in **volume** (volume is proportional to the radius cubed). Thus, to avoid mistakenly calling a slowly enlarging lesion "stable" on CT, we recommend a longer (3-year) follow-up for small lesions. In this context, however, we note that the analysis of very small chest nodules is relatively new, because the technology to study them has existed for only a few years; therefore, long-term longitudinal follow-up studies have not been completed. The guidelines are apt to undergo revision by 2006, but until then we have chosen to err on the conservative side, for the sake of patient safety.

▌ SUGGESTED READING

Erasmus JJ, Connolly JE, McAdams HP, Roggli VL: Solitary pulmonary nodules: Part I. Morphologic evaluation for differentiation of benign and malignant lesions. Radiographics 2000;20:43–58.

Erasmus JJ, McAdams HP, Connolly JE: Solitary pulmonary nodules: Part II. Evaluation of the indeterminate nodule. Radiographics 2000;20:59–66.

Gould MK, Sanders GD, Barnett PG, et al: Cost-effectiveness of alternative management strategies for patients with solitary pulmonary nodules. Ann Internal Med 2003;138:724–735.

Henschke CI, Yankelevitz DF, Naidich DP, et al: CT screening for lung cancer: suspiciousness of nodules according to size on baseline scans. Radiology 2004;231:164–168.

MacMahon H: Improvement in detection of pulmonary nodules: digital image processing and computer aided diagnosis. Radiographics 2000;20:1169–1177.

Patz EF: Evaluation of focal pulmonary abnormalities with FDG PET. Radiographics 2000;20:1182–1185.

Swensen SJ, Viggiano RW, Midthun DE, et al: Lung nodule enhancement at CT: multicenter study. Radiology 2000;214:73–80.

22 Mediastinal Mass

INTRODUCTION

Mediastinal masses may be symptomatic, suspected clinically but asymptomatic, or suspected because of incidental findings on chest radiography. Additional imaging can (1) confirm or exclude a lesion; (2) suggest a specific diagnosis; (3) help define the location of the mass in the mediastinum (i.e., anterior, middle, or posterior, which engenders an appropriate differential diagnosis); or (4) characterize the lesion sufficiently to guide biopsy or therapy.

Computed tomography (CT) and magnetic resonance (MR) imaging have made initial evaluation of the mediastinum safe and noninvasive. These cross-sectional techniques are sometimes diagnostically definitive (e.g., enlarged thyroid or aortic aneurysm), and both provide limited **tissue characterization** even without a specific histologic diagnosis (e.g., fat can be differentiated from other tissues). Some masses are clearly malignant (e.g., germ cell tumor that invades the mediastinal vessels and has spread to the lungs), but other lesions cannot be characterized as benign or malignant by their appearance.

CT can guide percutaneous needle biopsy of mediastinal masses (see **CHAPTER 60, Percutaneous Guided Biopsy and Imaging-Guided Therapy**), especially in the anterior mediastinum.

Relative Costs: CT, **$$$**; MR, **$$$$**.

PLAN AND RATIONALE

(A) GENERAL APPROACH

STEP 1: CHEST RADIOGRAPHY (PLAIN FILMS)

When evaluating a mediastinal mass **suspected on clinical grounds** (e.g., lymphoma or possible thymoma in myasthenia gravis), posteroanterior and lateral chest films are appropriate for a baseline determination, despite the need for additional imaging. The chest film is almost never specific, however, and **the next step is CT of the thorax, the most versatile and valuable imaging test for detecting, localizing, and characterizing a mediastinal mass.**

STEP 2: COMPUTED TOMOGRAPHY (CT), USUALLY WITH CONTRAST MEDIUM ("ENHANCED")

CT defines the location, size, density, and contour of a mediastinal mass, as well as its effects on adjacent structures. The lungs, hila, thoracic inlet, and chest wall are also examined. In general, CT for a known or suspected mediastinal mass (or process) is performed with peripheral intravenous contrast medium, tailored by the radiologist to the plain film findings and clinical information. For example, if an aneurysm of the aorta is suspected on plain films, the scan would usually be performed with intravenous contrast medium (and thin slices) to optimally define the relationship of the aneurysm to branch vessels and to the aortic lumen. Alternatively, if substernal extension of a goiter is suspected, iodinated contrast medium would be avoided, because it could interfere with subsequent radionuclide imaging (sometimes performed with radioactive iodine); the relationship of the substernal and cervical thyroid is usually clear without contrast medium. In some patients, CT may be required both without and then with contrast medium to define which portions and to what extent the mass "enhances" (see **INTRODUCTION** to the book for a discussion of the tumor "enhancement" phenomenon).

If CT proves that there is no mediastinal mass or provides an alternative explanation for an apparent mass on chest radiographs—such as prominent mediastinal fat or a tortuous but not substantially dilated aorta—the workup ends.

If a mass exists and is sufficiently defined for biopsy or therapy, CT may guide the biopsy (see Step 4) and then be used to follow up patients after appropriate therapy, if any.

If CT defines a mass but subtle relationships of the mass to the spine and neural foramina must be clarified, or if chest wall invasion needs to be analyzed in more detail, MR can be useful.

STEP 3: MAGNETIC RESONANCE (MR) IMAGING (IN SELECTED PATIENTS TO COMPLEMENT CT, OR AS AN ALTERNATIVE TO CT)

Modern CT has eliminated many former advantages of MR, because multidetector CT scanners readily create multiplanar images. The spatial resolution of CT is superior to MR, and MR does not show calcification as readily as CT. However, in some specific circumstances MR remains superior to CT: for showing (1) the exact relationship of a posterior mediastinal mass (which is frequently of neural origin) to the spine and neural foramina, and (2) the extent and characteristics of chest wall invasion.

MR is also an appropriate alternative for patients who cannot tolerate the iodinated contrast medium of CT and for children and pregnant women, who should avoid exposure to ionizing radiation. (See **IN-TRODUCTION** to this book for discussions of contrast medium intolerance and MR technology.)

STEP 3 OR 4: COMPUTED TOMOGRAPHY (CT)–GUIDED BIOPSY

The approach to biopsy of a mediastinal mass is made individually, considering the imaging findings, accessibility of the mass to a safe biopsy route, and clinical history. **Despite its value, CT-guided biopsy is not always possible or even preferable.**

For certain masses abutting the central airways, transbronchial biopsy can be performed through an endoscope by a pulmonologist (either "blindly," but using the CT as a road map, or using real-time guidance with fluoroscopy, CT, or, most recently, sonography).

If the mass is paraesophageal, transesophageal endoscopic ultrasound guidance by a gastroenterologist may be preferable, particularly for a subcarinal lesion.

For suspected lymphoma, surgical biopsy may be preferable to harvest a large volume of tissue for pathologic examination.

Thymic tumors usually undergo complete surgical excision.

(B) SPECIFIC SITUATIONS

SUSPECTED SUBSTERNAL GOITER

Mediastinal extension of thyroid tissue is a relatively common mediastinal mass. CT is the test of choice and confirms continuity of mediastinal and cervical thyroid tissue very well (Fig. 22-1). On nonenhanced CT, mediastinal thyroid tissue is usually relatively dense and often calcified.

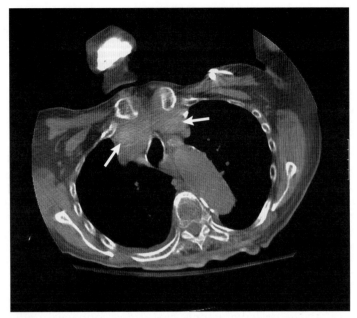

Figure 22-1. Chest CT in an 82-year-old woman with incidentally detected substernal intrathoracic goiter. Image from a CT without intravenous contrast medium shows significant enlargement of the thyroid (*arrows*), which surrounds the trachea, in the upper thorax.

HIATAL HERNIA

Although plain radiographic findings are usually diagnostic of a hiatal hernia, in selected cases a conventional barium swallow, performed under fluoroscopy, confirms the diagnosis. Alternatively, CT also definitively establishes whether the mass is a hiatal hernia (usually without the need for any contrast medium, although oral contrast medium could be given).

FATTY LESION

Fat **density** and **"signal"** are easily revealed on CT and MR, respectively. Many initially worrisome lesions on plain chest films can be classified as simple lipomatosis (e.g., in obese patients or in patients on steroids), lipoma, or mesenteric fat in a diaphragmatic hernia, ending the workup and concern. Fat may also be defined within a more complex anterior mediastinal mass—benign or malignant teratoma.

CYSTIC LESION

Mediastinal cystic masses have many etiologies, including bronchogenic cyst, pericardial cyst, lymphangioma, thymic cyst, and postsurgical fluid collection, all very well shown by both CT and MR. Further workup and management depend on the combination of imaging findings (size of the lesion, effect on adjacent structures) and the specific clinical history (particularly, whether the patient is symptomatic). Some patients should undergo no further workup (e.g., a presumed pericardial cyst in an asymptomatic patient whose lesion was detected incidentally), whereas others may benefit from aspiration under appropriate imaging guidance.

LYMPHADENOPATHY

Lymphadenopathy commonly causes a mass or masses in any part of the mediastinum. Differential diagnosis is extensive, including malignancy (e.g., lung cancer, lymphoma, and metastatic disease), infection (e.g., bacterial, tuberculous, fungal), and inflammatory/ immunologically mediated disorders (such as sarcoid). CT is invaluable for revealing and localizing adenopathy and guiding appropriate biopsy, as well as for follow-up—**but neither CT nor MR can reliably differentiate benign from malignant lymph nodes. Fluo-rodeoxyglucose–positron emission tomography (FDG-PET), or combined PET/CT, is very useful for characterizing the metabolic activity of thoracic adenopathy as an indicator of malignancy, especially in patients with lung cancer or lymphoma** (see **CHAPTER 61, PET and PET/CT in Cancer Staging**).

THE ENLARGED THYMUS

Thymic enlargement on CT or MR can be a diagnostic conundrum, especially in adults; the problem is to differentiate residual normal thymus, which can persist into the forties, from anterior mediastinal mass/disease, including thymic tumor or residual postchemotherapy lymphoma. The latter is complicated by the phenomenon of "thymic rebound," in which the thymus regrows rapidly after chemotherapy. FDG-PET can often differentiate between residual anterior mediastinal lymphoma and thymic rebound, because mediastinal lymphoma is usually more metabolically active.

SUMMARY AND CONCLUSIONS

1. CT is the best imaging test for confirming or excluding a mediastinal mass (or masses). CT also examines the lungs, which is critically important in patients who may have a thoracic neoplasm. Generally, for optimal imaging, CT is performed with intravenous contrast medium. MR has a decreased role given current CT scanner technology, but it remains an adjunctive examination that should be reserved for when questions unanswered by CT need to be resolved, when radiation exposure is a major concern, or when the patient cannot tolerate iodinated contrast medium.

2. CT findings may be diagnostic of a specific mediastinal mass, such as aortic aneurysm or intrathoracic extension of a thyroid goiter, or may show a grossly invasive mass consistent with malignancy, but often the mass has a nonspecific appearance and requires biopsy for definitive diagnosis.

3. Although mediastinal masses should be evaluated and managed on a case-by-case basis, CT is key to the decision-making process and commonly guides the biopsy.

4. FDG-PET and, when available, PET/CT are commonly used to help characterize mediastinal adenopathy, especially in patients undergoing staging and follow-up of lung cancer and lymphoma.

SUGGESTED READING

Erasmus JE, McAdams HP, Donnelly LF, Spritzer CE: MR imaging of mediastinal masses. MRI Clin North Am 2000;8:59–89.

Franco A, Mody NS, Meza MP: Imaging evaluation of pediatric mediastinal masses. Radiol Clin North Am 2005;43:325–353.

Panelli F, Erickson RA, Prasad VM: Evaluation of mediastinal masses by endoscopic ultrasound and endoscopic ultrasound-guided fine needle aspiration. Am J Gastroenterol 2001;96:401–408.

Yoneda KY, Louie S, Shelton DK: Mediastinal tumors. Curr Opinion Pulm Med 2001;7:226–233.

23 Pulmonary Embolism

INTRODUCTION

Pulmonary embolism (PE) is a common consideration whose true incidence, clinical manifestations, and natural history remain controversial. The "treatment" of pulmonary embolism is anticoagulation, a sometimes hazardous therapy. Anticoagulation does not treat pulmonary embolism per se; it prevents further thrombus formation and subsequent embolism. Thus, a diagnosis of PE raises the specter of future pulmonary emboli, and avoidance of that event is the benefit that clinicians balance against the risk of anticoagulation.

Patients referred to radiology for PE have chest-related symptoms (dyspnea, chest pain, hemoptysis), signs of deep venous thrombosis (DVT) in the legs, or a deterioration in blood gasses. The alarming nature and nonspecificity of these signs/symptoms and the danger of additional emboli are responsible for the enormous attention devoted to this problem.

Before any imaging studies are considered, a nonimaging screen, the quantitative plasma D-dimer assay, is prudent, where available. A normal D-dimer essentially excludes the diagnosis of PE in non–cancer patients and in those who are not chronically ill; **therefore, patients with normal D-dimer who are sent to radiology for a PE workup should have compelling signs/symptoms.**

Over the last decade the increased speed of CT scanners has caused a sea of change in the PE workup. CT angiography (CTA) is now almost universally considered the first-line test, unless contraindicated by massive obesity (patient cannot fit into the CT gantry), lack of good venous access for the intravenous contrast medium bolus injection, **extreme** dyspnea (patient cannot lie flat or breath-hold for 20 seconds), or contraindication to contrast medium. **This chapter assumes that diagnostic-quality CTA is available.**

The chest film, CT pulmonary angiogram (CTPA), CT venogram and pulmonary angiogram (CTVPA), Doppler ultrasound (US), and nuclear ventilation/perfusion (V̇/Q̇) scan are relevant.

Relative Costs: Chest films, posteroanterior and lateral, **$**; CTPA, **$$$**; CTVPA, **$$$**; V̇/Q̇ lung scan, **$$**; Doppler venous US of both legs, **$$**.

▋ PLAN AND RATIONALE

STEP 1: CHEST RADIOGRAPHY (PLAIN FILMS)

The chest film in patients with suspected PE is always normal or nonspecific. Suggestive findings such as an elevated hemidiaphragm, a small collection of pleural fluid, patches of atelectasis, and right ventricular enlargement have numerous causes. Thus, a more definitive study is required.

The chest film is nonetheless appropriate, because it sometimes reveals the cause of dyspnea and chest pain, for example rib fracture or pneumothorax.

If chest films elucidate the cause of symptoms/ signs, the workup ends.

If chest films are normal or nonspecific, two options are appropriate:

STEP 2A: CTA WITH A VENOUS STUDY (CTVPA)

CT angiography of the pulmonary arterial tree is known as CTPA (CT pulmonary angiography). A peripheral intravenous contrast medium injection is followed by a well-timed CT of the chest. The pulmonary arterial tree,

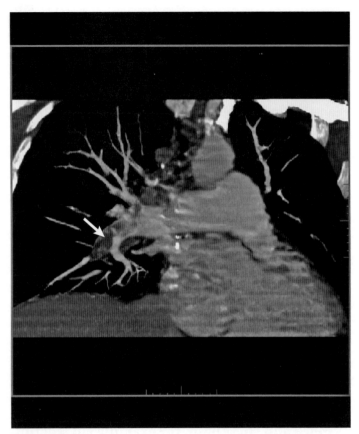

Figure 23-1. No, this is not a conventional pulmonary angiogram performed by injection of contrast medium into a pulmonary artery after a catheter has been introduced via percutaneous transfemoral puncture and threaded craniad into the superior vena cava, heart, and pulmonary artery. It is the coronal reconstruction of a CT after peripheral intravenous injection of contrast medium. Note the huge and obvious embolus in the lower lobe branch of the right pulmonary artery (*arrow*). The thrombus is an obvious dark "filling defect" that stands out against the background of white contrast medium.

down to segmental vessels, is defined (Fig. 23-1). An extension of the technique, CT venography and pulmonary arteriography (CTVPA), is gaining in popularity, because CTVPA studies the pulmonary arterial tree **and the entire venous system from the ankles to the**

diaphragm. Thus, CTVPA provides a picture of total thrombus burden, obviating the need for Doppler US of the legs.

CTVPA does **NOT** require a separate injection of contrast medium into the venous system. Rather, after the pulmonary arteries are scanned, the circulating contrast medium already injected for CTPA opacifies the venous system as the scanner traverses the legs, pelvis, and abdomen. There is no additional risk to the patient (aside from additional radiation exposure); the added examination time is less than 5 minutes.

If CTVPA findings are normal, the workup ends, because both the pulmonary circulation and the venous system of the abdomen, pelvis, and legs, have been exonerated.

Very often, CTPA reveals no emboli, but because the entire chest is scanned as the pulmonary arteries are studied, other key findings that explain the patient's symptoms and signs are identified; large studies have proven that more often than not these are nonembolic and include pneumothorax, pneumonia, pericardial effusion, pleuritis/effusion, subtle fractures, aortic dissection, mediastinal masses, and many others. The bulk of these findings escapes detection by the preliminary chest film.

Step 2b: CTPA (CT Pulmonary Angiography)

CTPA is the first half of CTVPA. The pulmonary arterial tree, down to segmental vessels, is defined, but subsegmental arteries are not seen, and the venous system of the pelvis and legs is not studied.

If CTPA reveals emboli, the workup ends.

Very often, CTPA reveals no emboli, but because the entire chest is scanned as the pulmonary arteries are studied, other key findings that explain the patient's symptoms and signs are identified; large studies have proven that more often than not these are nonembolic and include

pneumothorax, pneumonia, pericardial effusion, pleuritis/effusion, subtle fractures, aortic dissection, mediastinal masses, and many others. Many of these findings escape detection by the preliminary chest film.

If CTPA findings are normal, emboli are highly unlikely, but because subsegmental arteries are not defined, US of the legs may be appropriate to seek DVT. (Studies have shown that Doppler US and CT venography of the legs identify small thrombi after 1% to 8% of normal CTPA studies, implying that very small PEs may escape detection on CTPA.)

STEP 3: DOPPLER ULTRASOUND (US) OF THE LEGS

Although by definition US of the legs cannot directly address the issue of pulmonary embolism, thromboembolism is one disease, and thus peripheral thrombi and PE are part of one continuum. Because the vast majority of PEs originate in the legs, Doppler US is a reasonable, noninvasive choice to clarify the situation in the setting of a normal CTPA, especially when clinical suspicion of PE is high.

Doppler US is completely noninvasive and in experienced hands is both sensitive and specific. A normal Doppler US ends the workup.

When CTPA and CTVPA are contraindicated:

STEP 2: THE VENTILATION/PERFUSION LUNG SCAN

For a generation the radionuclide ventilation/perfusion ($\dot{V}/\dot{Q}$) scan was the backbone of PE diagnosis. Now, in most areas of the United States it is becoming a secondary procedure.

The $\dot{V}/\dot{Q}$ scan consists of two parts: a ventilation study that uses either aerosolized radioactive particles of technetium 99m–diethylenetriaminepentaacetic acid

(Tc-99m-DTPA) or a radioactive gas (Xenon-133 [Xe-133]) and a perfusion study using radiolabeled macro-aggregated albumin particles (Tc-99m-MAA).

The perfusion lung scan is safe and noninvasive; the peripheral intravenous injection of Tc-99m-MAA produces no physiologic effect, unless the pulmonary capillary bed is very severely compromised—a rare event that is almost unheard of—and the ventilation scan with either Xe-133 or Tc-99m-DTPA is harmless. Although the injection of Tc-99m-MAA does require venous access, any tiny peripheral vein (e.g., in the dorsum of the thumb) will suffice, unlike the venous access required for CTPA or CTVPA (usually an 18-gauge venous line).

CTPA or CTVPA define emboli or venous clots **directly,** by virtue of the "filling defect" they produce when compared with a column of opaque contrast medium (see Fig. 23-1), but the perfusion lung scan implies emboli **indirectly,** by filling the normal capillary bed with radioactivity, leaving a paucity of radioactive particles distal to an embolus. Thus, CTPA and CTVPA are highly specific, whereas the radioactivity void (perfusion deficit or "photopenic area") identified by a perfusion lung scan can be due to **any object (or event) that decreases perfusion.** Acute emboli, to be sure, block blood flow, but blood flow is also blocked by tumors, vascular hypoplasia, old emboli, vascular scar, and, most commonly, **vasoconstriction.** The latter is triggered in many (but not all) people by hypoxia, and the causes of hypoxia in the lung are legion. (Although beyond the scope of this basic text, we note for completeness that the purpose of vasoconstriction on a hypoxic basis is to equalize ventilation and perfusion to a hypoxic region of the lung; otherwise, unimpeded blood flow through a hypoxic area would result in unoxygenated blood returning to the left side of the heart, with subsequent peripheral oxygen desaturation.)

In an attempt to clarify the perfusion defects seen on many perfusion lung scans, a ventilation scan is always performed. The logic of combining the two imaging examinations is that a poorly perfused area that is well ventilated (unmatched) is likely the result of an embolus, whereas a poorly perfused region that is poorly ventilated (matched) is likely the result of local vasoconstriction.

Years of experience and hundreds of complex papers have demonstrated that **a normal perfusion lung scan reliably excludes a pulmonary embolus,** but there are many iterations and combinations of V̇/Q̇ scans that translate into probability estimates: "high probability," "intermediate probability," indeterminate, and "low probability." For the clinician, it is important to realize that an indeterminate examination means that no real information is provided, and **a "low probability" scan is NOT the same as "normal"—in many studies up to 15% of "low probability lung scans" are associated with pulmonary emboli**. A "high probability" scan is somewhere between 85% and 95% accurate.

Thus:

A normal V̇/Q̇ scan ends the workup.

A high probability scan, in the correct clinical setting, ends the workup.

An "indeterminate" or "intermediate probability" scan in any patient, and a "low probability" scan in a worrisome setting, often require a further step (see Step 3, Doppler US of the Legs).

SUMMARY AND CONCLUSIONS

1. Because it may reveal the cause of embolus-like symptoms, the chest film comes first.
2. In nonpregnant adults, we prefer CTVPA as the second step, **because it examines the pulmonary arterial tree and the venous system from the ankles to the diaphragm.** In children and pregnant women, pelvic irradiation should be avoided; therefore, either CTPA or a V̇/Q̇ scan is appropriate. (A V̇/Q̇ scan delivers less than one-hundredth the radiation dose of CTPA.)
3. **A normal CTVPA ends the workup,** but many thoughtful investigators recommend Doppler US of the legs after a normal CTPA.

4. A normal result on a V̇/Q̇ study or a "high probability" V̇/Q̇ scan ends the workup, but other classifications of the V̇/Q̇ scan should be followed by Doppler US of the legs. In this context, note that a "low probability" V̇/Q̇ scan is associated with PE in about 15% of cases.
5. The algorithm for PE is in flux, and a new generation of multidetector CT (MDCT) scanners will probably simplify the issue.

ADDITIONAL COMMENTS

- Doppler US after normal CTPA may become unnecessary as the new generation of 16-slice and even 32- to 64-slice multidetector CT (MDCT) scanners arrives. These scanners will be accurate down to the subsegmental arterial level.
- Some investigators have advocated Doppler US of the legs **after the initial chest film.** They reason that the goal of anticoagulation is not to dissolve pulmonary emboli but to prevent later catastrophic emboli; detection and treatment of DVT would accomplish that goal, because the anticoagulation regimen that treats DVT is the same as that used for PE. **The problem with this approach is that it does not address the issues of chest pain, dyspnea, and the other presenting signs and symptoms, so after DVT detection and treatment the clinician is left with the unexplained signs/symptoms that began the workup in the first place.** (DVT detected by US could be incidental.) Moreover, many Doppler US studies of the legs have normal results in patients with chest symptoms, a situation that then refocuses the diagnostic workup on the chest. **Therefore, we advocate an initial chest film followed by CTVPA or CTPA, because these modalities deal directly with the presenting chest problem.** However, if a patient **presents** with leg symptoms or

signs suggesting DVT or if the patient is pregnant or unable to undergo CTPA or even a $\dot{V}/\dot{Q}$ scan (no venous access without a surgical cut-down), then Doppler US of the legs would be appropriate and, if positive, would end the work up; if negative, surgical venous access would be required for a $\dot{V}/\dot{Q}$ study or CTPA, if feasible.

- The alert reader will have noted the large cost discrepancy between $\dot{V}/\dot{Q}$ scanning and CTVPA and may well ask how a book on **cost-effective** imaging can recommend the latter over the former. The answer: cost-effective imaging does NOT mean doing the cheapest test first (see line one, **PREFACE**).

  Although a normal result on $\dot{V}/\dot{Q}$ scan ends the workup **for PE,** it leaves the clinician with chest symptoms/signs that began the workup initially, and because these have not been elucidated by the chest film and presumably not by an electrocardiogram (which would come before a lung scan if the issue was chest pain), the clinician is left with **either no diagnosis or** the option of proceeding with the best imaging test for chest signs and symptoms—CT. Therefore, because few $\dot{V}/\dot{Q}$ scan findings are normal in a hospital population, we reason that CT is often likely to follow, so why not begin with CT?

  However, we concede that in a relatively healthy, ambulatory population (such as in the student health center of a college), when a patient has a normal chest film, no predisposing conditions (trauma, chronic illness, cancer), and perhaps even a normal D-dimer, the likelihood (pretest probability) of PE is low or very low, and the $\dot{V}/\dot{Q}$ scan is often normal; in this group one might rationally advocate the less expensive test first, knowing that after those few $\dot{V}/\dot{Q}$ examinations that are **not** normal a CT often follows, **or** the patient can be discharged with unexplained **but trivial symptoms.** Alas, most physicians who deal with PE do not work in such a disease-free world. Thus, the sicker the population, the fewer the number of normal radionuclide lung scans, and the larger the number of indeterminate, intermediate-probability, and low-probability studies, which are NOT sufficient to guide further therapy.

- Several recent, thoughtful articles (see Goldhaber and Quiroz and colleagues, below) advocate **CTA without the venous study for the diagnosis of PE**—that is, CTA but not CTVPA. Against this view we note that at the First World Congress of Thoracic Imaging and Diagnosis in Chest Disease, held in Florence, Italy, in May 2005, the most recent data from the PIOPED II (Prospective Investigation of Pulmonary Embolism Diagnosis II) study supported **CTVPA or CTA and US of the legs** as the best approach to the diagnosis of pulmonary embolism. In the view of the PIOPED II investigators, CTA (without the venous study and without US of the legs) **cannot stand alone** as the screening exam for PE.

SUGGESTED READING

Cham MD, Yankelevitz DF, Henschke CI: Thromboembolic disease detection at indirect CT venography versus CT pulmonary angiography. Radiology 2005;234:591–594.

Goldhaber SZ: Multislice computed tomography for pulmonary embolism—a technological marvel. N Engl J Med 2005;352; 1812–1814.

Katz DS, Loud PA, Bruce D, et al: Combined CT venography and pulmonary angiography: a comprehensive review. Radiographics 2002;22:S3–S24.

Katz DS, Loud PA, Klippenstein DL, et al: Extra-thoracic findings on the venous phase of combined computed tomographic venography and pulmonary angiography. Clin Radiol 2000;55:177–181.

Lee AY, Julian JA, Math M, et al: Clinical utility of a rapid whole-blood D-dimer assay in patients with cancer who present with suspected acute deep venous thrombosis. Ann Intern Med 1999;131:417–423.

Loud PA, Katz DS, Belfi L, Grossman ZD: Imaging of deep venous thrombosis in suspected pulmonary embolism. Semin Roentgenol 2005;40:33–40.

Loud PA, Katz DS, Bruce DA, et al: Deep venous thrombosis with suspected pulmonary embolism: detection with combined CT venography and pulmonary angiography. Radiology 2001;219:498–502.

Quiroz R, Kucher N, Zou KH, et al: Clinical validity of a negative computed tomography scan in patients with suspected pulmonary embolism: a systematic review. JAMA 2005;293:2012–2017.

Richman PB, Wood J, Kasper DM, et al: Contribution of indirect computed tomography venography to computed tomography angiography of the chest for the diagnosis of thromboembolic disease in two United States emergency departments. J Thromb Haemost 2003;1:652–657.

Schoepf UJ, Costello P: CT angiography for diagnosis of pulmonary embolism: state of the art. Radiology 2004;230:329–337.

Schoepf UJ, Goldhaber SZ, Costello P: Spiral computed tomography for acute pulmonary embolism. Circulation 2004;109:2160–2167.

Wu AS, Pezzullo JA, Cronan JJ, et al: CT pulmonary angiography: quantification of pulmonary embolus as a predictor of patient outcome—initial experience. Radiology 2004;230:831–835.

24 Aortic Dissection

INTRODUCTION

Thoracic aortic dissection is a potentially life-threatening disorder, especially when it involves the ascending aorta. Most patients have predisposing hypertension. Many of the clinical signs and symptoms of aortic dissection are nonspecific, complicating the diagnosis, and a high clinical index of suspicion is needed. Chest pain is most frequent, classically of abrupt onset and radiating to the back, depending upon the type and site of dissection. Other supportive findings include pulse deficit, the murmur of aortic insufficiency, and stroke. Aortic dissection involving the ascending aorta is often rapidly fatal if untreated, due to complications including rupture into the pericardium or mediastinum, acute aortic insufficiency, and compromise of the coronary arterial circulation, but appropriate medical and surgical therapy has increased both short- and long-term survival. Although associated with less morbidity and mortality, dissections that do not involve the ascending aorta can also have significant complications, including decreased blood flow to the kidneys, bowel, and lower extremities. Also, both acutely and chronically, the affected aorta may become significantly dilated (an aneurysm).

A dissection involving the ascending aorta is a "Stanford type A," whereas any other is "type B." Type A aortic dissections are surgical emergencies, but type B dissections can often be treated pharmacologically (blood pressure control). In complicated aortic dissections interventional radiologic procedures, such as stent placement and fenestration, may be indicated to restore blood flow.

A subset of aortic dissections may begin as (and sometimes remain) an intramural hematoma. In such situations, blood accumulates within the aortic wall, but there is no false lumen with demonstrable flow on imaging studies. Patients with aortic intramural hematoma should be treated as if they have a classic aortic dissection—that is, patients with type A intramural aortic hematoma should be treated surgically—because such patients are at risk for the same life-threatening complications as if they had a classic dissection with blood actively flowing in both the true and false lumina. Many patients with intramural hematomas, over time, do develop both true and false lumina. A minority of patients with acute aortic dissection, especially those with intramural hematoma, may have an underlying penetrating aortic ulcer that—along with hypertension—led to disruption of the aortic wall.

Chest films, computed tomography (CT) without and with intravenous contrast medium ("enhanced" and "nonenhanced"), magnetic resonance (MR) imaging usually without gadolinium-based contrast medium, and transesophageal echocardiography (TEE) all have roles in the workup. **Conventional catheter angiography was formerly used for suspected dissection, but it no longer plays a role in the diagnostic workup.** **Relative Costs:** CT, **$$$**; MR, **$$$**; TEE, **$$$**.

▌ PLAN AND RATIONALE

STEP 1: CHEST RADIOGRAPHY (PLAIN FILMS)

The chest radiograph, although usually nonspecific and nondiagnostic, can sometimes diagnose thoracic aortic dissection. Suspicious findings include widening of the superior mediastinum or aorta, disparity in the size of the ascending and descending aorta, and medial displacement of intimal aortic calcifications. (These findings are most helpful if comparison to a previous chest radiograph proves that they are new.) **Despite its insensitivity and poor specificity, the chest film should not be omitted, because it can define alternative conditions that explain the patient's pain. However, a normal chest radiograph does not exclude aortic dissection.**

If the patient has NO documented contraindication to intravenous iodinated contrast medium:

STEP 2: COMPUTED TOMOGRAPHY (CT) WITH (AND POSSIBLY INITIALLY WITHOUT) INTRAVENOUS CONTRAST MEDIUM

Some radiologists begin with nonenhanced CT of the chest, believing that contrast medium may obscure intramural hematoma or may be confused with nonacute atherosclerotic disease (i.e., plaque). However, in our experience, intramural hematoma is identifiable on enhanced CT; therefore, our preference is to proceed directly to **arterial-phase CT with contrast medium.** Because both types A and B commonly extend to the abdomen, **the scan should include the abdomen and perhaps the pelvis as well (dissection flaps may also involve the iliac and common femoral arteries).**

   CT has an extremely high accuracy for establishing or excluding the diagnosis.

   The aorta is easily defined in patients who can tolerate intravenous iodinated contrast medium. The entire chest, abdomen, and pelvis can be imaged with a single **peripheral intravenous bolus during a single breath-hold, in a matter of seconds.** The data can be reformatted, also in seconds, into images in other planes or into three-dimensional images, although review of the axial images remains the mainstay for diagnosis. **CT can define the presence or absence of an aortic dissection and the relationship of the aorta to its branch vessels, as well as**

complications such as pericardial hematoma or decreased abdominal organ perfusion.

CT is key to therapy planning, to following patients over time, and to revealing alternative diagnoses that may be causing the patient's symptoms (e.g., pulmonary embolism).

> **If the patient has a known contraindication to intravenous contrast medium and is in stable condition:**

STEP 2: MAGNETIC RESONANCE (MR) IMAGING

MR imaging of the thoracic and abdominal aorta is straightforward in the cooperative patient. A variety of acquisition sequences can be performed, including "cine" sequences that demonstrate blood flow in the aorta and heart, without the need for intravenous gadolinium-based contrast medium. The accuracy of MR is comparable to that of CT, and in younger patients a major **advantage** is that the examination can be repeated serially without exposure to ionizing radiation. The main **disadvantage** of MR is that even a limited examination of the chest and abdomen takes much longer than that for CT. Also, in contrast to CT, MR is difficult in borderline stable patients (who require monitoring devices that must be MR compatible; see the **INTRODUCTION** to this book). **MR is contra-indicated in patients with pacemakers/automatic implantable cardioverter-defibrillator (AICD) devices, and MR may not be readily available on an emergency basis.**

To diagnose or exclude aortic dissection, as noted above, intravenous gadolinium is not required. However, if there is a concern regarding the status of the branch vessels of the aorta if a dissection is present, or concern about possible perfusion abnormalities related to an aortic dissection (e.g., renal compromise due to decreased renal arterial flow), additional MR sequences can be performed with gadolinium administration.

SUMMARY AND CONCLUSIONS

1. A chest film is the recommended initial study in patients with chest pain or other symptoms that are suspicious for aortic dissection. The findings are usually normal or nonspecific but the film should not be bypassed, because it may reveal simple explanations for pain, such as rib fracture or pneumothorax.
2. CT is clearly the test of choice for patients who can tolerate iodinated contrast medium. **The study is extremely accurate and can image the entire chest and abdomen in a single breath-hold.**
3. If iodinated contrast medium is contraindicated, the patient is stable and cooperative, and there are no contraindications such as a pacemaker or AICD device, **MR is as effective as CT.** MR, however, may not be as readily available as CT on an emergency basis.
4. MR is particularly valuable for serially following younger patients, because ionizing radiation is not involved.

ADDITIONAL COMMENTS

- Conventional catheter aortography has **NO CURRENT ROLE** in the **diagnosis** of aortic dissection. In selected **therapeutic** situations, catheter angiography may apply in conjunction with interventional procedures, such as aortic fenestration or stent-stent or stent-graft placement.
- **Newer CT scanners present the option of imaging the coronary arteries (see CHAPTER 54, Coronary Artery Screening/Myocardial Ischemia) after a peripheral intravenous injection of contrast medium. Because aortic dissection, pulmonary emboli (see CHAPTER 23, Pulmonary Embolism), and myocardial ischemia all may present with acute chest**

pain, and because the latter two conditions are more common than aortic dissection (and its variants), CT can provide a practical "triple rule out" examination, in which the chest is screened with ONE EMERGENCY CT for all three conditions. This approach requires the newest generation of CT scanners, and many radiologists and emergency department physicians believe that it will dominate the emergency workup of acute chest pain in the future.

- Aortic dissection may be simulated by many other conditions, including pericardial disease, and even acute cholecystitis, and CT of the chest and abdomen can reveal most of these diagnoses.

- Transesophageal echocardiography (TEE) can demonstrate dissection of the thoracic aorta. An ultrasound transducer is introduced into the esophagus, and images of the heart and aorta are displayed on a monitor. The major advantage of this examination, if available on an emergency basis, is that patients who are not stable enough to undergo CT or MR can be imaged at the bedside, or even in the operating room. Unfortunately, there are blind spots within the thorax, including the great vessels, the procedure is somewhat invasive, and the procedure is very operator dependent. Patients also require sedation. Transthoracic echocardiography may also be used to identify aortic dissection, and may be performed immediately prior to TEE, although it is less accurate than TEE. Either transthoracic or transesophageal echocardiography supplements CT and MR when aortic regurgitation is suspected in a patient with a type A aortic dissection.

▌ SUGGESTED READING

Bhalla S, Menias CO, Heiken JP: CT of acute abdominal aortic disorders. Radiol Clin North Am 2003;41:1153–1169.

Hagan PG, Nienaber CA, Isselbacher EM, et al: The International Registry of Acute Aortic Dissection (IRAD). New insights into an old disease. JAMA 2000;283:897–903.

Khan IA, Chandra KN: Clinical, diagnostic, and management perspectives of aortic dissection. Chest 2002;122:311–328.

Macura KJ, Szarf G, Fishman EK, Bluemke DA: Role of computed tomography and magnetic resonance imaging in assessment of acute aortic syndromes. Semin Ultrasound CT MR 2003;24:232–254.

Moore AG, Eagle KA, Bruckman D, et al: Choice of computed tomography, transesophageal echocardiography, magnetic resonance imaging, and aortography in acute aortic dissection: International Registry of Acute Aortic Dissection (IRAD). Am J Cardiol 2002;89:1235–1238.

Nienaber CA, Eagle KA: Aortic dissection: new frontiers in diagnosis and management. Part I: From etiology to diagnostic strategies. Circulation 2003;108:628–635.

Quint LE, Williams DM, Francis IR, et al: Ulcerlike lesions of the aorta: imaging features and natural history. Radiology 2001;218:719–723.

Sebastia C, Pallisa E, Quiroga S, et al: Aortic dissection: diagnosis and follow-up with helical CT. Radiographics 1999;19:45–60.

Sommer T, Fehske W, Holzknecht N, et al: Aortic dissection: a comparative study of diagnosis with spiral CT, multiplanar transesophageal echocardiography, and MR imaging. Radiology 1996;199:347–352.

Yoshida S, Akiba H, Tamakawa M, et al: Thoracic involvement of type A aortic dissection and intramural hematoma: diagnostic accuracy—comparison of emergency helical CT and surgical findings. Radiology 2003;228:430–435.

25 Pleural Effusion

INTRODUCTION

A tiny amount of fluid normally exists between the visceral and parietal pleura. Abnormal fluid accumulates in a wide variety of conditions, including congestive heart failure, pulmonary embolism, ascites, collagen vascular or autoimmune diseases, pneumonia, sub-diaphragmatic inflammation (sympathetic effusion), hypoproteinemia, and malignancy. A pleural effusion may be suspected from the history and physical examination or may be discovered incidentally during imaging of the chest or upper abdomen.

Plain films, ultrasound (US), and computed tomography (CT) play a role in the workup and therapy.

Relative Costs: Plain films, **\$**; US, **\$\$**; CT, **\$\$\$**.

PLAN AND RATIONALE

STEP 1: CHEST RADIOGRAPHY (PLAIN FILMS)

Although pleural fluid can be suspected from diminished breath sounds and dullness to percussion over the lung base, the diagnosis should be confirmed and the size of the effusion estimated from frontal and lateral chest radiographs.

Small effusions appear as increased density blunting the normally sharp costophrenic angle or, when large, obscuring the contour of the diaphragm (Fig. 25-1). As little as 150 mL can be identified on a good quality chest radiograph (posteroanterior and lateral views), although occasionally subpulmonic effusion—situated between

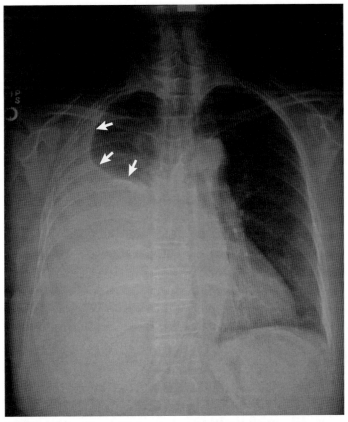

Figure 25-1. Pleural effusion. An upright chest film shows a large, homogeneous density characteristic of pleural effusion, occupying the mid and lower chest. The top of the effusion forms a meniscus extending to the lateral chest wall (*arrows*).

the lower lung and diaphragm—may not be readily apparent. If subpulmonic effusion or fluid trapped by pleural adhesions or septations is suspected, "lateral decubitus films" with the patient lying on his/her side will show an effusion as it layers along the dependent lateral thoracic wall. Such a free-flowing effusion is likely to be drainable.

The radiograph may indicate the **cause** of the effusion, although a large effusion frequently masks underlying pulmonary/pleural findings. Repeat radiographs **after thoracentesis** may then reveal underlying pulmonary or pleural disease.

STEP 2: ULTRASOUND (US)

Large effusions can be aspirated **without imaging guidance** by using percussion to identify the site to insert a thoracentesis catheter (usually 1 to 2 interspaces below the highest level of dullness with the patient sitting upright). Selective fluid analysis (chemistry, culture, and cytology) can help determine the effusion's cause. In previous generations, unguided taps were the rule, but readily available US guidance has recently engendered a shift toward guided taps among clinicians in developed countries. Moreover, US is commonly used to guide diagnostic or therapeutic thoracentesis when an effusion is small or complex and in technically difficult circumstances (e.g., unstable or ventilator-dependent patients).

Pleural fluid is easily seen sonographically, and the adjacent lung and diaphragm are easily avoided during catheter insertion. **Complications of thoracentesis, including pneumothorax, bleeding, and injury to liver or spleen, are uncommon with US-guided taps. US-guided thoracentesis can be performed safely if a layer of fluid greater than 1 cm is seen by US or on lateral decubitus films.**

If the cause of the effusion is clarified by chemistry, cytology, and culture, the diagnostic workup ends, but in some cases repeated therapeutic taps are required for the sake of respiratory comfort.

If the clinical presentation and analysis of pleural fluid do not reveal a cause for the effusion, pulmonary embolism should be excluded with CT pulmonary angiography (CTPA) (see CHAPTER 23, Pulmonary Embolism).

STEP 3: COMPUTED TOMOGRAPHIC PULMONARY ANGIOGRAPHY (CTPA)

CTPA is the best single screening examination for pulmonary embolism and should be the next step in the workup of a nonspecific effusion whose nature is not clarified by a tap.

At the time of CTPA, the entire chest is studied. Even if emboli are not detected, CT may reveal underlying pulmonary or pleural disease not visible on chest radiographs and define the cause of an effusion as well as the extent of complex, loculated pleural collections that can occur in patients with infected or malignant effusions and patients who are postsurgery or post-trauma.

Empyema is suggested by high fluid density and increased pleural thickening/enhancement. CT guidance is often required to drain complex collections in these patients. **Focal pleural thickening or nodularity** suggests pleural malignancy. Pleural biopsy, under CT or US guidance, or during thoracoscopy, is sometimes needed in cases of undiagnosed exudative pleural effusion.

SUMMARY AND CONCLUSIONS

1. Chest films are the first diagnostic study for suspected pleural effusions, to estimate the amount of fluid present and to look for underlying causes.
2. If a cause is not clinically or radiographically apparent, sampling and analysis of pleural fluid is the next step. Small or complex effusions, and effusions in unstable patients, can be safely drained under US guidance.
3. CT of the chest can exclude pulmonary embolism as a cause, optimally evaluate complex, loculated pleural collections, and seek a cause in underlying pulmonary, chest wall, and cardiovascular disease.

ADDITIONAL COMMENTS

- US and CT can reveal pleural effusions of only 10 to 20 mL, and, in this regard, are more sensitive than plain films. However, this degree of sensitivity is not required in the diagnostic workup.

SUGGESTED READING

Brant WE: The thorax. In Rumack CM, Wilson SR, Charboneau JW, Johnson JM (eds): Diagnostic Ultrasound. St. Louis, Elsevier-Mosby, 2005, pp 603–623.

Celli BR: Diseases of the diaphragm, chest wall, pleura, and mediastinum. In Goldman L, Ausiello D (eds): Cecil Textbook of Medicine, 22nd ed. Philadelphia, Saunders, 2004, pp 568–576.

Pleura, chest wall, and diaphragm. In Naidich DP, Muller NL, Zerhouni EA, et al (eds): Computed Tomography and Magnetic Resonance of the Thorax. Philadelphia, Lippincott-Raven, 1999, pp 657–754.

Part *IV*

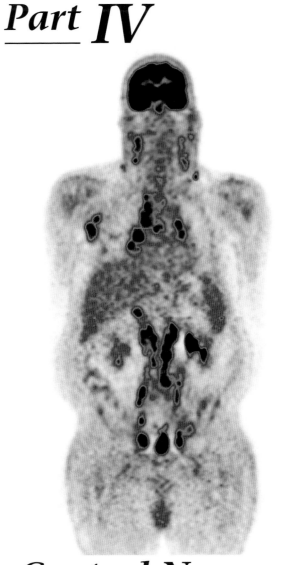

Central Nervous System/Head-Neck

26 Cerebral Metastases

INTRODUCTION

Throughout most of the 1980s, computed tomography (CT) was the modality of choice for the detection of cerebral metastases. However, magnetic resonance (MR) imaging has proven to be superior to CT in this regard, even when CT is "enhanced" with intravenous contrast medium. MR enhanced with intravenous contrast medium is particularly sensitive for leptomeningeal carcinomatosis, central nervous system bleeding, and hemorrhagic metastases.

Relative Costs: Brain CT, enhanced, **$$$**; brain MR, enhanced and unenhanced, **$$$$**.

PLAN AND RATIONALE

Where MR is available:

STEP 1: MAGNETIC RESONANCE (MR) IMAGING

A normal MR, enhanced **and** unenhanced, ends the cerebral metastatic workup.

The details of MR imaging are best left to the radiologist (or neuroradiologist), but for readers with a particular interest in technical specifics, axial precontrast T2-weighted images, with pre- and postcontrast axial T1-weighted images, are appropriate.

Where MR is not available:

STEP 1: COMPUTED TOMOGRAPHY (CT)

Contrast-enhanced CT is a less sensitive second choice screen for cerebral metastases. **However, CT without intravenous contrast medium (unenhanced CT) is unacceptable in modern radiologic practice, because it is much less sensitive; it should be considered only when even the least toxic nonionic contrast media (see INTRODUCTION to this book) cannot be tolerated.**

SUMMARY AND CONCLUSIONS

1. MR is the modality of choice for the detection of cerebral metastases.
2. Contrast-enhanced CT is not as sensitive as MR for cerebral metastatic screening, and if performed as a second choice it will inevitably miss some lesions.
3. If CT is the primary screen, in the absence of MR, every attempt should be made to augment the sensitivity of the examination with intravenous contrast medium. If no contrast medium is used, the sensitivity of the study declines severely.

ADDITIONAL COMMENTS

- Radionuclide brain scanning, even with fluorodeoxyglucose–positron emission tomography (FDG-PET), has no role **in the initial cerebral metastatic workup,** although the presence of residual tumor in an irradiated cerebral field can often be determined by FDG-PET.
- MR uses no ionizing radiation, but it **is incompatible with many life-support systems and with pacemakers** (see **INTRODUCTION** to this book for a discussion of the pacemaker issue).

SUGGESTED READING

Atlas SW, Grossman RI, Gomori JM, et al: Hemorrhagic intracranial malignant neoplasms: spin-echo MR imaging. Radiology 1987;164:71–77.

Atlas SW, Laui E, Fisher PG: Intraaxial brain tumors. In Atlas SW (ed): Magnetic Resonance Imaging of the Brain and Spine, 3rd ed. Philadelphia, Lippincott Williams & Wilkins, 2002, pp 565–774.

Davis PC, Hudgins PA, Peterman SB, Hoffman JC: Diagnosis of cerebral metastases: double-dose delayed CT vs. contrast-enhanced MR imaging. AJNR Am J Neuroradiol 1991;12:293–300.

Sze G, Milano E, Johnson C, Heier L: Detection of brain metastasis: comparison of contrast-enhanced MR with unenhanced MR and enhanced CT. AJNR Am J Neuroradiol 1990;11:785–791.

Sze G, Soletsky S, Bronen R, Krol G: MR imaging of the cranial meninges with emphasis on contrast enhancement and meningeal carcinomatosis. AJNR Am J Neuroradiol 1989;10:965–975.

Yuh WT, Engelken JD, Muhonen MG, et al: Experience with high-dose gadolinium MR imaging in the evaluation of brain metastases. AJNR Am J Neuroradiol 1992;13:335–345.

Acute Head Trauma

INTRODUCTION

Computed tomography (CT) without intravenous contrast medium (unenhanced) has long been—and remains—the primary imaging modality for the evaluation of acute head trauma.

The study clearly and rapidly defines lesions that may require immediate surgical intervention—depressed fractures, extracerebral blood collections, and intracerebral hematoma. Although superior to CT for many central nervous system (CNS) problems, **magnetic resonance (MR) imaging is less effective than CT for fractures and subarachnoid hemorrhage.** Also, the need for special MR-compatible life-support equipment and long scanning time preclude MR as a first-line test in acute head trauma.

Relative Costs: Head CT, unenhanced, **$$**; head MR, unenhanced, **$$$**.

PLAN AND RATIONALE

STEP 1: COMPUTED TOMOGRAPHY (CT), UNENHANCED

CT images are electronically adjusted to reveal details of brain parenchyma, the subdural spaces, and bone—in the technical jargon of radiology three "window settings." In almost all cases, CT alone is sufficient to end the imaging workup. **However, if the patient's neuro-**

logical status is unexplained by a normal CT, then MR should follow.

Although nondepressed fractures in the plane of section can be inconspicuous on axial CT images, the preliminary planar or "scout" images, which are produced on the CT scanner but resemble classic "skull films" and are used to plan the subsequent CT, usually define **nondepressed fractures. Depressed skull fractures** are almost universally conspicuous on CT.

STEP 2: MAGNETIC RESONANCE (MR) IMAGING

MR defines a small number of important acute CNS injuries, **notably brain stem hemorrhagic and nonhemorrhagic contusions and diffuse axonal injuries, that CT can miss.** Moreover, in the **sub-acute** and **chronic** setting, MR is invaluable; chronic nonhemorrhagic and hemorrhagic contusions, diffuse axonal injuries, and small subdural hematomas are better delineated by MR than by CT.

SUMMARY AND CONCLUSIONS

---

1. CT is the modality of choice for the evaluation of acute head injury and almost always ends the imaging workup. The study is performed without contrast medium (unenhanced).
2. MR is **inappropriate** as a first-line study in the setting of acute head trauma but is sometimes indicated as a follow-up to normal CT **when clinical symptomology remains unexplained;** brain stem contusions, axonal injuries, and post-traumatic strokes are better defined by MR than by CT.
3. In the subacute and chronic setting, MR is invaluable; it is superior for nonhemorrhagic and hemorrhagic contusions, diffuse axonal injuries, and small subdural hematomas.

ADDITIONAL COMMENTS

- Cervical spine injury may accompany closed head trauma (see **CHAPTER 28, Acute Spine Trauma**).
- **Plain skull films have no role in the contemporary evaluation of head trauma.**
- CT angiography delineates vascular injuries after trauma in the head and neck and, where available, can acutely exclude dissection or pseudoaneurysm.
- If acute stroke is a clinical concern after trauma, MR is best for detection of the infarct and evaluation of cervical/intracranial vessels for traumatic dissection or occlusion.

SUGGESTED READING

Dublin AB, French BN, Rennick JM: Computed tomography in head trauma. Radiology 1977;122:365–369.

Gentry LR, Godersky JC, Thompson BH, Dunn VD: Prospective comparative study of intermediate-field MR and CT in the evaluation of closed head trauma. AJNR Am J Neuroradiol 1988;9:91–100.

Hesselink JR, Dowd CF, Healy ME, et al: MR imaging of brain contusions: a comparative study with CT. AJNR Am J Neuroradiol 1988;9:269–278.

Koo AH, LaRoque RL: Evaluation of head trauma by computed tomography. Radiology 1977;123:345–350.

Osborn AG: Intracranial hemorrhage. In Osborn AG (ed): Diagnostic Neuroradiology. Boston, Mosby, 1994, pp 154–247.

Zimmerman RA, Bilaniuk LT, Hackney DB, et al: Head injury: early results of comparing CT and high-field MR. AJNR Am J Neuroradiol 1986;7:757–764.

28 Acute Spine Trauma

INTRODUCTION

The potentially injured spine must be imaged with the patient immobilized to prevent damage to the spinal cord. Plain films, computed tomography (CT), and magnetic resonance (MR) imaging are used.

Relative Costs: Cervical spine plain films, **$**; thoracic spine plain films, **$**; lumbar spine plain films, **$**; cervical spine CT, unenhanced, **$$–$$$**; thoracic spine CT, unenhanced, **$$–$$$**; lumbar spine CT, unenhanced, **$$–$$$**; cervical spine MR, unenhanced, **$$$**; thoracic spine MR, unenhanced, **$$$**; lumbar spine MR, unenhanced, **$$$**.

PLAN AND RATIONALE

Cervical spine:

STEP 1: RADIOGRAPHY (PLAIN FILMS)

A lateral plain film is the first step.

If a fracture is demonstrated, CT is next in the evaluation (see **Step 2A, Computed Tomography,** below).

If no fracture is defined by the initial lateral film, additional plain films are appropriate: anteroposterior (AP), "swimmer's," oblique, and open-mouth views. (The patient's neck is immobilized by a special collar during positioning for these films to prevent spinal injury.)

If a fracture is detected by any of these additional views, CT is next (see **Step 2A, Computed Tomography,** below).

If the additional views are normal and there is **focal pain** without other related neurologic signs or symptoms, views in **flexion and extension,** with the immobilizing collar removed, are an essential next step. (Flexion and extension views may identify ligamentous injury that can induce instability of the cervical spine and, if undetected, cause major cervical cord injury later.)

If the additional views are normal and there is no focal pain yet symptoms or signs suggest spinal cord trauma, MR is next (see **Step 2B, Magnetic Resonance Imaging,** below).

In the comatose patient, who cannot cooperate for additional views after the initial lateral film or communicate symptoms, **MR can help exclude spinal cord and ligament injury** (see **Step 2B, Magnetic Resonance Imaging,** below).

Thoracic and lumbar spine:

STEP 1: RADIOGRAPHY (PLAIN FILMS)

AP and lateral films are the first step.

If the initial films are normal and there are no significant symptoms or signs of spine trauma, the workup ends.

If there are significant symptoms or signs of spine trauma despite normal initial plain films, MR is appropriate to exclude injury to the spinal cord itself or an adjacent traumatic lesion, such as hematoma encroaching upon the cord (see **Step 2B, Magnetic Resonance Imaging,** below).

If the initial AP and lateral films reveal a fracture or are equivocal, CT is appropriate (see **Step 2A, Computed Tomography,** below).

STEP 2A: COMPUTED TOMOGRAPHY (CT)

CT displays the bony spine in exquisite detail in the axial projection. Fracture fragments and their relationship to the spinal cord and nerve roots are well defined, and fractures missed by plain films are sometimes detected. Images can be "reformatted" in the sagittal and coronal projections, as well as into three-dimensional models, augmenting their diagnostic value. The study is rapid and for spine trauma requires no intravenous contrast medium.

If CT is abnormal and explains the patient's symptoms/signs, the workup ends. If CT is normal despite clear symptoms of spinal injury, or if CT findings do not explain the patient's signs/symptoms, MR should follow (see **Step 2B, Magnetic Resonance Imaging**, below).

STEP 2B: MAGNETIC RESONANCE (MR) IMAGING

The multiplanar imaging capability of MR and its **direct** visualization of the spinal cord, ligaments, and cerebrospinal fluid allow it to define the relationship of fracture fragments to the thecal sac and spinal cord, the presence of spinal cord compression, ligamentous injuries, disk herniation, epidural hematoma, and nonhemorrhagic and hemorrhagic spinal cord contusion. **With the sole exception of fractures, virtually all significant spinal injures are better defined by MR than by CT.** Nonetheless, MR is not appropriate as a first-line study because CT is superior for fracture detection.

SUMMARY AND CONCLUSIONS

1. Plain films are the initial study.
2. CT is the appropriate second examination if plain films are equivocal or if a fracture requires further study. MR is the appropriate second study if initial

plain films are normal, yet signs or symptoms of significant spinal cord injury persist.

3. In the comatose patient who cannot cooperate for additional views of the cervical spine, MR can exclude spinal cord injury.

ADDITIONAL COMMENTS

• For a generation CT required patient immobility for several minutes to generate an adequate scan, and if the patient was uncooperative, general anesthesia was sometimes necessary. Newer scanners now installed in virtually all American radiology departments can create high-resolution images in less than 1 second, so anesthesia is rarely, if ever, required.

SUGGESTED READING

Brandt-Zawadski M, Miller EM, Federle MP: CT in the evaluation of spine trauma. AJR Am J Roentgenol 1981;136:369–375.

Flanders AE, Croul SE: Spinal trauma. In Atlas SW (ed): Magnetic Resonance Imaging of the Brain and Spine, vol 2. Philadelphia: Lippincott Williams & Wilkins, 2002, pp 1769–1824.

Kulkarni MV, McArdle CB, Kopanicky D, et al: Acute spinal cord injury: MR imaging at 1.5T. Radiology 1987;164:837–843.

McArdle CB, Crofford MJ, Mirfakhraee M, et al: Surface coil MR of spinal trauma: preliminary experience. AJNR Am J Neuroradiol 1986;7:885–893.

Mirvis SE, Geisler FH, Jelinek JJ, et al: Acute cervical spine trauma: evaluation with 1.5-T MR imaging. Radiology 1988;166:807–816.

Post MD, Green BA: The use of computed tomography in spinal trauma. Radiol Clin North Am 1983;21:327–375.

Tarr RW, Drolshagen LF, Kerner TC, et al: MR imaging of recent spinal trauma. J Comput Assist Tomogr 1987;11:412–417.

29 Normal Pressure Hydrocephalus

INTRODUCTION

Although uncommon, normal pressure hydrocephalus (NPH) is of considerable importance and interest because it is one of the few treatable dementias. The clinical hallmarks of the syndrome are early dementia, unsteadiness of gait, and urinary incontinence. The imaging hallmarks of NPH are large ventricles and abnormal cerebrospinal fluid (CSF) migration. Paradoxically, some cases of NPH are associated with normal ventricles.

NPH has several possible etiologies: (1) obstruction to CSF flow at the level of the basal cisterns or arachnoid villi from previous inflammatory disease or subarachnoid hemorrhage; (2) ischemic damage to the periventricular white matter with decreased ventricular wall tensile strength; (3) intermittent-but-undetected obstruction in the aqueduct; and (4) poor absorption of CSF in the arachnoid granulations.

Magnetic resonance (MR) imaging produces superb images of the ventricles, easily confirming or excluding ventricular enlargement, **but a conclusive diagnosis of NPH requires analysis of CSF flow.** Therefore, although a rough idea of CSF movement can be gleaned from MR in some cases, reliable analysis of CSF migration requires gamma cisternography—a test that entails installation of radioactive material into the subarachnoid space, followed by serial gamma camera images.

Relative Costs: Head MR, unenhanced, **$$$**; gamma cisternogram, including lumbar puncture, **$$$$**.

■ PLAN AND RATIONALE

STEP 1: MAGNETIC RESONANCE (MR) IMAGING

MR is the best initial study in suspected NPH to confirm the presence of hydrocephalus and **to exclude other causes of the neurologic symptoms.** NPH typically produces large ventricles and compressed sulci, but in some cases the ventricles and sulci are both enlarged, mimicking the appearance of atrophy. However, because occasional cases of NPH are associated with ventricles of normal size, MR cannot firmly exclude the diagnosis.

MR can detect changes in CSF "signal" that relate to CSF flow rates. Normally, bright signal is detected in the ventricles on T2-weighted images, because of the CSF. The CSF flow void sign (CFVS) seen in the aqueduct of Sylvius and the third and fourth ventricles results from rapid and/or turbulent CSF flow. Although the CFVS can indicate that there is CSF movement, the specific pattern that is characteristic of NPH—failure of CSF to migrate over the cerebral convexities—cannot be solidly confirmed by MR.

If MR is normal and the initial clinical index of suspicion is relatively low, the workup usually ends, but if MR confirms hydrocephalus and excludes other causes of symptoms, a nuclear cisternogram (gamma cisternogram) is appropriate. Moreover, if clinical suspicion is high, even a normal MR should be followed by gamma cisternography.

STEP 2: GAMMA CISTERNOGRAM

Gamma cisternography involves installation of a radiopharmaceutical into the subarachnoid space by lumbar puncture. Indium-111–diethylenetriamine pentaacetic acid (In-111-DTPA) is used, because its half-life permits 72 hours of imaging, it is nontoxic, and it is not absorbed from the CSF. Images at 24, 48, and even 72 hours define ventricular filling and emptying as well as CSF migration over the cerebral convexities. Normal lateral ventricles may fill transiently at 24 hours but should be essentially clear of radiopharmaceutical at 48 hours, whereas continued ventricular radioactivity at 48 hours and afterward indicates NPH. **Failure of radiopharmaceutical to migrate normally over the convexities is confirmatory.**

A normal gamma cisternogram excludes NPH.

SUMMARY AND CONCLUSIONS

1. MR is the appropriate screening exam for NPH, to confirm hydrocephalus and exclude other causes of symptoms.
2. MR can sometimes suggest NPH, by means of the CFVS, but a gamma cisternogram is required for a firm diagnosis.
3. Some cases of NPH are associated with ventricles of normal size. If there is strong clinical suspicion of NPH, a **normal** MR result should be followed by a gamma cisternogram. If the initial clinical index of suspicion is low, a normal MR result usually ends the workup.

ADDITIONAL COMMENTS

- A computed tomography (CT) cisternogram can be performed with intrathecal injection of nonionic contrast medium. The contrast medium follows CSF flow. This examination is cumbersome and costly relative to the gamma cisternogram and has no clear-cut advantages.
- CT, as well as MR, defines the ventricles, but the initial study should be MR, because the latter better defines white matter characteristics as well as parts of the ventricular system.
- Persons with proven NPH often experience dramatic improvement after the placement of a ventriculo-peritoneal shunt.

30 Cerebrospinal Fluid Leak

INTRODUCTION

When a post-traumatic or postsurgical cerebrospinal fluid (CSF) leak is suspected, imaging focuses on proving that a CSF leak exists and detecting the bony discontinuity through which CSF escapes. Meningitis may occur if the leak is not spontaneously or surgically closed.

In patients with a **suspected but unconfirmed CSF leak,** a screening procedure is indicated. In patients with a **proven CSF leak through an unknown site,** a high-resolution technique to define the responsible anatomic defect is appropriate. The nuclear gamma cisternogram and computed tomography (CT) apply respectively.

Relative Costs: Gamma cisternogram, including lumbar puncture, **$$$$**; CT, skull base, **$$$**.

PLAN AND RATIONALE

When a CSF leak is suspected but no specific site is known:

STEP 1: GAMMA CISTERNOGRAM

The gamma cisternogram is a sensitive screen for leaking CSF. Although some centers prefer a relatively short study, which examines the suspected region for 24 hours, many prefer to image the skull base and face for

48 hours. Thus, a short-lived technetium 99m (Tc-99m) or a longer-lived indium 111 (In-111) is the radionuclide of choice, chelated to diethylenetriamine pentaacetic acid (DTPA). The radiopharmaceutical is injected intrathecally via lumbar puncture. Over the next 24 to 48 hours, images of the head and neck can reveal passage of radioactive CSF outside of its normal confines. This technique can detect CSF leaks in many sites, including the middle ear, nose, and pharynx, **yet the study can detect only leaks that are active.** Occasionally, cotton pledgets placed in the nasopharynx are later assayed in a sensitive radiation counter to confirm radioactive CSF in the nose.

When the approximate site of a CSF leak is known:

STEP 1: COMPUTED TOMOGRAPHY (CT) OR CT CISTERNOGRAPHY

CT provides superb images of the skull base, where minor bony discontinuities can provide an egress point for CSF into the sinuses, nose, nasopharynx, or even the middle ear.

In former years, CT cisternography was a more common method of defining the leak site. A few mL of contrast medium were injected into the lumbar sub-arachnoid space, and the patient was positioned prone, head down, for several minutes, so that the contrast medium would migrate craniad. The patient was then scanned. (However, the examination could be "customized," so that the suspected site of leakage would be dependent.) The resolution of CT cisternography is exquisite, but, like the gamma cisternogram, it can detect only active leaks.

The superb resolution of modern CT scanners has made the need for intrathecal contrast medium uncommon, if not rare.

SUMMARY AND CONCLUSIONS

1. A gamma cisternogram is the initial screening study for a suspected but unconfirmed CSF leak.
2. When a CSF leak is known, CT can often identify the bony defect responsible, as a road map for surgical repair. Uncommonly, a gamma cisternogram may be performed to identify the leaking site.

ADDITIONAL COMMENTS

- Magnetic resonance (MR) imaging demonstrates the central nervous system and its coverings in exquisite detail. CSF is particularly well demonstrated, because of its high signal intensity on T2-weighted images. However, MR does not adequately display the bony anatomy of the paranasal sinuses and skull base; therefore, **bony discontinuities through which CSF can leak will not be detected.** Nonetheless, if all else fails, some neuroradiologists attempt an MR cisternogram, in which the MR contrast medium containing gadolinium is introduced into the lumbar subarachnoid space and then directed craniad by carefully positioning the patient. The passage of small amounts of gadolinium through bony defects can sometimes be detected.
- CSF leaks are often intermittent, and multiple examinations may be necessary to "catch" an ongoing leak. **Sometimes no leak is demonstrated, even in the presence of overwhelming clinical evidence.**

Encephalitis

INTRODUCTION

The differentiation of encephalitis from lesions that may, in unusual circumstances, mimic encephalitis (hemorrhage, abscess, or tumor) is important, **because their management differs radically.**

Current techniques do not differentiate herpes encephalitis from other acute encephalitides. Magnetic resonance (MR) imaging with intravenous contrast medium (enhanced) and computed tomography (CT) with intravenous contrast medium (enhanced) apply.

Relative Costs: Brain MR, enhanced, **\$\$\$–\$\$\$\$**; head CT, enhanced, **\$\$\$**.

PLAN AND RATIONALE

Where MR is feasible and available:

STEP 1: MAGNETIC RESONANCE (MR) IMAGING

Enhanced MR is the modality of choice for the evaluation of suspected encephalitis, **but MR is not feasible in the presence of certain life-support systems.**

In herpes encephalitis, subtle areas of hyperintense signal on T2-weighted images combined with diffusion signal abnormality and enhancement with or without hemorrhage are evident in the temporal lobes as early as 2 days after the onset of symptoms. The temporal lobes are better defined by MR than CT, because MR has a higher soft tissue contrast resolution and is not affected by temporal bone artifacts that degrade CT. The sensitivity of MR is augmented by the intravenous administration of contrast medium.

A normal or abnormal finding on MR scan ends **the imaging workup for encephalitis,** but correlation with cerebrospinal fluid (CSF) sampling is still required, because MR imaging can be normal in some cases of early encephalitis.

Where MR is not feasible or is unavailable:

STEP 1: COMPUTED TOMOGRAPHY (CT)

Enhanced CT can diagnose encephalitis. In herpes encephalitis, characteristic hypodense lesions that enhance after the intravenous injection of contrast medium are visualized in the temporal lobes. **However, a normal CT does not exclude encephalitis.** If CT findings are normal or equivocal and herpes encephalitis is suspected on clinical grounds, every effort should be made to procure an MR study of the brain.

SUMMARY AND CONCLUSIONS

1. MR is the procedure of choice for encephalitis.
2. When MR is unfeasible or unavailable, contrast-enhanced CT is appropriate. Although CT is less effective than MR for visualizing the temporal lobes, which are the site of most findings in herpes encephalitis, a positive CT finding ends the imaging workup.
3. A normal CT scan does not exclude encephalitis, and if there is compelling clinical evidence, every effort should be made to scan with MR.

ADDITIONAL COMMENTS

• MR with diffusion-weighted imaging or MR spectroscopy can differentiate abscess from cystic metastases. (Abscesses can mimic encephalitis, and the ability to differentiate abscess from cystic metastases can be valuable in the cancer population.)

SUGGESTED READING

Benator RM, Magill LH, Gerald B, et al: Herpes simplex encephalitis: CT findings in the neonate and young infant. AJNR Am J Neuroradiol 1985;6:539–543.

Davidson HD, Steiner RE: Magnetic resonance imaging of infections of the central nervous system. AJNR Am J Neuroradiol 1985;6:499–504.

Herman TE, Cleveland RH, Kushner DC, Taveras JM: CT of neonatal herpes encephalitis. AJNR Am J Neuroradiol 1985;6:773–775.

Holmes RA: Conventional brain imaging. In Freeman LM (ed): Freeman and Johnson's Clinical Radionuclide Imaging, 3rd ed. Orlando, Grune & Stratton, 1984, pp 611–663.

Kim EE, Deland FH, Mantebello J: Sensitivity of radionuclide brain scan and computed tomography in early detection of viral meningoencephalitis. Radiology 1979;132:425–429.

Meyer, MA: Focal high uptake of HMPAO in brain perfusion studies: a clue in the diagnosis of encephalitis. J Nucl Med 1990;31: 1094–1098.

Schroth G, Kretzschmar K, Gawehn J, Voigt K: Advantage of magnetic resonance imaging in the diagnosis of cerebral infections. Neuroradiology 1987;29:120–126.

Zimmerman RA, Bilaniuk LT, Sze G: Intracranial infection. In Brandt-Zawadzki M, Norman D (eds): Magnetic Resonance Imaging of the Central Nervous System. New York, Raven Press, 1987, pp 235–257.

Zimmerman RD, Russell EJ, Leeds NE, Kaufman D: CT in the early diagnosis of herpes simplex encephalitis. AJR Am J Roentgenol 1980;134:61–66.

32 New Onset Seizures in the Adult

INTRODUCTION

The patient with seizures of new onset may have a surgical lesion, so cerebral imaging is mandatory. Two techniques apply to screening this population: magnetic resonance (MR) imaging without and with intravenous contrast medium (unenhanced and enhanced) and computed tomography (CT) without and with intravenous contrast medium (unenhanced and enhanced). MR better detects many small lesions and is unaffected by artifacts that degrade CT. MR or CT angiography is useful to further characterize some lesions.

Relative Costs: Brain MR, unenhanced, **$$$**; brain MR, enhanced and unenhanced, **$$$$**; head CT, unenhanced and enhanced, **$$$**; cerebral angiography, complete "four-vessel study," **$$$$$$**.

PLAN AND RATIONALE

Where MR is available:

STEP 1: MAGNETIC RESONANCE (MR) IMAGING

Because of its superior contrast resolution and multiplanar imaging capacity, **MR is the preferred study for evaluation of new seizures.** Intravenous contrast medium is usually **not** required but is reserved for select cases to better define abnormalities seen on the unenhanced study.

Where MR is not available:

STEP 1: COMPUTED TOMOGRAPHY WITH AND WITHOUT INTRAVENOUS CONTRAST MEDIUM (UNENHANCED AND ENHANCED)

For maximum sensitivity, CT is performed without and with intravenous contrast medium. Although CT exquisitely defines intracranial anatomy, it is less sensitive than MR. Calcified lesions can be differentiated from uncalcified lesions by including the noncontrast scan.

If a vascular lesion detected by CT or MR requires further study:

STEP 2: CEREBRAL ANGIOGRAPHY

Imaging of the blood vessels (a cerebral angiogram) that lead to and create a vascular lesion—aneurysm or arteriovenous malformation—is indicated for interventional/surgical planning. Conventional catheter angiography involves injection of contrast medium directly into blood vessels of the head or neck through a catheter threaded retrograde up the aorta, introduced via percutaneous femoral arterial puncture. An x-ray beam passes through the head-neck as contrast medium is injected, producing radiographs with exquisite resolution of blood vessels. The procedure is uncomfortable, time consuming, and expensive, although invariably effective.

CT and computer analysis have improved to the point that a **peripheral intravenous injection of contrast medium can be followed by CT as it enters the blood vessels of the neck and head, and the individual CT "slices" can be reconstructed to produce a vascular image that rivals a conventional cerebral angiogram; in most cases, the CT** angiogram (CTA) provides information equivalent to that of a conventional cerebral angiogram, without the associated risk and expense. Therefore, if CTA is available, catheter angiography should be reserved for interventional endovascular procedures.

MR angiography is also useful but is more limited because of certain flow-related artifacts and longer imaging times.

SUMMARY AND CONCLUSIONS

1. MR is the best initial imaging method for screening the patient with seizures of new onset.
2. CT without and with enhancement is an adequate screen where MR is not available.
3. CT angiography can characterize most vascular lesions anatomically.

ADDITIONAL COMMENTS

- Plain skull films have no value in the evaluation of patients with new onset seizures.
- Although CTA can beautifully characterize the anatomy of cerebral vascular lesions, some large arteriovenous malformations require flow measurements, which necessitate a catheter in place; thus, when specialized flow information or endovascular intervention is planned, conventional angiography is appropriate.
- Positron emission tomography with fluorodeoxyglucose (FDG-PET) nuclear brain scanning has a place in the study of certain seizure patients. The goal of FDG-PET is to define hypermetabolic areas of brain that are suitable for stereotaxic or surgical ablation. If successful, ablation may eliminate seizures and a lifetime of medication. These methods are usually applied to the study of chronic,

intractable epilepsy, rather than to adults with new onset seizures.

- A surgical lesion is unlikely in patients younger than 30 years of age with a normal neurologic examination and typical primary, idiopathic, generalized seizures; however, many clinicians choose to exclude a surgical lesion before committing the patient to anticonvulsant therapy.

- In children, congenital "cortical dysplasias" or "gray matter heterotopias" can cause seizures that begin shortly after birth or years later. These lesions are often cured by surgery, and MR is appropriate for evaluation (see **CHAPTER 33, Chronic, Intractable Epilepsy**).

SUGGESTED READING

Blom RJ, Vinuela F, Fox AJ, et al: Computed tomography in temporal lobe epilepsy. J Comput Assist Tomogr 1984;8:401–405.

Elster AD, Mirza W: MR imaging in chronic partial epilepsy: role of contrast enhancement. AJNR Am J Neuroradiol 1991;12:165–170.

Grattan SJ, Harvey AS, Desmond PM, et al: Hippocampal sclerosis in children with intractable epilepsy: pathologic correlation and prognostic importance. AJR Am J Roentgenol 1993;161:1045–1048.

Lee DH, Gao FQ, Rogers JM, et al: MR in temporal lobe epilepsy: analysis with pathologic confirmation. AJNR Am J Neuroradiol 1998;19:19–27.

Schîrner W, Meencke HJ, Felix R: Temporal-lobe epilepsy: comparison of CT and MR imaging. AJR Am J Roentgenol 1987;149:1231–1239.

Triulzi F, Franceshi M, Fazio F, Del Maschio A: Nonrefractory temporal lobe epilepsy: 1.5-T MR imaging. Radiology 1988;166:181–185.

33 Chronic, Intractable Epilepsy

INTRODUCTION

Chronic, intractable epilepsy often results from a temporal lobe condition called mesial temporal sclerosis, which occurs in the body of the hippocampus. Mesial temporal sclerosis is usually associated with a subtle change in local brain volume and also with abnormal metabolism—increased blood flow during a seizure (ictally) and decreased blood flow between seizures (interictally). Magnetic resonance (MR) imaging without and with intravenous contrast medium (unenhanced and enhanced) is best able to detect the volumetric changes, and nuclear brain scanning with fluorodeoxyglucose–positron emission tomography (FDG-PET) best evaluates the brain's metabolic status. Neoplasms and vascular malformations less commonly cause seizures in this population; for the latter, computed tomographic angiography (CTA)—or if endovascular intervention is considered, catheter angiography—is definitive.

Relative Costs: Brain MR, unenhanced, **\$\$\$**; brain MR, unenhanced and enhanced, **\$\$\$\$**; FDG-PET nuclear brain scan, **\$\$\$\$\$**; CTA, **\$\$\$**; cerebral angiography, complete "four-vessel study," **\$\$\$\$\$\$**.

PLAN AND RATIONALE

STEP 1: MAGNETIC RESONANCE (MR) IMAGING, INITIALLY WITHOUT CONTRAST MEDIUM (UNENHANCED)

MR is the modality of choice for the initial evaluation of chronic intractable epilepsy,

212

because it effectively studies the temporal lobes for mesial temporal sclerosis and also excludes neoplasms and vascular malformations (Fig. 33-1). MR is superior to CT in this regard because of its multiplanar imaging capability, superior contrast resolution, and freedom from temporal bone artifacts. Intravenous contrast medium is sometimes used to better characterize an abnormality detected on the initial unenhanced study.

Hippocampal volume measurements derived from three-dimensional MR are extremely useful. Some neuroradiologists believe that abnormal hippocampal volume measurements are sufficiently specific to end the workup and justify surgical or stereotactic intervention, but most believe that one or more additional signs, such as associated white matter atrophy, increased "signal" on T2-weighted images, and increased volume of the ipsilateral temporal ventricular horn, are also necessary. **A small percentage of patients with chronic intractable epilepsy has a normal finding on MR. In these cases, FDG-PET may define metabolically abnormal foci that are morphologically normal.**

If MR reveals a vascular malformation that requires better definition before intervention, catheter angiography is appropriate.

When MR findings are normal:

STEP 2: FLUORODEOXYGLUCOSE–POSITRON EMISSION TOMOGRAPHY (FDG-PET)

FDG is a glucose analogue in which a fluorine atom has replaced a hydroxyl group; the altered molecule is taken up by cells and phosphorylated but cannot complete either the aerobic (Krebs) cycle or the anaerobic cycle. The accumulation rate of FDG mirrors the metabolic state of a tissue, **and an image of FDG is thus a "metabolic" rather than an anatomic image.** Because the radioactive atom fluorine 18 (Fl-18) is a positron emitter, a camera that detects positron emitters is required—that is, a PET unit.

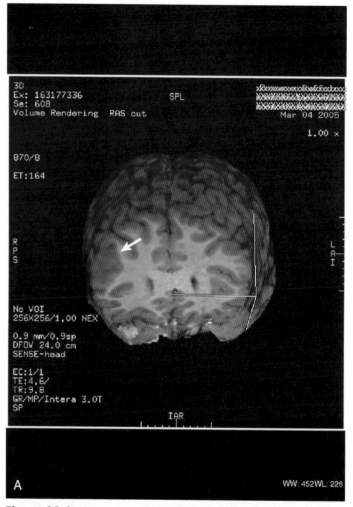

Figure 33-1. Three-dimensional MR images of a 4-year-old boy with intractable epilepsy. The asymmetry of the right frontal gyrus is a developmental disorder that was appreciated with multiplanar and three-dimensional imaging available only on MR. **A,** Note the thickened gyrus in the cut-away view of the right frontal lobe (*arrow*).

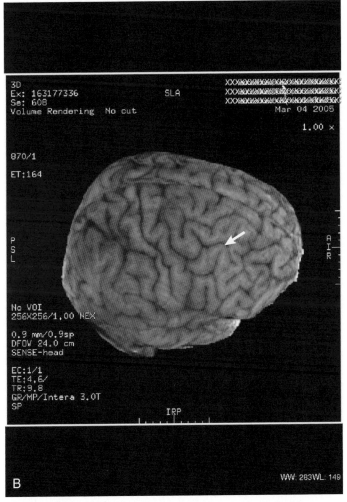

Figure 33-1. *Continued.* **B** and **C,** Three-dimensional computer-derived models, created from standard "slices," help guide the surgeon to the proper gyrus for surgical treatment of epilepsy (*arrows*).

Continued

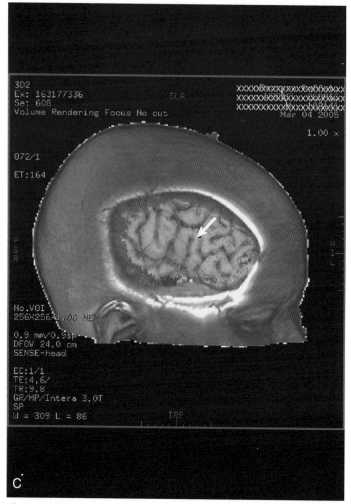

Figure 33-1. *Continued.*

FDG-PET is applicable to the problem of chronic, intractable epilepsy because both interictal hypometabolism and ictal/post-ictal hypermetabolism have been documented in seizure foci.

When FDG-PET reveals a seizure focus, **even in the absence of abnormalities on MR scan,** the imaging workup ends; **FDG-PET data are usually considered sufficiently strong to support surgical or stereotactic intervention.**

When MR reveals a vascular malformation or a neoplasm associated with large vessels:

STEP 2: COMPUTED TOMOGRAPHIC ANGIOGRAPHY (CTA)

CTA requires only **peripheral intravenous injection** of contrast medium followed by rapid CT of the head and/or neck; computer software then "reconstructs" and "reformats" the cross-sectional CT "slices" to generate three-dimensional images **of the intracranial or cervical circulation.** CTA exquisitely reveal aneurysms, dural sinus thrombosis, arteriovenous malformations, and vessel stenosis or occlusion—without the risk and discomfort associated with conventional catheter angiography.

When vascular flow information or endovascular therapy is needed:

STEP 3: CATHETER ANGIOGRAPHY

When transcatheter blood flow measurements are required before therapy of highly vascular lesions (usually for arteriovenous malformations), catheter angiography is required. The study involves injection of contrast medium into blood vessels of the head or neck through a catheter that has been threaded retrograde up the aorta, introduced via percutaneous femoral arterial puncture. In addition to flow measurements, the vascular images provide a road map for surgical or angiographic intervention.

SUMMARY AND CONCLUSIONS

1. MR is the modality of choice for the initial evaluation of chronic, intractable epilepsy. In many cases MR is sufficient to end the imaging workup.
2. A normal MR scan should be followed by FDG-PET.
3. FDG-PET results can be clearly abnormal when MR findings are normal.
4. CTA can further characterize vascular lesions detected by MR, without the expense and risk of conventional catheter angiography.
5. Catheter angiography is appropriate for blood flow measurements in certain highly vascular lesions.

ADDITIONAL COMMENTS

- Although CT is effective for many intracranial lesions, it is poorly suited to study of the temporal lobes, the site of mesial temporal sclerosis. **Therefore, if only CT is available, the patient should be referred elsewhere for MR and possibly subsequent FDG-PET.**
- MR angiography is sometimes considered an alternative to CTA for intracerebral vascular lesions. Although in some hands the two studies are competitive, the consensus among neuroradiologists is that CTA produces better spatial resolution than MR angiography in the brain.
- Many vascular abnormalities can be treated with a transcatheter approach, without the need for "open" neurosurgery.
- In addition to mesial temporal sclerosis, other congenital cortical dysplasias or "gray matter heterotopias" can cause seizures, beginning shortly

after birth or years later; MR is the imaging procedure of choice for all of these conditions.

SUGGESTED READING

Bronen RA, Cheung G, Charles JT, et al: Imaging findings in hippocampal sclerosis: correlation with pathology. AJNR Am J Neuroradiol 1991;12:933–940.

Elster AD, Mirza W: MR imaging in chronic partial epilepsy: role of contrast enhancement. AJNR Am J Neuroradiol 1991;12:165–170.

Fisher RS, Frost JJ: Epilepsy. J Nucl Med 1991;32:651–659.

Grattan SJ, Harvey AS, Desmond PM, et al: Hippocampal sclerosis in children with intractable epilepsy: pathologic correlation and prognostic importance. AJR Am J Roentgenol 1993;161:1045–1048.

Jack CR, Sharbrough FW, Twomey CK, et al: Temporal lobe seizures: lateralization with MR volume measurements of the hippocampal formation. Radiology 1990;175:423–429.

Jackson GD, Berkovic SF, Duncan JS, Connelly A: Optimizing the diagnosis of hippocampal sclerosis using MR imaging. AJNR Am J Neuroradiol 1993;14:753–762.

Lee DH, Gao FQ, Rogers JM, et al: MR in temporal lobe epilepsy: analysis with pathologic confirmation. AJNR Am J Neuroradiol 1998;19:19–27.

Triulzi F, Franceschi M, Fazio F, Del Maschio A: Nonrefractory temporal lobe epilepsy: 1.5-T MR imaging. Radiology 1988;166:181–185.

34 Aneurysms and Arteriovenous Malformations

INTRODUCTION

Aneurysms and arteriovenous malformations (AVMs) are common anomalies of the central nervous system. Both often present acutely—aneurysms with headache, cranial nerve palsies, and subarachnoid hemorrhage; AVMs with seizures or intracerebral hematomas. Computed tomography (CT) with and without intravenous contrast medium (enhanced and unenhanced), computed tomographic angiography (CTA), magnetic resonance (MR) imaging with intravenous contrast medium (enhanced), magnetic resonance angiography (MRA), and catheter angiography effectively study aneurysms and AVMs.

Relative Costs: Head CT, enhanced and unenhanced, **$$$**; CTA, **$$$**; MRA, excluding standard MR, **$$$**; conventional cerebral angiography, complete "four-vessel study," **$$$$$**.

PLAN AND RATIONALE

For the acutely ill patient with possible subarachnoid hemorrhage or intracerebral hematoma:

STEP 1: COMPUTED TOMOGRAPHY (CT)/COMPUTED TOMOGRAPHIC ANGIOGRAPHY (CTA)

CT is the initial study of choice for the assessment of aneurysms and AVMs that present acutely, because their presenting complications—

subarachnoid hemorrhage and intracerebral hematoma—are clearly demonstrated by CT.

Also, unlike MR, CT is compatible with virtually all life-support systems, and scanning times are so short that the study is almost always feasible in an acutely ill, unstable, or moving patient.

In addition to defining the sequelae—hemorrhage or hematoma—of ruptured aneurysms or AVMs, **enhanced CT can often detect the AVM or aneurysm itself.** Enhanced CT can be augmented with CTA, if available, **which visualizes aneurysms nearly as well as catheter angiography (Fig. 34-1).** CTA requires only a **peripheral intravenous injection of contrast medium,** after which the standard "slice images" are reconstructed and reformatted into vascular images of the head and neck. The images reveal and characterize almost all aneurysms and AVMs, providing necessary preoperative anatomic detail, without the expense and discomfort of conventional catheter angiography. (Similar vascular imaging is possible with MRA, but the resolution is not quite as good, the technique is more difficult, the examination is more time consuming, and very ill patients often cannot tolerate its longer scanning times.)

When CT or CTA defines an AVM that may be amenable to transcatheter endovascular therapy—as opposed to "open" neurosurgery—a catheter angiogram is appropriate, because the catheter can measure blood flow within the lesion and across its nidus.

STEP 2: CATHETER ANGIOGRAPHY AND ENDOVASCULAR THERAPY

A catheter introduced by femoral arterial puncture is threaded retrograde up the aorta and passed through the arterial circulation of the neck into the brain. Contrast medium is injected, and the lesion is located; appropriate flow measurements are followed by the transcatheter introduction of various therapeutic substances (e.g., glue, thrombogenic coils, inflatable balloons, Gelfoam) to stabilize and/or obliterate the lesion.

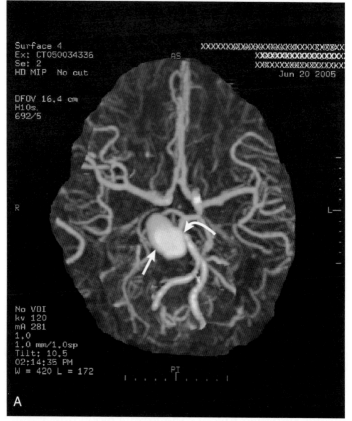

Figure 34-1. A, CTA of a 6-year-old child with a large basilar artery aneurysm (*arrow*). The aneurysm neck is clearly seen (*curved arrow*).

For the elective evaluation of suspected AVMs and aneurysms:

STEP 1: COMPUTED TOMOGRAPHIC ANGIOGRAPHY (CTA)

CTA has become the modality of choice for detection of intracranial vascular lesions; it is faster and more sensitive than MR and also visualizes bony landmarks for surgical planning. (See **Step 1**, above, under **the acutely ill patient with possible subarachnoid**

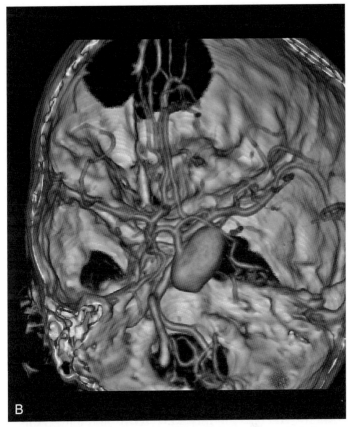

Figure 34-1. B, This "volume rendering" of the same patient allows **simultaneous views of the skull and the vessels.** The images were created from a CT scan that required less than 60 seconds, after a peripheral intravenous injection of contrast medium. **Sedation was not required.**

hemorrhage or intracerebral hematoma, for a discussion of CTA technique.)

Notwithstanding the above, MR is appropriate as a screen for intracranial vascular lesions **when there is a major contraindication to CTA** (see the **INTRODUCTION of this book** for a discussion of contraindications to contrast medium). If clinical suspicion is low for a vascular abnormality, MRA may also be preferable to CTA, particularly for children, because MRA lacks the ionizing radiation of CT and the gadolinium-based contrast medium of MRA is less likely to produce a reaction than that of CT/CTA.

STEP 2: CATHETER ANGIOGRAPHY AND ENDOVASCULAR THERAPY

In the patient with a legitimate contraindication to CTA, a lesion defined by MR then proceeds to catheter angiography; special precautions must be taken to prevent reactions to contrast medium (see **INTRODUCTION** to this book).

(See **Step 2,** above, under **the acutely ill patient with possible subarachnoid hemorrhage or intracerebral hematoma,** for a discussion of endovascular therapy technique.)

SUMMARY AND CONCLUSIONS

1. CT/CTA is the initial study of choice in the emergency evaluation of aneurysms and AVMs, because the hemorrhagic consequences of these lesions are clearly identified, and the vascular etiology of the bleed can be assessed during the same scan.
2. CTA can also identify some AVMs and aneurysms that have **not** bled and is more sensitive and specific than MR for this purpose.
3. MR is a good alternative to CTA for evaluating AVMs and aneurysms but is less sensitive and should be reserved for patients with contraindications to CTA.
4. Catheter angiography is the definitive study for AVMs and is equivalent to—or slightly better than—CTA for aneurysms; it is too invasive to compete with CTA as a screening examination, but it is currently required before endovascular treatment.

ADDITIONAL COMMENTS

- In patients who are studied by MR/MRA because of contraindications to the contrast medium required for CT/CTA, symptoms may persist after a normal good quality study. Such patients deserve a conventional catheter angiogram, because MRA can miss very small aneurysms.

SUGGESTED READING

Alberico RA, Patel M, Casey S, et al: Evaluation of the circle of Willis with three-dimensional CT angiography in patients with suspected intracranial aneurysms. AJNR Am J Neuroradiol 1995;16:1571–1578.

Atlas SW, Grossman RI, Goldberg HI, et al: Partially thrombosed giant intracranial aneurysms: correlation of MR and pathologic findings. Radiology 1987;162:111–114.

Hope JK, Wilson JL, Thomson FJ: Three-dimensional CT angiography in the detection and characterization of intracranial berry aneurysms. AJNR Am J Neuroradiol 1996;17:439–445.

Huston J, Rufenacht DA, Ehman RL, Wiebers DO: Intracranial aneurysms and vascular malformations: comparison of time-of-flight and phase-contrast MR angiography. Radiology 1991;181:721–730.

Kucharczyk W, Lemme-Pleghos L, Uske A, et al: Intracranial vascular malformations: MR and CT imaging. Radiology 1985;156:383–389.

Liang EY, Chan M, Hsiang JHK, et al: Detection and assessment of intracranial aneurysms: value of CT angiography with shaded surface display. AJR Am J Roentgenol 1995;165:1497–1502.

Masaryk TJ, Modic MT, Ross JS, et al: Intracranial circulation: preliminary clinical results with three-dimensional (volume) MR angiography. Radiology 1989;171:793–799.

Ogawa T, Okudera T, Noguchi K, et al: Cerebral aneurysms: evaluation with three-dimensional CT angiography. AJNR Am J Neuroradiol 1996;17:447–454.

Vieco PT, Shuman WP, Alsoform GF, Gross CE: Detection of circle of Willis aneurysms in patients with acute subarachnoid hemorrhage: a comparison of CT angiography and digital subtraction angiography. AJR Am J Roentgenol 1995;165:425–430.

35 Spinal Cord Compression from Metastases

INTRODUCTION

Spinal cord compression from metastases can progress rapidly to profound and irreversible neurologic damage. Imaging can define the level, extent, and cause of the compression.

Spinal cord studies are often requested on an emergency basis, reinforcing the need for rapid, accurate diagnosis. Several techniques apply: myelography, computed tomography (CT) with intrathecal contrast medium (CT myelography), and magnetic resonance (MR) imaging with and without intravenous contrast medium (enhanced and unenhanced). The choice may depend on availability, particularly in an emergency.

Relative Costs: Cervical MR, unenhanced and enhanced, **$$$$**; thoracic MR, unenhanced and enhanced, **$$$$**; lumbar MR, unenhanced and enhanced, **$$$$**; cervical CT myelography, **$$$**; thoracic CT myelography, **$$$**; lumbar CT myelography, **$$$**; conventional cervical, thoracic, and lumbar myelography, **$$–$$$**.

PLAN AND RATIONALE

Where MR is available:

STEP 1: MAGNETIC RESONANCE (MR) IMAGING

MR is the examination of choice for evaluating suspected spinal cord compression.

MR images the spine in multiple planes, clearly defining the cerebrospinal fluid, spinal cord, nerve roots, intervertebral disks, and vertebral bodies. The location and extent of lesions and their relationship to the spinal cord and dura are well delineated. MR is noninvasive and better tolerated than myelography, which requires a lumbar puncture. Intravenous contrast medium can augment lesion conspicuity and better define the extent of disease.

Where emergency MR is unavailable:

STEP 1: COMPUTED TOMOGRAPHIC MYELOGRAPHY (CT MYELOGRAPHY)

CT myelography is an acceptable alternative if MR is unavailable. The technique is almost as sensitive as MR for defining the cause of spinal cord compression. Contrast medium is injected into the lumbar subarachnoid space, and the patient is positioned head down. The contrast medium usually flows beyond the level of an obstruction, defining its craniad extent. **CT without intrathecal contrast medium is usually insufficient.**

Where MR and CT are unavailable or unfeasible:

STEP 1: PLAIN FILM MYELOGRAPHY

In a few hospitals, emergency MR and CT are unavailable; moreover, these studies may be unfeasible because of (1) massive patient obesity, which exceeds the weight tolerances of the CT and MR tables or prevents the patient from fitting into the opening of the machine (the gantry); or (2) metal "hardware" from spinal surgery that produces artifacts on CT and MR.

Before the advent of CT and MR, conventional myelography was the standard study for spinal cord compression, and this generally obsolete study remains useful in rare, special circumstances. Contrast medium is injected into the subarachnoid space, and the patient is placed head down, so that the contrast medium migrates craniad. When the contrast medium encounters a block, radiographs reveal the outline of the lower end of the lesion, and sometimes contrast medium passes around it to reveal the lesion's general shape. Although the study can demonstrate spinal cord compression, the offending lesion itself **is inferred,** and the superior extent of the block may not be visualized at all. (Sometimes a separate cervical puncture may be necessary to define the superior extent of the block, as contrast medium moves downward toward the lower end of the thecal sac.) **Clearly, conventional myelography is inferior to MR or CT myelography.**

SUMMARY AND CONCLUSIONS

1. MR is the modality of choice for evaluating suspected spinal cord compression from metastatic tumor.
2. If MR is unavailable, CT myelography is an acceptable alternative.
3. If MR and CT are unavailable or unfeasible, conventional plain film myelography can define the level of a spinal cord compression, but the study is clearly inferior to MR or CT myelography.

SUGGESTED READING

Carmody RF, Yang PJ, Seeley GW, et al: Spinal cord compression due to metastatic disease: diagnosis with MR imaging versus myelography. Radiology 1989;173:225–229.

Dublin AB, McGahan JP, Reid MH: The value of computed tomographic metrizamide myelography in the neuroradiological evaluation of the spine. Radiology 1977;146:79–86.

Fink IJ, Garra BS, Zabell A, Doppman JL: Computed tomography with metrizamide myelography to define the extent of spinal canal block due to tumor. J Comput Assist Tomogr 1984;8:1072–1075.

Gilbert RW, Kim JH, Posner JB: Epidural spinal cord compression from metastatic tumor: diagnosis and treatment. Ann Neurol 1978;3:40–51.

Kelly WM, Badami P, Dillon W: Epidural block: myelographic evaluation with a single-puncture technique using metrizamide. Radiology 1984;151:417–419.

Le Bihan DJ: Differentiation of benign vs. pathologic compression fractures with diffusion-weighted MR imaging: a closer step toward the "holy grail" of tissue characterization? Editorial. Radiology 1998;207:305–307.

Smoker WR, Godersky JC, Knutzon RK, et al: The role of MR imaging in evaluating metastatic spinal disease. AJR Am J Roentgenol 1987;149:1241–1248.

Sze G, Krol G, Zimmerman RD, Deck MD: Malignant extradural spinal tumors: MR imaging with Gd-DTPA. Radiology 1988;67:217–223.

36 Demyelinating Disease

INTRODUCTION

Traditionally, multiple sclerosis (MS) has been a clinical diagnosis. The previous role of imaging was to exclude other diseases that might simulate MS, but **magnetic resonance (MR) imaging with and without intravenous contrast medium (enhanced and unenhanced) is now capable of confirming the diagnosis of MS and excluding other diseases.** Other causes of demyelination—radiation-induced leukoencephalopathy, acute disseminated encephalomyelitis, and metabolic abnormalities—can also be investigated by MR.

Relative Costs: Brain MR, unenhanced, **$$$**; brain MR, enhanced and unenhanced, **$$$$**.

PLAN AND RATIONALE

STEP 1: MAGNETIC RESONANCE (MR) IMAGING

MR has replaced computed tomography (CT) as the modality of choice for the evaluation of MS and other demyelinating diseases.

The multiplanar imaging capability of MR demonstrates lesions that are specific for MS. Intravenous contrast medium increases both the sensitivity and the specificity of the study. Lesions that are more conspicuous on the enhanced study sometimes correlate with specific symptoms.

230

SUMMARY AND CONCLUSIONS

1. MR is the modality of choice for the evaluation of demyelinating disease.
2. Computed tomography (CT) can exclude other diseases that mimic MS, but CT is not recommended in the workup of MS, because a normal CT must be followed by MR, unnecessarily increasing the cost of the workup.

ADDITIONAL COMMENTS

- Special MR techniques such as "fat suppression" may augment detection of optic nerve lesions in patients with optic neuritis, a common presenting symptom of MS.
- Demyelinating lesions of the spinal cord are visualized by MR but rarely by CT.

SUGGESTED READING

Bruck W, Bitsch A, Kolenda H, et al: Inflammatory central nervous system demyelination: correlation of magnetic resonance imaging findings with pathology. Ann Neurol 1997;42:783–793.

Gean-Marton AD, Vezina LG, Marton KI, et al: Abnormal corpus callosum: a sensitive and specific indicator of multiple sclerosis. Radiology 1991;180:215–221.

Gebarski SS, Gabrielsen TO, Gilman S, et al: The initial diagnosis of multiple sclerosis: clinical impact of magnetic resonance imaging. Ann Neurol 1985;17:469–474.

Grossman RI, Gonzalez-Scarano F, Atlas SW, et al: Multiple sclerosis: gadolinium enhancement in MR imaging. Radiology 1986;161:721–725.

Horowith AL, Kaplan RD, Grewe G, et al: The ovoid lesion: a new MR observation in patients with multiple sclerosis. AJNR Am J Neuroradiol 1989;10:303–305.

Kirshner HS, Tsai SI, Runge VM, Price AC: Magnetic resonance imaging and other techniques in the diagnosis of multiple sclerosis. Arch Neurol 1985;42:859–863.

Rocco MA, Mastronardo G, Horsfield MA, et al: Comparison of three MR sequences for the detection of cervical cord lesions in patients with multiple sclerosis. AJNR Am J Neuroradiol 1999;20:1710–1716.

Simon JH: Neuroimaging of multiple sclerosis. Radiol Clin North Am 1993;3:229–246.

Zagzag D, Miller DC, Kleinman GM, et al: Demyelinating disease vs. tumor in surgical neuropathology. Clues to correct pathologic diagnosis. Am J Surg Pathol 1993;17:537–545.

37 Sellar and Juxtasellar Lesions

INTRODUCTION

Sellar and juxtasellar lesions usually present with endocrine syndromes, such as amenorrhea/galactorrhea, diabetes insipidus, and acromegaly, or with neurologic syndromes, such as visual loss. The goal of imaging is to determine whether a significant lesion exists and, if so, to localize and characterize it for therapy. Magnetic resonance (MR) imaging with and without intravenous contrast medium (enhanced and unenhanced), computed tomography (CT) with and without intravenous contrast medium (enhanced and unenhanced), and angiography can play roles in the workup.

Relative Costs: Brain MR, unenhanced, **$$$**; brain MR, enhanced and unenhanced, **$$$$**; head CT, enhanced and unenhanced, **$$$**; CT angiogram, **$$$**; catheter cerebral angiogram, complete "four-vessel study," **$$$$$$**.

PLAN AND RATIONALE

Where MR is available:

STEP 1: MAGNETIC RESONANCE (MR) IMAGING

MR is the modality of choice for the evaluation of sellar and juxtasellar lesions. The study is superior to CT because of its multiplanar imaging capability, lack of bone-induced artifact, and superior spatial resolution. MR clearly delineates sellar and juxtasellar masses and their relationship to adjacent structures such as the optic

233

chiasm, hypothalamus, carotid arteries, and cavernous sinus. Studies with intravenous contrast medium better characterize pituitary macroadenomas and microadenomas. **Very often a firm diagnosis is possible without surgery or biopsy.**

When bone destruction and calcifications must be further defined, CT can be helpful (see **Step 1: Computed Tomography,** below). When vascular lesions require study before surgical or angiographic intervention, cerebral angiography is effective (see **Step 2: Catheter Angiography,** below).

Where MR is not available:

STEP 1: COMPUTED TOMOGRAPHY (CT)

CT with and without intravenous contrast medium (enhanced and unenhanced) can evaluate most sellar and juxtasellar lesions. Unenhanced CT clearly reveals soft tissue abnormalities, cortical bone, and calcifications. Enhanced CT helps to characterize juxtasellar vascular masses such as carotid artery aneurysms. The findings in some lesions, particularly meningiomas, are pathognomonic. **Normal findings on CT exclude all but very small lesions, such as isodense pituitary microadenomas. Frequently, a definite diagnosis is possible.**

CT is superior to MR in defining bone destruction and calcifications; nonetheless, these advantages do not fully compensate for its important weaknesses relative to MR. Thus, **MR remains the examination of choice.**

If CT findings are normal, the workup usually ends, but if a lesion is nonetheless suspected on clinical grounds, the patient should be referred to a facility that has MR. When vascular lesions require further study, computed tomographic angiography (CTA) can be used to define vessels and aneurysms. CTA requires only a peripheral intravenous injection of contrast medium, after which the standard "slice images" of the head and neck are reformatted and computer manipulated to create vascular images in the head and neck, without the expense and trauma of conventional catheter angiography. The vascular images are virtually equivalent to those provided by catheter angiography (see **Step 2,** below). If vascular lesions are identified that may require endovascular therapy or if CTA is not available, catheter angiography is appropriate.

STEP 2: CATHETER ANGIOGRAPHY

A catheter is threaded retrograde up the aorta following percutaneous femoral artery puncture, and the catheter tip is positioned in one of the great vessels of the neck. Contrast medium is injected as serial films are exposed, revealing the vascular components of a lesion and the vascularity of adjacent brain. Some vascular lesions can be treated by "endovascular therapy," eliminating the need for "open" neurologic surgery. Angiography is useful in the evaluation of vascular lesions, such as aneurysms and arteriovenous malformations, and certain tumors, like meningiomas, before surgical resection or as a method of treatment using embolic material, such as detachable metallic coils.

SUMMARY AND CONCLUSIONS

1. MR is the best initial study for suspected sellar and juxtasellar lesions.
2. If MR is unavailable, CT is a reasonable alternative, although CT is not as sensitive for small lesions.
3. CT may be a useful adjunct to MR in the evaluation of bone destruction and in the detection of calcification.
4. Angiography has limited **diagnostic** value but is helpful to further characterize vascular lesions, provide a presurgical "vascular road map," or be a part of endovascular therapy.

ADDITIONAL COMMENTS

• Newer MR software—"gradient recall echo techniques"—increases the sensitivity of MR for calcification, eliminating the need for CT in most cases.

SUGGESTED READING

Chakeres DW, Curtin A, Ford G: Magnetic resonance imaging of pituitary and parasellar abnormalities. Radiol Clin North Am 1989;27:265–281.

Davis PC, Hoffman JC Jr, Malko JA, et al: Gadolinium-DTPA and MR imaging of pituitary adenoma: a preliminary report. AJNR Am J Neuroradiol 1987;8:817–823.

Kucharczyk W, David DO, Kelly WM, et al: Pituitary adenomas: high-resolution MR imaging at 1.5T. Radiology 1986;161:761–765.

Sartor K, Karnaze MG, Winthrop JD, et al: MR imaging in infra-, para- and retrosellar mass lesions. Neuroradiology 1987;29:19–29.

Taylor S: High resolution computed tomography of the sella. Radiol Clin North Am 1982;20:207–236.

38 Stroke

INTRODUCTION

Stroke is a major cause of morbidity and mortality in the developed world. Computed tomography (CT) without intravenous contrast medium (unenhanced), magnetic resonance (MR) imaging with and without intravenous contrast medium (enhanced and unenhanced), and angiography each play a role.

Over the past 5 years neurologists, neuroradiologists, and neurosurgeons have come to realize that the brain damage caused by stroke can be limited by timely intervention and that sophisticated diagnostic imaging with special MR techniques, particularly "diffusion-weighted imaging" (DWI), can define brain tissue not yet irreversibly injured but at risk. Therefore, in many cities, "stroke teams" have been created; the skills of these multidisciplinary teams include emergency MR with DWI, MR angiography (MRA), and transcatheter therapy. **Where available, stroke teams perform first-line evaluation and therapy for stroke. Effective life-altering therapy usually must be applied within 3 hours of symptom onset.**

Relative Costs: Head CT, enhanced and unenhanced, **$$$**; brain MR, enhanced and unenhanced, **$$$$**; cerebral angiogram, carotid catheterizations only, **$$$$$–$$$$$$**.

PLAN AND RATIONALE

STEP 1: COMPUTED TOMOGRAPHY (CT)

CT is the current modality of choice for the evaluation of acute stroke.

The study can easily exclude lesions—such as tumor and abscess—that simulate stroke and can often differentiate between ischemic and hemorrhagic infarction; hemorrhagic infarction is seen immediately, whereas ischemic infarction usually appears by 24 hours. Intravenous contrast medium is usually not required, because the majority of infarctions are evident without it. In the setting of potential thrombolytic therapy, CT serves the major role of excluding intracerebral hemorrhage (which would contraindicate thrombolytic therapy).

When CT reveals a non-stroke cause of symptoms, or when stroke is diagnosed but the temporal "window" for effective intervention has passed, the diagnostic workup ends.

When CT fails to differentiate infarction from another disease process, when posterior fossa infarction is suspected, or when CT does not explain the clinical findings, MR, if feasible, is next. Furthermore, in the presence of a normal CT but strong clinical evidence of stroke, when time is short and/or the patient cannot tolerate the longer scanning times of MR, direct intervention via angiography is appropriate.

STEP 2: MAGNETIC RESONANCE (MR) IMAGING

MR better visualizes the posterior fossa because it is not hampered by occipital bone artifacts that sometimes degrade CT of this anatomic region, especially older CT scanners. MR is more sensitive than CT for early infarction, and the greater sensitivity of MR can be further augmented by diffusion-weighted imaging (DWI). DWI is an MR technique that detects areas of restricted movement of **extracellular** water. (In acute stroke, cellular edema occurs almost immediately, creating an impediment to flow of extracellular water). As a consequence, DWI is very sensitive for detection of stroke **within minutes of the event**. MR perfusion imaging uses a fast MR scan with a 2 to 3 mL/second peripheral intravenous bolus injection of gadolinium-based contrast medium. MR perfusion imaging can define areas of **hypoperfusion** as well as areas with **no perfusion. DWI, when combined with perfusion-weighted imaging, can define areas of viable brain tissue at risk for infarction adjacent to an acute infarct. These crucial areas can be salvaged if a good blood supply can be reestablished.**

Despite its advantages, MR is not always feasible in the acute setting, because most life-support systems are not MR compatible, **and the acutely ill patient often cannot tolerate the relatively long scanning times of most MR units.** Also, MR can be time consuming, and in acute stroke delay can be fatal or permanently disabling.

When MR and/or CT reveals lesions that may be caused by carotid or vertebral artery disease, or when MR directly visualizes vascular flow abnormalities, and when interventional therapy is contemplated, angiography is next.

STEP 2 OR 3: ANGIOGRAPHY

Angiography involves percutaneous femoral artery puncture, passage of a catheter up the aorta, and catheterization of one of the neck arteries. Contrast medium is injected as serial films are exposed. The technique exquisitely demonstrates narrowed areas that restrict blood flow. **Intra-arterial injection of thrombolytic agents or the acute application of vascular stents and/or angioplasty (balloon dilation of a vessel) can reverse the devastating effects of stroke in some circumstances.** Years—even a lifetime—of disability can be avoided in some patients.

All interventions work best if applied quickly, because, in the parlance of stroke teams, "time is brain tissue."

SUMMARY AND CONCLUSIONS

1. CT is the modality of choice for the evaluation of stroke.
2. In some cases MR is required after CT, particularly to better image the posterior fossa on older CT scanners and/or to detect early infarction. A normal CT finding in the presence of strong clinical evidence of stroke can be followed by MR, if feasible, and if time permits.
3. Enhanced MR can detect stoke earlier than CT. However, MR is not always practical in the evaluation of acute stroke because of relatively long scanning times and MR-incompatible life-support systems.
4. Angiography is appropriate in the presence of a normal CT and strong clinical indications of stroke; the procedure can demonstrate arterial narrowing in the neck that restricts blood flow to the brain.
5. Endovascular therapy, through a catheter, can reverse the effects of stroke and prevent further infarction if applied within a few hours of the stroke onset.
6. When stroke is a clinical possibility, emergency imaging is essential. The age-old belief that rapid diagnosis does not count, because brain destruction is inevitable and irreversible, has been completely discredited.
7. **THE STROKE TEAM, IF ONE IS AVAILABLE, SHOULD BE NOTIFIED OF THE CASE EVEN BEFORE IMAGING BEGINS.**

ADDITIONAL COMMENTS

- Newer MR units are markedly faster than older ones. Moreover, more and more life-support systems are

MR compatible. **Therefore, eventually MR may replace CT as the procedure of choice in acute stroke.**

SUGGESTED READING

Adams HP, Brott TG, Furlan AJ, et al: Guidelines for thrombolytic therapy for acute stroke: a supplement to the guidelines for the management of patients with acute ischemic stroke. Stroke 1996;27:1711–1718.

Bryan RN, Levy LM, Whitlow WD, et al: Diagnosis of acute cerebral infarction: comparison of CT and MR imaging. AJNR Am J Neuroradiol 1991;12:611–620.

Crain MR, Yu WT, Greene GM, et al: Cerebral ischemia: evaluation with contrast-enhanced MR imaging. AJNR Am J Neuroradiol 1991;12:631–639.

Elster AD, Moody DM: Early cerebral infarction: gadopentetate dimeglumine enhancement. Radiology 1990;177:627–632.

Ginsberg MD: The new language of cerebral ischemia. AJNR Am J Neuroradiol 1997;18:1435–1445.

Inoue Y, Takemoto K, Miyamoto T, et al: Sequential computed tomography scans in acute cerebral infarction. Radiology 1980;135:655–662.

Yuh WT, Crain MR, Loes DJ, et al: MR imaging of cerebral ischemia: findings in the first 24 hours. AJNR Am J Neuroradiol 1991;12:621–629.

Sinusitis

39

INTRODUCTION

"Sinusitis" is infection, usually bacterial but sometimes fungal, of one or more of the paranasal sinuses. The condition is common and seldom requires imaging for confirmation.

In the general population, acute bacterial sinusitis follows a viral upper respiratory infection and presents with fever, rhinorrhea, facial pain, and purulent nasal secretions. Similar but less acute symptoms occur in recurrent or chronic disease. However, in the cancer population, or in any population that is immunosuppressed, acute sinusitis can develop without a known antecedent viral "cold"; whether a viral infection goes undetected in such persons or the bacterial sinusitis develops spontaneously from overgrowth of preexisting flora, or whether seeding from bacteremia is responsible, remains unclear.

For more than 60 years plain "sinus films" were the mainstay of diagnostic imaging for this disease. However, plain films are operator dependent and often poorly define the sphenoid sinus, the lower-lateral ethmoid air cells, and the frontal sinuses. Complex and/or subtle cases can be completely missed by plain films, and, overwhelmingly, head-neck radiologists as well as otolaryngologists have come to prefer computed tomography (CT). Our view is that in the hospitalized population, or in any population that is immunosuppressed or at risk for serious infection, plain films should be skipped in favor of CT.

Relative Costs: Sinus series, complete, **$**; sinus series, limited (three views or less), **.5$**; sinus CT, unenhanced,

$$$; sinus CT, enhanced, $$$; sinus CT, unenhanced and enhanced, $$$; MR, unenhanced, $$$$.

PLAN AND RATIONALE

For adults or adolescents who are NOT immunosuppressed, with questionable acute sinusitis:

STEP 1: STANDARD SINUS SERIES

A standard four-view sinus series is simple and relatively inexpensive. Unfortunately, the accuracy of this study is limited. An air-fluid level is the only completely reliable radiographic sign of acute sinusitis. Moreover, the ethmoid sinuses, which are most commonly affected, are inadequately evaluated. **Thus, a negative sinus series does not completely exclude sinusitis.**

If the study is positive, the disease is treated with antibiotics, and follow-up imaging is rarely required. If the study is negative or equivocal, symptoms persist for weeks to months, and empirical antibiotic therapy is ineffective, chronic sinusitis may have developed and CT is usually definitive.

For young children who are NOT immunosuppressed, with questionable acute sinusitis:

In a general hospital or in an imaging center with limited pediatric experience:

STEP 1: LIMITED PLAIN FILM SINUS SERIES

Sinusitis is particularly common in small children. The signs and symptoms of acute sinusitis in these patients are different than those in adults and older children; fever may be absent and otitis media is frequently present. A two-view study (a Waters view—a frontal view with the x-ray beam angled upward—and a lateral view) is inexpensive, limits radiation, and is helpful for confirmation. Even in children as young as 1 year of age, an air-fluid level in the maxillary sinus is a reliable indicator of acute sinusitis. Usually no further imaging is necessary. However, if the study findings are negative or equivocal, symptoms persist for weeks to months, and empirical antibiotic therapy is ineffective, chronic sinusitis may have developed and CT is usually definitive.

In a pediatric hospital or an imaging center with extensive pediatric experience:

STEP 1: THICK-SECTION, LIMITED SINUS COMPUTED TOMOGRAPHY (CT)

A limited sinus CT can provide more information than a limited plain films sinus series with no more radiation but a greater cost. If this study is normal, sinusitis is excluded.

As a follow-up to equivocal plain sinus films:

For adults or children with complicated acute sinusitis and for any immunocompromised patient with suspected sinusitis:

STEP 1: COMPUTED TOMOGRAPHY (CT)

As a purely diagnostic procedure for the sinuses only, when plain films are equivocal or in the immunosuppressed patient, contrast medium is usually not required. However, in suspected complications of acute sinusitis, contrast medium is mandatory, because the complications of acute sinusitis may be serious and even life-

threatening and adjacent structures must be defined. Infection may spread to the orbit and the intracranial cavity, causing meningitis, abscess, subdural empyema, and thrombophlebitis.

In most cases of complicated sinusitis, CT is sufficient, but when aggressive fungal infection, meningitis, or vascular thrombosis is suspected, additional MR may be required.

STEP 2: MAGNETIC RESONANCE (MR) IMAGING WITH CONTRAST MEDIUM (ENHANCED)

Especially in cases of aggressive fungal infection, MR is superior to CT for the evaluation of meningeal infection and vascular thrombosis. However, MR should not precede CT, because CT better displays the complex bony anatomy of the paranasal sinuses, orbits, and skull base; the infection originates in and propagates from bony cavities. **In severe chronic sinusitis MR can actually be falsely negative, so starting with CT is essential.**

SUMMARY AND CONCLUSIONS

1. Acute uncomplicated sinusitis in adults and older children is usually apparent clinically, and imaging is uncommonly required. In equivocal cases, a standard sinus series is helpful, although the accuracy of sinus radiographs is somewhat limited.
2. Imaging is seldom necessary in children with suspected acute sinusitis, although a limited sinus series may be helpful, particularly because the diagnosis of sinusitis in children may be more difficult than in adults and older children. **If the radiologist or hospital has sufficient pediatric experience, a thick-section limited sinus CT is the ideal choice for children.**
3. In the immunocompromised population, **the initial study should be CT,** because this population is at high risk for serious complications, and

the lower sensitivity of a plain films sinus series is inappropriate.

4. Adults or children with suspected or definite complications of acute sinusitis should undergo CT with intravenous contrast medium and, for some further complications, MR. CT and MR are complementary in this setting.

SUGGESTED READING

Naidech TP, Zimmerman RA, Bauer BS, et al: Midface: Embryology and congenital lesions. In Som PM, Curtin H (eds): Head and Neck Imaging. Boston, Mosby, 1996, pp 1–126.

Zinreich S: Imaging of inflammatory sinus disease. Otolaryngol Clin North Am 1993;26:535–547.

Zinreich S, Kennedy D, Rosenbaum A, et al: Paranasal sinuses: CT imaging requirements for endoscopic surgery. Radiology 1987;163:769–775.

40 Acute and Chronic Back Pain

INTRODUCTION

Back pain affects nearly all of us during our lives. It probably began when our proto-hominid ancestors first stood erect, or possibly when we were cast out of Eden to hoe the dry earth of the Middle East in a semi-upright position, like our proto-hominid ancestors, with a spine that had just evolved for erect walking. ("In the sweat of thy brow shalt thou eat thy daily bread...") Whatever your belief, you will likely sooner or later experience back pain.

The less fortunate among us may experience back pain on a chronic basis, for years or even decades. The following diagnostic options apply in the setting of acute or chronic back pain **unrelated to known acute trauma.** (For trauma-related back pain, **see CHAPTER 28, Acute Spine Trauma.**)

In every imaging workup, history and physical examination are important, but particularly so in back pain. Radiculopathy can define the level of interest and the appropriate imaging test. Tenderness is key. Immune compromise, diabetes, previous surgery, fever, elevated C-reactive protein, and malignancy also influence the imaging workup.

Relative Costs: Cervical spine plain films, **$**; thoracic spine plain films, **$**; lumbar spine plain films, **$**; cervical spine computed tomography (CT), unenhanced, **$$$**; thoracic spine CT, unenhanced, **$$$**; lumbar spine CT, unenhanced, **$$$**; cervical spine magnetic resonance (MR), unenhanced, **$$$**; thoracic spine MR, unenhanced, **$$$**; lumbar spine MR, unenhanced, **$$$–$$$$**.

▎PLAN AND RATIONALE

> **In patients with no contraindications to MR (see INTRODUCTION to this book for a discussion of contraindications):**

STEP 1: MAGNETIC RESONANCE (MR) IMAGING, SOMETIMES WITH GADOLINIUM-BASED CONTRAST MEDIUM (ENHANCED)

MR is the study of choice for evaluation of acute and chronic back pain—cervical, thoracic, and lumbar. MR accurately assesses disk-related causes of pain (herniations and protrusions), spinal stenosis, and arthritic changes such as facet joint arthritis and bony impingement on neural structures due to osteophytes.

In the setting of chronic progressive pain with or without fever, especially with tenderness, diskitis/osteomyelitis must be considered and MR should be gadolinium "enhanced." **This is key for patients with elevated C-reactive protein or erythrocyte sedimentation rate or with immune compromise.** But for patients without known malignancy or previous surgery and no sign or suspicion of infection, contrast medium is not necessary.

In the lumbar spine enhanced MR can be useful after previous back surgery to help differentiate recurrent disk disease from scar tissue and/or arachnoiditis. (Due to the large normal epidural venous plexus in the cervical spine, contrast medium does not have a similar value in the postoperative cervical spine.)

If MR findings are normal, plain films may nonetheless be useful.

> **In patients who cannot tolerate MR, or when MR reveals a lesion of bone that requires further evaluation:**

STEP 1 OR 2: COMPUTED TOMOGRAPHY (CT), SOMETIMES WITH INTRATHECAL CONTRAST MEDIUM (CT MYELOGRAPHY)

CT is rarely the first test for evaluation of back pain unless MR is contraindicated by a cardiac pacemaker, intracranial aneurysm clips (which endanger the patient in the magnetic field), or implanted surgical hardware in the spine (which creates artifacts that severely compromise the images). However, when MR demonstrates a bone lesion, **CT is often more useful for demonstrating its extent and nature, as well as guiding biopsy** (see **CHAPTER 60, Percutaneous Guided Biopsy and Imaging-Guided Therapy**).

When screening for disk herniation, contrast medium is usually not required, but in patients with a high clinical suspicion of other disease (malignancy or mass in the spinal canal) for whom CT without contrast medium is normal, the study can be repeated after translumbar percutaneous instillation of contrast medium into the subarachnoid space; the contrast medium is then directed to the level of interest by tilting the table so that it flows to the dependent anatomy. This examination, a CT myelogram, is more invasive than MR but is highly accurate for detecting sources of nerve root compression or intrathecal mass lesions. CT myelography may be better than MR in postoperative patients who have had considerable surgical hardware implanted. The hardware creates artifacts that distort MR images more than in CT images in some cases.

After MR and/or CT (with or without CT myelography) have excluded disk disease, plain films may nonetheless be useful.

STEP 2 OR 3: PLAIN FILMS OF THE SPINE

Lowly, old-fashioned plain films can be useful for patients whose MR or CT imaging does not explain symptoms. Simple degenerative change of the posterior joints that exist between the facets of vertebra (apophyseal joints) can be a significant cause of pain, and plain films during flexion and extension can demonstrate that a vertebral body moves forward abnormally, causing pain by positional compression of nerve roots in the foramen or simply by direct irritation of the joint.

Normal results on plain films, following normal results on MR or CT imaging, end the workup, unless there is good evidence of an unrelated malignancy (see **Additional Comments** regarding a bone scan).

> **When multiple disks are abnormal on MR or CT, surgery is contemplated, and a particular level must be selected for repair:**

STEP 3 OR 4: DISKOGRAPHY

Diskography is an invasive, provocative test that involves the insertion of a needle directly into an intervertebral disk followed by contrast medium injection. During the injection pain is elicited, and the patient is questioned as to whether the pain mimics the pain for which the evaluation is performed.

The hope is that diskography will identify the disks that cause pain, which surgery will mitigate. **The technique remains controversial, because it has never been definitively associated with improved surgical outcome. It has a 2% to 3% incidence of complication, including diskitis/osteomyelitis, and is most controversial in the cervical and thoracic spine.** Except in a small subset of patients with severe lumbar back pain and ambiguous findings on MR, CT, and plain films, diskography is unlikely to be of value and should be performed only in a department that has wide experience with the procedure.

SUMMARY AND CONCLUSIONS

1. MR is the cornerstone of the workup for back pain.
2. CT is the appropriate second examination if MR is not possible or to further define bony lesions that need further evaluation or biopsy.
3. Plain films and myelography may add information in a subset of patients and enable evaluation in flexion and extension.
4. Diskography is not usually useful and is especially risky in the cervical or thoracic spine, but it may be useful in a small subset of patients in the lumbar spine—but **only if surgery is a definite consideration.**

ADDITIONAL COMMENTS

- MR **in normal asymptomatic volunteers** is positive for disk herniation in 65% of cases. Disk herniations that do not specifically correlate with symptoms are a frequent finding. **Disk surgery should be reserved for patients with functional deficits and/or pain that correlates with imaging findings.**
- Although it seems counterintuitive, we prefer to begin the workup of back pain with MR, a much more expensive test than plain radiography, because plain films do not address the key issues of disk protrusion and herniation. Thus, the much less expensive plain films are usually noncontributory and represent a waste of effort and resources.
- A bone scan is often prudent after a bone lesion has been defined by MR, CT, or plain films, because the demonstration of additional lesions (the bone scan is a total body study) can radically change the workup. Furthermore, normal findings on plain films after normal findings on MR and/or CT can occasionally miss a bony malignancy; therefore, if the patient has a known malignant lesion elsewhere, a bone scan is prudent (see **CHAPTER 44, Skeletal Metastases**).

- CT myelography is also accurate for defining compression of the spinal cord and is appropriate if MR is not possible (see **CHAPTER 35, Spinal Cord Compression from Metastases**).

SUGGESTED READING

Czervionke LF, Haughton VM: Degenerative disease of the spine. In Atlas SW (ed): Magnetic Resonance Imaging of the Brain and Spine, 3rd ed. Philadelphia, Lippincott Williams & Wilkins, 2002, pp 1633–1714.

Grossman RI, Yousem DM: Neuroradiology: the Requisites. Boston, Mosby, 1994, pp 447–476.

Osborn AG: Diagnostic Neuroradiology. Boston, Mosby, 1994, pp 836–872.

41 Thyroid Nodule(s)/ Thyroid Enlargement

INTRODUCTION

The workup of thyroid nodules and diffuse thyroid enlargement differs. In nodular disease, the central issue is to differentiate benign from malignant conditions, whereas in diffuse thyroid enlargement imaging helps to narrow a wide range of usually benign diagnostic options.

(This chapter, unlike others, includes fairly extensive descriptions of various scan patterns and correlates these patterns with clinical syndromes; although we have avoided this approach elsewhere, we have found that such a condensed synopsis of thyroid disease **simply cannot be found elsewhere:** the key data can be gleaned only by exhaustive searching through large endocrinology and nuclear medicine texts. Therefore, the busy clinician should use the detailed descriptions as a reference to better understand the thyroid scan report and should concentrate on the most appropriate testing sequence.)

ONE OR MORE THYROID NODULES, WITHOUT OVERALL THYROID ENLARGEMENT

Traditionally, imaging was used to establish whether nodular lesions "in the thyroid region" were actually part of the thyroid gland and, if so, what they probably represented. However, in recent years, fine-needle aspiration biopsy (FNAB) has largely supplanted imaging. A thorough discussion of FNAB is beyond the scope of this book; nonetheless, ample evidence supports the view that in the patient who is **not** hyperthyroid,

253

nodules that are clearly in the thyroid gland on palpation should undergo initial FNAB rather than imaging. Patients with malignant nodules go directly to surgery, whereas those with benign nodules are followed clinically; re-aspiration of benign lesions is necessary only if the lesion grows. "Suspicious" cytology is associated with malignancy about 20% of the time and also mandates surgery. **Thus, the role of imaging is to clarify those cases in which the cytologic specimen is nondiagnostic, to work up a thyroid mass when expert cytopathology is unavailable, to establish whether a nodule is actually in the thyroid (when localization by palpation is unclear), and to follow some benign nodules during treatment.**

LARGE THYROID GLAND

Nodular
Such patients require thyroid function tests, often followed by a radioiodine uptake and thyroid scan. In select cases, ultrasound (US)-guided biopsy is then appropriate.

Non-Nodular Enlargement
The initial workup involves thyroid function tests, and imaging then often is unnecessary. However, in borderline or ambivalent cases a thyroid uptake and scan can be a useful adjunct to lab values.

    Relative Costs: Radionuclide thyroid uptake, **\$\$\$**; radionuclide thyroid scan, **\$\$\$**; thyroid US, **\$\$**; US-guided thyroid biopsy, **\$\$\$**.

▌ PLAN AND RATIONALE

(A) NODULAR THYROID DISEASE

> **If a nodule or nodules are thought to be in the thyroid on palpation and the thyroid is not enlarged overall:**

STEP 1: FINE-NEEDLE ASPIRATION BIOPSY (FNAB), UNGUIDED

FNAB usually requires no imaging guidance. It is safe, minimally invasive, and productive, yielding diagnostic material about 85% of the time. The cytopathologic interpretation, in good hands, is 95% accurate. Therefore, malignant and "suspicious" lesions are directed to surgery, whereas benign lesions are followed. Indeterminate or nondiagnostic specimens can be referred for re-biopsy, usually under US guidance.

STEP 2: ULTRASOUND (US)-GUIDED FINE-NEEDLE ASPIRATION BIOPSY (FNAB)

The majority of nodules that are re-biopsied under ultrasound guidance yield diagnostic material. To provide a more diagnostic specimen, some sonographers have opted for larger needles that produce a "core biopsy."

A small minority of nodules remains indeterminate, and for these cases radionuclide scanning can be helpful (see **Step 1,** below).

> If even US-guided biopsy of a thyroid nodule is inconclusive, if the procedure and/or expert cytopathology is unavailable, or if the patient is hyperthyroid:

STEP 1: NUCLEAR THYROID SCAN

Traditionally, nuclear thyroid scans used the radiopharmaceutical technetium 99m–pertechnetate (TcO_4^-), a molecule with the same charge (–1) and approximate ionic radius as iodide (I^-). Therefore, the trap mechanism of thyroid tissue traps TcO_4^-, although the trapped TcO_4^- is not subsequently organified or incorporated into thyroid hormone. Nonetheless, a TcO_4^- scan provides physiologic information about nodules, because well-differentiated thyroid tissue can trap the pharmaceutical, whereas poorly differentiated tissue (malignant neoplasm) cannot; and, of course, cysts, scar, and hemorrhage contain no functioning tissue, differentiated or otherwise.

As cyclotrons have proliferated, the radionuclide I-123 has become more readily available. I-123 is trapped, organified, and then incorporated into thyroid hormone, providing more physiologic data on nodules than TcO_4^- does.

Both TcO_4^- and I-123 produce excellent images of the thyroid gland, and pharmaceutical uptake can be quantitated for an "uptake value" with either pharmaceutical.

After thyroid images are generated, the neck is usually reimaged as a nuclear physician places a marker on any palpable lesion to confirm that what is visualized indeed corresponds to what is clinically palpable. This maneuver is key, because in clinical practice it is common to find that a lesion that was allegedly intrathyroid is, in fact, not part of the thyroid gland at all; in that event, the workup moves in a different direction (mass in the neck), and the thyroid workup is over.

If the palpable lesion is indeed in the thyroid, the workup diverges according to the nuclear findings. By and large, truly functional (hot) nodules can safely be considered benign and do not require surgery, whereas nonfunctional or poorly functioning (cold or cool nodules) may be cysts or neoplasms and require a tissue diagnosis.

Solitary Cold or Cool Nodule

A solitary nonfunctioning nodule is ominous, especially if it is hard. Depending on the size of the lesion and the patient population, the likelihood of malignant neoplasm is between 15% and 40%. Benign cold nodules are cysts, scar, old hemorrhage/scar, nonfunctioning adenomas, or partly cystic and partly solid benign lesions such as degenerating adenomas. **With the exception of simple cysts, sonographic patterns cannot establish benignity with a high degree of confidence, and a histologic or cytologic diagnosis is mandatory. Therefore, we do not**

recommend sonography without biopsy as the next step, although sonographically guided biopsy can be definitive.

Multiple Cold and/or Cool Nodules

Multiple well-defined hypofunctioning nodules in an otherwise normal gland may also represent malignant neoplasm and should be pursued histologically, especially if the nodules are hard on palpation. Most of these lesions are benign adenomas or cysts superimposed on a finely multinodular adenomatous goiter, too subtle to detect by palpation or nuclear scanning.

Irregular Cold or Cool Area

A hard, irregular cold area or a hard, cold area distorting the gland is ominous and could indicate either malignant neoplasm, scar (secondary to previous inflammation, hemorrhage, or trauma), or atypical adenoma. Histologic diagnosis is required.

Solitary Hyperfunctioning Nodule

A solitary hot nodule is usually a hyperfunctioning benign adenoma, especially if it suppresses the remainder of the gland by producing enough thyroxine (T_4) to reduce thyroid-stimulating hormone (TSH) by feedback inhibition. Although the chance of malignancy in a single hyperfunctioning nodule is very, very low, a few cases have been reported when the pattern of "hyperfuction" is based on a TcO_4^- scan. Nonetheless, most endocrinologists prefer to follow such cases clinically and, if indicated, treat with radioiodine to ablate the nodule and repeat the thyroid scan only if the lesion enlarges. If the pattern of hyperfunction is based on an I-123 scan, the hyperfunction indicates both trapping and organification; the degree of differentiation required to **trap and organify iodine** is virtually certain to indicate benignity, and tissue diagnosis is generally not required.

Multiple Hot Nodules

Multiple, clearly hyperfunctioning nodules and faint or absent visualization of the remainder of the thyroid gland indicate Plummer's disease. In this condition several separate areas of the thyroid develop autonomy, producing sufficient thyroid hormone to suppress the remainder of the gland by reducing TSH (feedback inhibition). The hyperfunctioning lesions may or may not produce enough hormone to cause clinical hyperthyroidism. Autonomy of these nodules may be proved by re-imaging after a course of triiodothyronine (T_3 suppression test). Statistically, the chance of malignancy in one of several hyperfunctioning (hot) nodules is virtually nil, so further imaging is unnecessary, except to follow their regression after radioiodine therapy. Histologic diagnosis is not appropriate.

If a nodule "in the thyroid region" may or may not be intrathyroidal and the thyroid is not enlarged overall:

STEP 1: SONOGRAPHY

Sonography clearly defines the thyroid gland and establishes whether a palpable nodule is intra- or extrathyroidal. Not infrequently, the sonogram proves that a palpable "thyroid nodule" is, in fact, a prominent lobe of the normal thyroid gland, ending the workup.

Sonography can establish whether a nodule is solid, cystic, or "complex" (mixed solid and cystic). Although multiple nodules, simple cysts, and peripheral calcifications favor benignity, the pattern is generally nonspecific, **and malignancy usually cannot be excluded with a high degree of confidence.**

If the nodule is extrathyroidal, it is worked up like any other soft tissue mass in the neck. If a true intrathyroidal nodule is located, FNAB is appropriate, and the workup proceeds as described above.

(B) ENLARGED THYROID

STEP 1: NUCLEAR THYROID SCAN

Before any imaging, thyroid function tests are appropriate. Often, these are conclusive, obviating the need for any imaging. However, in ambiguous cases, a nuclear thyroid scan and uptake can be useful.

An intravenous injection of technetium 99m–pertechnetate (TcO_4^-) or I-123 is followed by images of the neck. The typical patterns observed when the gland is enlarged include the following:

Enlarged Homogeneous Hot Gland

A diffusely enlarged homogeneous gland with **increased** TcO_4^- or I-123 accumulation strongly suggests Graves' disease. Elevated serum hormone levels, low TSH levels, and a high radioiodine uptake are confirmatory. Graves' disease requires neither further imaging nor histology.

Rarely, however, this scan pattern may result from a metabolic defect in thyroid hormone synthesis after iodide is trapped (e.g., an organification or coupling defect). In these cases, serum thyroid hormone levels are low and the patient is euthyroid or hypothyroid; TSH is accordingly high, with subsequent enlargement of the gland (compensatory goiter) and intense radiopharmaceutical trapping. (The radioiodine uptake may be low or high, depending on the site of the metabolic defect: if iodine is properly organified, the uptake is high, but if organification is defective, the uptake is normal to low, because any trapped radioiodine soon leaves the thyroid.)

Synthesis defects may be idiopathic or may accompany Hashimoto's thyroiditis or recovering subacute thyroiditis. Further imaging usually is not required.

Enlarged Homogeneous Gland with Normal Radiopharmaceutical Uptake

A diffusely enlarged, homogeneous gland with **normal** radiopharmaceutical accumulation could represent early, developing Graves' disease (euthyroid Graves' disease), in which the gland is in a borderline state between normal function and autonomous hyperfunction and may later progress to flagrant hyperthyroidism. Radio-iodine uptake usually is "upper normal." Correlation with serum thyroid hormone levels is useful to confirm developing hyperthyroidism, but a test of thyroid autonomy, the TRH (thyrotropin-releasing hormone) level, is virtually diagnostic.

A diffusely large, homogeneous gland could also represent a stage of Hashimoto's disease, recovering sub-acute thyroiditis, a normal variant, or simply a very finely multinodular colloid goiter, in which the nodules are so small as to be unpalpable and beyond the resolution threshold of the nuclear camera. None of these conditions warrants histologic diagnosis.

Large Faint Gland

A large, tender gland with poor radiopharmaceutical uptake, barely visualized on the scan, is characteristic of subacute thyroiditis. Usually serum thyroid hormone levels are high, whereas radioiodine uptake is low (or virtually absent). Further imaging or histology is unnecessary.

Enlarged Inhomogeneous Gland

An enlarged, inhomogeneous gland with multiple patchy, poorly defined areas of increased and decreased function is frequently termed a "multinodular goiter." "Multinodular goiter" literally means "an enlarged gland with many nodules," and, strictly speaking, it is a descriptive rather than a diagnostic term. In common medical usage, however, "multinodular goiter" has become synonymous with "multinodular colloid adenomatous goiter," a patho-logic entity in which the thyroid gland is partly replaced by cysts, poorly functioning normal tissue resembling adenomas, fibrosis-compressed normal tissue, and, possibly, calcification or hemorrhage. The condition is frequently familial and typical on palpation (rubbery and nodular), with a characteristic imaging appearance: an enlarged, inhomogeneous gland with areas of hypofunction interspersed between areas of normal function. The poorly functioning (cold) areas in multinodular colloid adenomatous goiter have traditionally been considered to have a very, very low incidence of malignancy, but recent evidence suggests that as many as 15% to 20% may become malignant. **Therefore, histologic diagnosis of a cold lesion that is hard, growing, or dominant is prudent in a multinodular gland. Serial FNAB-guided follow-up biopsies, sometimes US-guided, may be required.**

A condition that may mimic multinodular colloid adenomatous goiter on imaging is chronic (Hashimoto's) thyroiditis, which merits no further imaging.

SUMMARY AND CONCLUSIONS

1. **When a palpable nodule is almost certainly in the thyroid, FNAB should precede all imaging.** The cytopathologic results of FNAB can direct patients to surgery or nonsurgical follow-up.
2. When FNAB yields nondiagnostic material, US-guided FNAB is usually successful.
3. US can precede FNAB **when it is important to determine whether a lesion is actually in the thyroid.**
4. Where FNAB and expert cytopathology are unavailable or when repeat guided FNAB is nondiagnostic, radionuclide scanning of a nodule can be helpful.
5. Functioning or hyperfunctioning nodules (hot or warm) on I-123 scans are **virtually certain** to be benign, because they both trap and organify radio-

pharmaceutical. They are **very likely** benign on TcO_4^- scans.

6. In the hyperthyroid patient with one or more nodules, a thyroid scan after basic thyroid function tests is usually more valuable than FNAB, because the thyroid often contains one or more hot nodules that do not require biopsy and because the scan pattern is a helpful guide to proper therapy.

7. Radionuclide scanning is the procedure of choice for workup of an enlarged thyroid, but guided FNAB is sometimes required to follow cold or cool nodules.

ADDITIONAL COMMENTS

- The population exposed to childhood head and neck radiation is at a higher risk for thyroid malignancy than is the general population. US can effectively screen this population for subtle, nonpalpable lesions. These radiation-induced malignancies sometimes present as multiple cold nodules. **Therefore, ANY cold nodule, or multiple cold nodules, in a previously radiated patient always requires a tissue diagnosis.**

- Occasionally, two thyroid diseases can coexist (e.g., Graves' disease superimposed upon a preexistent colloid adenomatous goiter). In these cases FNAB can exclude malignancy, but a radionuclide thyroid scan may also be necessary to arrive at an endocrinologic diagnosis.

- Incidentally discovered nonpalpable thyroid nodules are common findings on computed tomography (CT) of the neck or chest or on US of the neck for carotid disease or hyperparathyroidism. Incidentally discovered small (<1.5-cm) nodules without suspicious features should be followed, because the vast majority are benign. Growth, of course, mandates a tissue diagnosis.

SUGGESTED READING

Belfiore A, La Rosa GL, La Porta GA, et al: Cancer risk in patients with cold thyroid nodules: relevance of iodine intake, sex, age, and multinodularity. Am J Med 1992;93:363–369.

Katz JF, Kane RA, Reyes J, et al: Thyroid nodules: sonographic-pathologic correlation. Radiology 1984;151:741–745.

Rausch, P, Nowels K, Jeffrey, RB Jr: Ultrasonographically guided thyroid biopsy: a review with emphasis on technique. J Ultrasound Med 2001;20:79–85.

Topliss D: Thyroid incidentaloma: the ignorant in pursuit of the impalpable. Clin Endocrinol (Oxf) 2004;60:18–20.

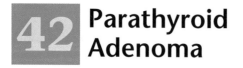

42 Parathyroid Adenoma

INTRODUCTION

Clinical and laboratory findings almost always raise the suspicion of parathyroid adenoma; usually there is no palpable mass in the neck. For generations surgeons were content to explore the neck without any imaging guidance, and their success rate was high—often reported in the classic literature as 90% to 95%. However, current practice favors imaging first, which raises the operative localization rate to greater than 95%. Because computed tomography (CT), magnetic resonance (MR) imaging, ultrasound (US), and technetium 99m (Tc-99m)–sestamibi (MIBI) with single-photon emission computed tomography (SPECT) are all readily available, the choice is not a priori clear. Fortunately, comparative studies have established a clear "winner": **MIBI.**

Relative Costs: MIBI with SPECT, **$$$–$$$$**; US of the neck, **$$**; MR of the neck, enhanced and unenhanced, **$$$$**.

PLAN AND RATIONALE

STEP 1: TECHNETIUM 99M–SESTAMIBI (MIBI)

MIBI is the acronym for **m**ethoxy**i**so**b**utyl-**is**onitrile, a nuclear medicine technique. Originally developed for myocardial perfusion imaging, this compound, when labeled with technetium 99m (Tc-99m), concentrates in certain well-perfused noncardiac tissues, including some neoplasms, **particularly parathyroid adenomas.**

The thyroid gland itself also accumulates MIBI, but the pharmacodynamics of MIBI differ in thyroid and parathyroid tissue; early (almost immediate) nuclear images of the thoracic inlet reveal uptake **in the thyroid gland and parathyroid adenomas, whereas images 1 hour later reveal only parathyroid adenomas.**

If MIBI results are positive, most surgeons operate without further imaging, and the workup ends.

If MIBI results are negative, US is the appropriate follow-up.

STEP 2: ULTRASOUND (US)

Despite its high sensitivity, MIBI can be falsely negative for very small nodules (<1 cm) and for nodules that are necrotic and/or associated with low metabolic activity. US can sometimes localize these, but US techniques for such lesions are highly operator dependent; therefore, US cannot be recommended unless an experienced operator is involved. **The clinician should be aware that any reluctance to undertake the search with US is an indirect indication that the sonographer is inexperienced, and in that case US will be of little value and should be skipped.**

A positive US result ends the workup.

A negative ultrasound result, even in experienced hands, does not **absolutely** exclude a parathyroid adenoma, but in the face of a normal MIBI and a normal US, most surgeons proceed directly to exploration. However, if the surgeon is reluctant to operate without imaging evidence, then MR is appropriate.

STEP 3: MAGNETIC RESONANCE (MR) IMAGING

MR has a lower sensitivity and specificity than MIBI and US for parathyroid lesions and should NOT be a first- or even a second-line examination.

Nonetheless, MR can be positive in the event of negative findings on MIBI and US, especially if the US operator is inexperienced in this highly specialized type of examination or if the parathyroid adenoma is in an atypical location (such as the mediastinum).

Whether the findings are positive or negative, MR ends the workup.

SUMMARY AND CONCLUSIONS

1. MIBI is the procedure of choice for detecting parathyroid adenomas.
2. Many surgeons operate on the basis of a MIBI scan alone, in the proper clinical context.
3. A negative MIBI study in the face of strong clinical evidence should be followed by US rather than MR, assuming the US operator is experienced in this type of examination.
4. Rarely, MR can define a parathyroid lesion in the presence of negative findings on MIBI and US, especially if the US is suboptimal.

ADDITIONAL COMMENTS

- Despite its excellence in many clinical settings, CT is NOT appropriate to this clinical problem, and the combination of MIBI and CT is weaker than MIBI and US. This point bears emphasis, because on many clinical services the knee-jerk response to any issue is "get a CT." Furthermore, in the presence of failed MIBI/US, MR is a better third option than CT.
- MIBI has also successfully defined parathyroid carcinomas and hyperplasia, in addition to adenomas.

SUGGESTED READING

De Feo ML, Colagrande S, Biagini C, et al: Parathyroid glands: combination of 99mTc MIBI scintigraphy and US for demonstration of parathyroid glands and nodules. Radiology 2000;214:393–402.
Nguyen BD: Parathyroid imaging with Tc-99m sestamibi planar and SPECT scintigraphy. Radiographics 1999;19:601–614.

Part V

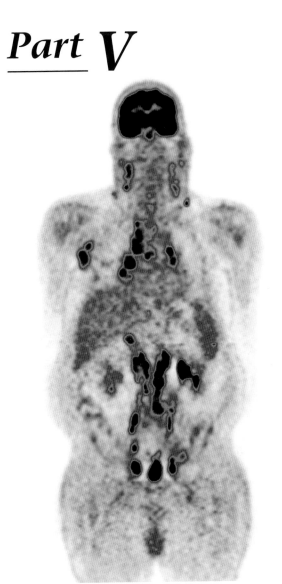

Musculoskeletal

43 Osteomyelitis

INTRODUCTION

Plain radiographs, conventional nuclear scans, fluorodeoxyglucose–positron emission tomography (FDG-PET), computed tomography (CT), PET/CT, ultrasound (US), and magnetic resonance (MR) imaging can all address four issues regarding bone inflammation: (1) Is acute osteomyelitis present in previously normal bone? (2) Is there new osteomyelitis superimposed upon preexistent bone disease? (3) Is there an associated soft tissue pus collection or subcutaneous sinus tract? (4) Can an etiology like a foreign body be defined?

Relative Costs: Plain bone films, **$**; conventional bone scan, without SPECT, **$$$**; three-phase bone scan, **$$$**; cervical MR, **$$$$**; thoracic MR, **$$$$**; lumbosacral MR, **$$$$**; upper extremity MR, **$$$$**; lower extremity MR, **$$$$**; nuclear WBC scan, with In-111-oxine or Tc-99m-HMPAO, **$$$$–$$$$$$**, depending on the number of days required for complete imaging; Ga-67 scan, with SPECT, **$$$**; FDG-PET, **$$$$$**.

PLAN AND RATIONALE

(A) When Acute Osteomyelitis Is Suspected in Previously Normal Bone

Step 1: Plain Radiography (Plain Films)

In the presence of osteomyelitis, typical radiographic signs appear in about 1 week. Earlier, plain films are usually normal or nonspecific, and further imaging is needed. However, plain films should not be skipped during the first week, because they can exclude other causes of symptoms, such as fracture, tumor, or radiopaque soft tissue foreign body, **and sometimes they can be diagnostic of osteomyelitis during the first week, especially if the infection is aggressive.**

In the appropriate clinical context, plain films can be specific for osteomyelitis and end the workup, but all too often, despite worrisome signs and symptoms, the findings are normal.

When findings on initial plain films are normal:

STEP 2: CONVENTIONAL NUCLEAR BONE SCAN

The typical nuclear bone scan for osteomyelitis is a "three-phase" study, involving a peripheral intravenous bolus injection of technetium 99m (Tc-99m)–labeled methylene diphosphonate (MDP), rapid-sequence "flow" images of the area of interest, immediate "static" or "blood pool" images, and images of the entire skeleton after 1 to 2 hours. The bone scan in osteomyelitis usually becomes abnormal by 24 hours, **much earlier than plain films.**

MDP accumulates in the crystalline structure of bone, according to local bone blood flow, and areas of osteomyelitis almost always appear "hot." In the patient **without preexisting bone disease** (i.e., normal result on plain radiographs), a focal abnormality at the symptomatic site on a three-phase bone scan is quite specific. Thus, **a positive scan is diagnostic of osteomyelitis in the proper clinical context** (e.g., in the presence of fever, leukocytosis, and local pain). However, an abnormal bone scan in the presence of concomitant bone lesions—including old or recent trauma, primary or metastatic bone tumor, arthritis, metabolic bone disease, and Paget's disease—is nonspecific; further imaging is usually needed.

In patients older than 3 years of age, **a normal scan almost always excludes osteomyelitis and ends the workup;** rarely, if the patient has been scanned within a few hours of onset, the scan may be falsely negative, because the infected bone has had insufficient time to react; a follow-up scan in 24 hours is usually conclusive. Moreover, in patients younger than 3 years of age, the bone scan is less sensitive, and in children younger than 3 months, it is often falsely negative.

When the scan is negative in young children or nonspecific or equivocal in older children and adults, additional imaging may help, and the choice of test **depends upon the suspected site.**

When the initial bone scan is negative in young children or nonspecific or equivocal in older children or adults and osteomyelitis of the spine is suspected:

Step 3: Magnetic Resonance (MR) Imaging

MR produces "sectional" images that can be displayed in any plane; it excels in early detection of **bone marrow edema,** an early change in osteomyelitis. For this condition it is as sensitive and specific as the bone scan, especially in the spine, which has abundant red marrow. (Some investigators even suggest that a faster generation of MR scanners could eventually replace conventional bone scanning as a screen.)

Bony and soft tissue involvement, including sinus tracts and soft tissue abscesses, are clearly defined, **and MR reveals the relationship of an infectious**

process to the subarachnoid space, the spinal cord, and nerve roots.

The specificity of MR decreases in patients with pre-existing bone disease (i.e., fracture, surgery, or neoplasm).

When the initial bone scan is negative in young children or nonspecific or equivocal in older children and adults and extraspinal osteomyelitis is suspected:

STEP 3: WHITE BLOOD CELL (WBC) SCAN (LABELED AUTOLOGOUS LEUKOCYTES) OR GALLIUM-67 (GA-67) CITRATE SCAN

A WBC scan involves harvesting leukocytes from a small sample of the patient's blood, labeling them with indium-111-oxine (In-111-oxine) or technetium 99m–hexamethylpropyleneamine oxime (Tc-99m-HMPAO), and injecting them intravenously. The labeled cells accumulate in sites of purulent infection, especially in the appendicular skeleton. The study is highly specific for osteomyelitis and when positive ends the imaging workup. **Tc-99m-HMPAO is often preferred to In-111-oxine,** because it produces images of much higher quality. Furthermore, the skeleton is imaged only 3 hours after Tc-99m-HMPAO injection, whereas an 18- to 24-hour interval between injection and imaging is required for In-111-oxine. In the setting of suspected osteomyelitis, an 18- to 24-hour delay is undesirable.

Gallium-67 accumulates in various inflammatory (and sometimes neoplastic) foci 2 to 3 days after intravenous injection. The mechanism of gallium accumulation has not been established but probably relates to its affinity for lactoferrin released by polymorphonuclear neutrophilic leukocytes. Gallium is less sensitive and specific for osteomyelitis than WBC scanning is; however, gallium is a reasonable alternative when a WBC study is unavailable.

(B) WHEN ACUTE OSTEOMYELITIS IS SUSPECTED IN THE CONTEXT OF PREEXISTENT BONE DISEASE (TRAUMATIC, POSTSURGICAL, NEOPLASTIC, OR POSTINFLAMMATORY)

STEP 1: PLAIN RADIOGRAPHY (PLAIN FILMS)

Even in the presence of preexistent bone disease, plain films are appropriate, because they often reveal changes that indicate new infection. (Obviously, old films for comparison are critical to this effort.) However, if plain films are not diagnostic, a WBC scan may be helpful.

STEP 2: WHITE BLOOD CELL (WBC) SCAN (LABELED AUTOLOGOUS LEUKOCYTES) OR GALLIUM-67 (GA-67) CITRATE SCAN (see Step 3, above, for technique)

In the presence of preexisting bone abnormalities—surgical, traumatic, or neoplastic—**the conventional Tc-99m-MDP bone scan findings are virtually always abnormal but, unfortunately, nonspecific.** (The "three-phase" bone scan was designed to prevent this problem, because the "flow" portion of the study reflects perfusion; lesions that hyperperfuse are theoretically inflammatory, rather than traumatic, postsurgical, or neoplastic, but all too often the distinction between infectious and noninfectious lesions blurs.) Thus, **many nuclear imagers prefer to skip the bone scan when there is significant preexisting bone disease and proceed directly to WBC or gallium scans** (see above, under **When the initial bone scan is negative in young children or nonspecific or equivocal in older children and adults and extraspinal osteomyelitis is suspected**).

A normal WBC or gallium scan in an area of radiographically abnormal bone excludes osteomyelitis with high degree of probability, especially in the appendicular skeleton. However, WBC or gallium accumulation, unless intense, may be nonspecific. **In such cases, it may be necessary to compare the WBC or gallium scan to a conventional bone scan to determine for sure whether the abnormal accumulation is in bone or soft tissue.**

STEP 3: BONE SCAN

(See above, under **When findings on initial plain films are normal**.) The side-by-side comparison of plain films, a WBC or gallium study, and a bone scan is usually sufficient. **In very unusual cases, both WBC and gallium studies are appropriate to clarify equivocal situations. In practical terms, however, if conventional radiographs, a WBC scan, and a bone scan cannot solidify the diagnosis, many clinicians proceed directly to bone biopsy. Depending on the anatomic site, CT, US, or MR may be required.**

STEP 4: COMPUTED TOMOGRAPHY (CT), ULTRASOUND (US), OR MAGNETIC RESONANCE (MR) IMAGING

CT and US can accurately define sequestra, soft tissue abscesses, and bone destruction before surgery. In some centers the biopsy itself is performed under CT guidance. MR is superior to CT in depicting the extent of bone marrow and soft tissue involvement, including sinus tracts and soft tissue abscesses, but it is intrinsically less well suited to biopsy guidance. US provides real-time evaluation of soft tissue pus collection/abscess drainage. Also, US is a highly specific examination for the investigation of subcutaneous foreign bodies, unless they are too deep for the ultrasound beam to effectively visualize. Each case should be discussed with the musculoskeletal or interventional radiologist before biopsy.

SUMMARY AND CONCLUSIONS

1. Plain films are the first examination in the investigation of osteomyelitis; although 7 days usually pass before signs become manifest, the plain films exclude many other causes of symptoms and reveal any preexisting bone disease.

2. A Tc-99m-MDP bone scan is the most appropriate next examination when there is no preexisting bone disease.

3. A normal bone scan in patients older than 3 years of age usually ends the osteomyelitis workup. In patients younger than 3 years of age, or when new disease may be superimposed on old disease, further imaging may be required.

4. In the presence of preexisting bone disease, many imagers proceed directly from the plain films to a WBC study or MR. This sequence is also often justified when the initial bone scan is normal in a patient **younger than 3 years of age.**

5. For suspected **osteomyelitis of the spine, MR is highly effective. Elsewhere, radiolabeled WBCs are preferred to clarify an abnormal but nonspecific bone scan, in acute or chronic osteomyelitis,** or to reveal osteomyelitis in very young patients with falsely negative bone scans. Tc-99m-HMPAO–labeled cells produce superior images that are generated within 3 hours of intravenous cell injection.

6. Ga-67 citrate is a viable alternative if WBC scanning is not available. Uncommonly both studies are required.

7. When the exact extent of bony or soft tissue involvement must be known, MR, CT, or US apply. **MR is superior for soft tissue definition but is less suited to biopsy guidance. US is very effective in diagnosing associated soft tissue pus collections or finding adjacent foreign bodies, but it is limited by its inability to penetrate deep structures with adequate**

resolution. CT defines bone disease quite well but is inferior to MR for soft tissue definition; however, CT biopsy guidance is highly effective.

ADDITIONAL COMMENTS

- AT THE PRESENT TIME, FDG-PET IS NOT APPROVED BY THE U.S. FOOD AND DRUG ADMINISTRATION OR MEDICARE FOR THE STUDY OF OSTEOMYELITIS, BUT SEVERAL RECENT STUDIES HAVE DEMONSTRATED EXCELLENT SENSITIVITY OF FDG-PET IN OSTEOMYELITIS. SPECIFICITY OF FDG-PET IS LIMITED, HOWEVER, BECAUSE OF OVERLYING SOFT TISSUE, BUT WHEN IT IS COMBINED WITH CT IN A SINGLE EXAM (PET/CT), DIFFERENTIATING INFECTION IN BONE FROM INFECTION IN SURROUNDING SOFT TISSUE IS NOT DIFFICULT (see CHAPTER 61, PET and PET/CT in Cancer Staging).
- In the authors' judgment, COMBINED PET/CT will eventually dominate the diagnostic algorithm for many cases of suspected osteomyelitis, but at the present time we hesitate to recommend a $2200 test that must be billed directly to the patient or absorbed by a healthcare provider; notwithstanding these financial concerns, the fact is that in difficult cases (e.g., the diabetic patient with soft tissue edema but without confounding additional lesions such as fractures or metastases), FDG-PET/CT is very likely the most sensitive and specific examination for osteomyelitis of an extremity.
- MR is excellent for the detection of marrow edema in the long bones as well as in the spine. If MR were faster and less costly, the study could compete effectively with total body bone scanning.

SUGGESTED READING

Keidar Z, Militianu D, Melamed E, et al: The diabetic foot: initial experience with Fl-18-FDG PET/CT. J Nucl Med 2005;46:444–449.

Kipper SL, Rypins EB, Evans DG, et al: Neutrophil-specific ^{99m}Tc-labeled anti-CD14 monoclonal antibody imaging for diagnosis of equivocal appendicitis. J Nucl Med 2000;41:449–455.

Palestro CJ, Caprioli R, Love C, et al: Rapid diagnosis of pedal osteomyelitis in diabetics with a technetium-99m-labeled monoclonal antigranulocyte antibody. J Foot Ankle Surg 2003;42:2–8.

Palestro CJ, Kipper SL, Weiland FL, et al: Osteomyelitis: diagnosis with ^{99m}Tc-labeled antigranulocyte antibodies compared with diagnosis with ^{111}In-labeled leukocytes—initial experience. Radiology 2002;223:758–764.

Rypins EB, Klipper SL: Scintigraphic determination of equivocal appendicitis. Am Surg 2000;66:891–895.

44 Skeletal Metastases

INTRODUCTION

Four imaging techniques are frequently involved in the search for bone metastases: (1) conventional radiography, which largely reflects alterations in skeletal structure; (2) conventional nuclear bone scanning, which largely reflects alterations in bone perfusion; (3) magnetic resonance (MR) imaging, which reveals replacement of bone marrow by tumor and to a lesser extent by destruction of skeletal structure; and (4) fluorodeoxyglucose–positron emission tomography (FDG-PET), which reflects uptake of radiolabeled glucose and, thus, metabolic rate of the bone marrow.

The goal of imaging is to demonstrate metastatic lesions as early as possible or to exclude them with a high degree of confidence. Both the clinician and the imager should recall that **skeletal metastases are not necessarily painful or symptomatic.**

Patients **without** known skeletal metastases are usually studied to stage their disease, because the disease stage determines resectability in potential surgical candidates and may influence medical and/or radiation therapy in nonsurgical cancers. Patients **with** known skeletal metastases are studied to explain new or changed symptoms and to monitor therapeutic efficacy.

When patients with a known cancer are staged, both FDG-PET and a bone scan are usually considered in the staging process; **for tumors that are Medicare approved for FDG-PET, we recommend that FDG-PET be performed first, because FDG-PET is a multiorgan, multisystem examination (see CHAPTER 61, PET and PET/CT in Cancer Staging), whereas conventional bone scanning is limited,** virtually always, to providing data only on the skeleton. Thus, FDG-PET is much more likely to provide definitive staging information that directs therapy.

Notwithstanding the above, in clinical practice most bone scans are ordered on patients who have already been staged and are on therapy but require follow-up or are being followed after therapy, or on those who have known metastases but develop new bone pain. With the exception of lymphoma, for which FDG-PET is virtually always superior, these circumstances are best approached by standard radionuclide bone scanning.

Relative Costs: Plain bone films, variable cost according to area radiographed, **$**; total body nuclear bone scan, without SPECT, **$$**; total body bone scan, with SPECT of one region, **$$**; MR, enhanced, variable cost according to area studied, **$$$**; bone biopsy, CT-guided, "superficial lesion," **$$$$**; bone biopsy, CT-guided, "deep lesion," **$$$**; FDG-PET, **$$$$$**.

PLAN AND RATIONALE

When no skeletal metastases are known, and the patient is not scheduled for FDG-PET as part of initial cancer staging:

STEP 1: CONVENTIONAL RADIONUCLIDE BONE SCAN, POSSIBLY WITH SINGLE-PHOTON EMISSION COMPUTED TOMOGRAPHY (SPECT)

Bone scanning involves peripheral intravenous injection of technetium 99m–methylene diphosphonate (Tc-99m-MDP). One to two hours later, the skeleton is scanned from head to foot. Most of the radiopharmaceutical accumulates in the crystalline structure of bone proportional to local bone blood flow. Skeletal metastases usually accumulate more radioactivity than adjacent normal bone and appear "hot." However, most other bone lesions—including old or recent trauma, primary benign or malignant neoplasm, acute or chronic osteomyelitis, inflammatory or degenerative arthritis, metabolic bone disease, and Paget's disease—also appear "hot." Thus **an abnormal bone scan is nonspecific.**

In most malignancies, the bone scan is more sensitive than plain radiographs; neither is foolproof. Overall, about 30% of metastases detected by bone scans are missed by bone radiographs; conversely, 2% of metastases detected by radiographs are missed by scans. The sensitivity of bone scanning is somewhat enhanced by SPECT, a technological enhancement of the conventional nuclear scan that uses the same pharmaceutical but produces higher-resolution "slice" images. SPECT is especially useful in the study of lesions of the bony spine.

If the bone scan is abnormal, revealing a "hot" lesion (or lesions), typical of metastases, the workup ends.

If the bone scan is abnormal, and findings are (1) atypical for metastatic disease; (2) consistent with a variety of conditions (such as metastatic disease, benign degenerative change, or trauma); or (3) inconsistent with clinical status, follow-up radiographs (plain films) are required for clarification.

If the bone scan is normal and there is no bone pain, skeletal metastases are unlikely, and the workup ends.

If the bone scan is normal yet there is bone pain, further imaging is appropriate, because no test is perfect and even a good-quality bone scan can be falsely negative. MR is then appropriate.

STEP 2: SKELETAL RADIOGRAPHY OR X-RAYS (PLAIN FILMS)

If radiographs reveal benign lesions like degenerative or rheumatoid arthritis that explain the bone scan findings, the imaging workup ends.

If benign lesions that do not necessarily account for the bone scan findings are defined, leaving the issue of bone metastases unresolved, the patient can be rescanned in 6 to 8 weeks to look for lesion growth (which would support a malignant etiology), proceed to biopsy, or undergo MR.

STEP 2 OR 3: MAGNETIC RESONANCE (MR) IMAGING

MR beautifully demonstrates bone marrow and can usually differentiate normal marrow from tumor. Because most metastatic disease to bone begins in the marrow space at least as early as it destroys the crystalline structure, MR is often helpful in confirming or excluding metastatic disease.

(MR is particularly effective in back pain, because it demonstrates the spinal cord itself, nerve roots, and subarachnoid space; the status of these vital structures and spaces is determined along with the presence or absence of marrow replacement.)

If MR reveals metastatic disease, the workup ends.

If MR is normal or reveals a non-bony cause of pain, the workup usually ends, but in occasional cases the cause of a bone scan abnormality remains unresolved, even after radiographs and MR. In this event, biopsy (see below) is the sole remaining option.

STEP 4: BONE BIOPSY

Percutaneous biopsy under computed tomography (CT) guidance (see **CHAPTER 60, Percutaneous Guided Biopsy and Imaging-Guided Therapy**) with a large-bore biopsy needle is often feasible.

When no skeletal metastases are known and the patient is scheduled for FDG-PET as part of initial cancer staging:

STEP 1: FLUORODEOXYGLUCOSE–POSITRON EMISSION TOMOGRAPHY (FDG-PET)

FDG-PET has become a cornerstone in the staging of many cancers, including non–small cell lung, colorectal, melanoma, breast, esophageal, head-neck, and lymphoma. Applications to Medicare for many others, including ovarian, hepatoma, follicular thyroid carcinoma, multiple myeloma, and high-grade prostate, are pending. Because the PET camera "looks at" the body from the mid head to the mid thighs, it is inevitable that the scan includes much of the skeleton; therefore, the impact of PET on the workup for skeletal metastases is growing by leaps and bounds. Nonetheless, the implications of skeletal findings on PET are not widely understood among clinicians and diagnostic radiologists alike.

PET is an outgrowth of nuclear medicine. PET cameras detect the gamma rays produced when a positron encounters an electron. Both the cameras that can "see" these gamma rays and fluorine 18 (Fl-18), the most common radionuclide used for PET imaging, have become readily available only within the past 3 to 5 years. Fl-18 can substitute for an –OH radical in the glucose molecule, forming FDG, which mimics the biodistribution of glucose—to a point; it is taken up and trapped by cells but not metabolized. The degree to which a tissue uses glucose determines its FDG uptake; thus, cancers (and other major metabolic organs: the brain and heart) are clearly identified by FDG-PET.

Originally, the focus of FDG-PET was on soft tissue tumors. Bone lesions were a secondary consideration, especially given the fact that multiple other technologies—particularly the conventional bone scan—were adept at defining them. However, as experience with FDG-PET has burgeoned, scan after scan has defined focally increased FDG in bone, and the clinician is often left with a diagnostic conundrum: does intense, focal, skeletal uptake on FDG-PET indicate skeletal metastases, and which test, if any, is appropriate for confirmation?

Experience has now established that focal, intense skeletal FDG uptake is strong evidence for skeletal metastatic disease that is equivalent to—if not better than—a conventional Tc-99m bone scan. Therefore, when the FDG-PET study is strongly positive in focal areas that are not suspicious for other hypermetabolic states (such as osteomyelitis or rheumatoid arthritis), the workup for skeletal metastases ends.

If FDG-PET reveals lesions in the skeleton whose pattern is probably, but not certainly, degenerative change:

STEP 2: SKELETAL RADIOGRAPHY OR X-RAYS (PLAIN FILMS), FOR CONFIRMATION OF DEGENERATIVE CHANGE

Plain films of the skeleton are a hundred-year-old technique that remains useful to this day, because plain films produce excellent visualization of joints and establish easily the presence or absence of "degenerative change"—that is, joint-space narrowing (from loss of cartilage), subchondral sclerosis, and degenerative spur formation. Thus, a suspicious area of increased FDG accumulation that could represent degenerative change (especially near a joint or in the bony spine) can usually be clarified by plain films.

If extensive degenerative change is documented at a site of FDG uptake, the FDG uptake is attributed to this degenerative change and metastatic disease need not be postulated. The workup ends.

If **no** degenerative change is documented, **metastatic disease is a very worrisome possibility.** Although an increasing number of nuclear imagers currently believe that the workup should end if no degenerative change is seen, majority opinion at the time of this writing is that further confirmation is appropriate **because the presence or absence of skeletal metastatic disease is critical for cancer staging.** Opinion is currently divided between a conventional Tc-99m bone scan and MR imaging for follow-up clarification. Overall, the majority favors a Tc-99m bone scan, **but in our experience a better study is usually MR imaging.**

STEP 3: CONVENTIONAL BONE SCAN OR MAGNETIC RESONANCE (MR) IMAGING

Conventional Bone Scan (The Most Common Next Choice)
Bone scanning involves peripheral intravenous injection of Tc-99m-MDP. One to two hours later, the skeleton is scanned from head to foot. Most of the radio-pharmaceutical accumulates in the crystalline structure of bone proportional to local bone blood flow. Skeletal metastases usually accumulate more radioactivity than adjacent normal bone and appear "hot." However, most other bone lesions—including old or recent trauma, primary benign or malignant neoplasm, acute or chronic osteomyelitis, inflammatory or degenerative arthritis, metabolic bone disease, and Paget's disease—also appear "hot." Thus, **an abnormal bone scan is nonspecific.**

In most malignancies, the bone scan is more sensitive than plain radiographs; neither is foolproof. Overall, about 30% of metastases detected by bone scans are missed by bone radiographs; conversely, 2% of metastases detected by radiographs are missed by scans. The sensitivity of bone scanning is somewhat enhanced by SPECT, a technological enhancement of the conventional bone scan that uses the same pharmaceutical but produces higher-resolution "slice" images. SPECT is especially useful in the study of lesions of the bony spine.

If the bone scan confirms abnormal Tc-99m-MDP uptake in the area of enhanced FDG accumulation, metastases are assumed to exist, and the workup ends.

If the bone scan reveals no abnormal Tc-99m-MDP uptake in the area of enhanced FDG accumulation and if no worrisome lesions elsewhere are defined, many nuclear imagers would stop the workup, but evidence is increasing that FDG-PET is frequently more sensitive than a Tc-99m scan for some skeletal lesions, particularly in the bony spine; because MR excels in this area, we proceed to MR as a "tie breaker"; in fact, for most other suspicious areas on FDG-PET, we proceed directly to MR for clarification, bypassing the conventional bone scan.

Magnetic Resonance (MR) Imaging (Our Preferred Choice, Especially for the Bony Spine)
Normal bone marrow is beautifully demonstrated by MR and usually can be differentiated from tumor. Because most metastatic disease of bone begins in the marrow space at least as early as it destroys the crystalline structure, MR is often helpful in confirming or excluding metastatic disease.

(MR is particularly effective in back pain, because it demonstrates the spinal cord itself, nerve roots, and subarachnoid space; the status of these vital structures and spaces is determined along with the presence or absence of marrow replacement.)

Normal or abnormal, MR ends the workup.

When FDG-PET defines lesions in the skeleton that may represent metastases and are not suspicious for degenerative change, plain films can be skipped and the workup proceeds to the conventional bone scan or MR (see above).

When skeletal metastases are known:

STEP 1: SKELETAL RADIOGRAPHY (PLAIN FILMS)

When one or more bone metastases are already known, by means of previous imaging studies, confirmation of additional lesions in areas of new, worsening, or recurrent pain is sought most expeditiously with radiographs, because these are less expensive and simpler than a bone scan (unless the new suspected areas are so widespread that a scan would be simpler). **Positive, confirmatory radiographs need not be followed by a bone scan, because a search for additional asymptomatic lesions in a patient already known to have bone metastases often serves no purpose, unless an overall assessment of the skeletal status is important for determining the choice/efficacy of chemotherapy. However, negative radiographs in the face of persistent pain are followed by a scan.**

STEP 2: CONVENTIONAL RADIONUCLIDE BONE SCAN

Bone scanning involves peripheral intravenous injection of Tc-99m-MDP. One to two hours later, the skeleton is scanned from head to foot. Most of the radiopharmaceutical accumulates in the crystalline structure of bone proportional to local bone blood flow. Skeletal metastases usually accumulate more radioactivity than adjacent normal bone and appear "hot." However, most other bone lesions—including old or recent trauma, primary benign or malignant neoplasm, acute or chronic osteomyelitis, inflammatory or degenerative arthritis, metabolic bone disease, and Paget's disease—also appear "hot." Thus, **an abnormal bone scan is nonspecific.**

In most malignancies, the bone scan is more sensitive than plain radiographs; neither is foolproof. Overall, about 30% of metastases detected by bone scans are missed by bone radiographs; conversely, 2% of metastases detected by radiographs are missed by scans. The sensitivity of bone scanning is somewhat enhanced by SPECT, a technological enhancement of the conventional bone scan that uses the same pharmaceutical but produces higher-resolution "slice" images. SPECT is especially useful in the study of lesions of the bony spine.

If both radiographs and a bone scan are negative, a follow-up scan in 6 to 8 weeks is often helpful. When it is crucial to establish the presence or absence of a lesion in a symptomatic site **and both the scan and radiographs are normal,** the remaining options are MR and biopsy.

STEP 3: MAGNETIC RESONANCE (MR) IMAGING

MR beautifully demonstrates bone marrow and can usually differentiate normal marrow from tumor. Because most metastatic disease to bone begins in the marrow space at least as early as it destroys the crystalline structure, MR is often helpful in confirming or excluding metastatic disease.

(MR is particularly effective in back pain, because it demonstrates the spinal cord itself, nerve roots, and subarachnoid space; the status of these vital structures and spaces is determined along with the presence or absence of marrow replacement.)

If MR reveals metastatic disease, the workup ends.

If MR is normal or reveals a non-bony cause of pain, the workup usually ends, but in occasional cases the cause of a bone scan abnormality remains unresolved, even after radiographs and MR. In this event, biopsy is the sole remaining option.

STEP 4: BONE BIOPSY

Percutaneous biopsy under CT guidance (see **CHAPTER 60, Percutaneous Guided Biopsy and Imaging-Guided Therapy**) with a large-bore biopsy needle is often feasible.

SUMMARY AND CONCLUSIONS

1. When FDG-PET is **not** scheduled and no metastases are known, a conventional nuclear bone scan is the best screen for metastases in the asymptomatic skeleton; it is more sensitive than radiographs, and it images the entire body.

2. FDG-PET has changed the paradigm for seeking metastatic disease in the skeleton, when the scan is scheduled as part of the cancer staging process. Many PET studies reveal skeletal lesions that are clearly metastatic. Plain films for clarification may be necessary when degenerative change is a consideration, and if the FDG-PET study is equivocal, most imagers select a conventional bone scan for confirmation. We have found that MR is more often a better study, especially in the bony spine.

3. Normal or abnormal bone scans that are consistent with the patient's clinical status end the metastatic skeletal workup, unless the patient was referred for a bone scan because of a suspicious FDG-PET. In that event, a normal bone scan may be followed by MR, especially if the site is symptomatic, particularly in the bony spine.

4. **A symptomatic site** that is normal on a conventional bone scan and radiograph can be rescanned in 6 to 8 weeks; metastatic lesions may progress during that interval, declaring themselves on the second scan. Alternatively, MR is often definitive.

5. MR frequently defines marrow infiltration by tumor and often reveals soft tissue lesions causing apparent bone pain. MR is particularly effective for the spine and often avoids the need for biopsy.

6. **When metastases are known,** a new, painful site is probably best studied first by radiographs, because these are simpler and less expensive than a bone scan. Many times, however, the radiographs are normal, and a bone scan is also necessary. If **many** new, painful sites develop, the scan should come before radiographs, to ensure that the entire skeleton is covered.

ADDITIONAL COMMENTS

- In multiple myeloma of bone, the bone scan is often falsely negative. Plain radiographs are the best way to detect and follow the course of this disease, but when there is bone pain, radiographs and the bone scan are often necessary, because neither is extremely sensitive. The value of FDG-PET in multiple myeloma is unknown; anecdotal reports indicate that the technique is very promising.

- Patients with follicular thyroid carcinoma may have bone metastases, and these lesions, like multiple myeloma, are usually missed by bone scans. Late in the disease, radiographs may be positive. **An iodine-131 total body metastatic thyroid carcinoma search is the best conventional diagnostic procedure.** This study requires careful preparation, and, therefore, patients with follicular thyroid carcinoma should be discussed individually with the nuclear medicine physician. FDG-PET has recently been approved for metastatic thyroid cancer to bone and soft tissue, but the study requires an injection of recombinant DNA human thyroid-stimulating hormone (TSH; Thyrogen) several days before imaging; Thyrogen stimulates TSH-dependent metastases; the stimulated lesions become hypermetabolic and glucose-avid, thereby accumulating more radiolabeled glucose and appearing on the scan (see **CHAPTER 61, PET and PET/CT in Cancer Staging**).

- Occasionally, a metastasis seen on a plain radiograph is uncharacteristic of the primary cancer (e.g., a lytic lesion in a patient with prostate carcinoma). When this occurs, the possibility of a second primary cancer should be considered. Often the most expedient way to resolve the question is bone biopsy.

- The "flare" phenomenon, an increase in lesion intensity on the bone scan following therapy, **accompanying clinical improvement** may rarely cause confusion. A follow-up scan in 2 to 3 months clarifies the situation.

- Sometimes a very abnormal bone scan is followed by a request for skeletal radiographs, even when the findings are unequivocal, particularly when the metastatic lesions are in weight-bearing bones, especially the femora or the acetabula. **The purpose of the request is not to confirm the bone scan (which is far more sensitive than radiographs) but to establish whether there is sufficient osteolysis to precipitate disabling and unexpected pathologic fractures.** (The bone scan can be flagrantly abnormal when lesions are **osteolytic or osteoblastic,** but old-fashioned bone x-rays can reveal huge holes in a bone that is ready to collapse.) **The alert interpreter of nuclear bone scans will suggest x-rays if weight-bearing sites are heavily involved, but if he/she does not, the clinician should be alert to this issue and order plain films.**

SUGGESTED READING

Haywood RB, Frazier TG: A reevaluation of bone scans in breast cancer. J Surg Oncol 1985;28:111–113.

Kagan AR, Bassett LW, Steckel RJ, Gold RH: Radiologic contributions to cancer management. Bone metastases. AJR Am J Roentgenol 1986;147:305–312.

McNeil BJ: Value of bone scanning in neoplastic disease. Semin Nucl Med 1984;14:277–286.

O'Mara RE, Weber DA: The osseous system. In Freeman LM (ed): Freeman and Johnson's Clinical Radionuclide Imaging, 3rd ed. Orlando, Grune & Stratton, 1984, pp 1141–1239.

Pagani JJ, Libshitz HI: Imaging bone metastases. Radiol Clin North Am 1982;20:545–560.

45 Fracture, Stress Fracture, "Shin Splints"

INTRODUCTION

The majority of serious fractures are detected by conventional radiographs. Sometimes, however, major fractures can be radiographically occult, requiring more sophisticated techniques for detection. Moreover, pain after sports-related injuries, although often trivial compared to major trauma, often causes disability, necessitating further investigation. Effective techniques for the detection of skeletal injury include conventional radiography, bone scanning, computed tomography (CT), and magnetic resonance (MR) imaging.

Relative Costs: Plain films, **$**; MR, unenhanced, upper extremity, **$$$**; MR, lower extremity, unenhanced and enhanced, **$$$$**; facial bones CT, unenhanced, **$$$**; skull CT, unenhanced, **$$$**; pelvic CT, unenhanced, **$$$**; bone scan, without SPECT, **$$**.

PLAN AND RATIONALE

STEP 1: CONVENTIONAL RADIOGRAPHY (PLAIN FILMS)

In virtually all cases in which musculoskeletal pain, trauma, or neurologic deficit suggests bony injury, radiographs are the appropriate first study.

A fracture or another cause of pain is often defined by plain films, **but in the presence of continued pain and/or disability without a radiographic lesion, further imaging is appropriate.**

When fracture is clinically suspected but initial radiographs are normal, and **when delay in definitive**

diagnosis is acceptable (e.g., suspected undisplaced fracture of a phalanx, a rib, or other long tubular bones), follow-up films in 10 to 14 days are the most practical and cost-effective option. After this interval, telltale fracture healing is often manifested by periosteal reaction. Sometimes, however, rapid diagnosis is mandatory—for example, in serious trauma with suspected fracture of the spine (see **CHAPTER 28, Acute Spine Trauma**) or when athletic training cannot easily be interrupted. In other cases follow-up films are not definitive or would examine the site of interest ineffectively. Finally, sometimes supplementary imaging is required to detect important **additional** fractures, even when conventional radiographs reveal one fracture. In these situations, a bone scan, MR, or CT can be decisive.

For fractures of the femoral neck in the elderly:

STEP 2: MAGNETIC RESONANCE (MR) IMAGING

MR produces "sectional" images that can be displayed in any plane. Although calcium is not directly detected, the bony cortex is seen as a "signal void" and the bone marrow is well seen; soft tissues are exquisitely defined.

Although the nuclear bone scan is highly sensitive for detection of fractures (see below, **For fractures elsewhere, or when stress injury or "shin splints" are suspected**), nuclear findings may be delayed and nonspecific in elderly patients, owing to physiologic differences and the higher incidence of preexisting bone/joint disease in this population. Theoretically, a follow-up bone scan in 3 or 4 days would be a viable option, but in view of the cost of hospitalization and the high morbidity and mortality associated with undiagnosed hip fracture in the elderly, MR is a more appropriate follow-up to normal or equivocal plain radiographs when hip fracture is suspected. **The precise anatomic**

extent of the fracture as well as associated soft tissue injuries are readily demonstrated by MR, in addition to other radiographically occult injuries, such as bone bruise or ligamentous/ tendinous injury.

For most fractures other than the femoral neck (facial bones, spine, base of skull, pelvis, scapula, and calcaneus):

STEP 2: COMPUTED TOMOGRAPHY (CT)

CT detects fractures in these sites much more effectively than do conventional films; moreover, for the skull and facial bones, CT is appropriate to define additional radiographically occult fractures, even when conventional films reveal one or more fractures. Each case should be discussed with the radiologist, because CT can be "customized" for a given anatomic area.

In the spine, conventional radiographs and CT may reveal no fracture, yet underlying injury to the spinal cord itself and supporting ligaments may exist (see **CHAPTER 28, Acute Spine Trauma**). **Therefore, if CT is equivocal or normal and fails to explain trauma-related cord symptoms, MR is appropriate.**

STEP 3: MAGNETIC RESONANCE (MR) IMAGING

MR clearly defines spinal cord compression, ligamentous injuries, disk herniation(s), epidural hematoma, and non-hemorrhagic and hemorrhagic spinal cord contusion. With the sole exception of fractures, virtually all significant spinal injuries are better defined by MR than CT. Nonetheless, MR should not precede CT, because of the superiority of CT in fracture detection.

For fractures elsewhere, or when stress injury or "shin splints" are suspected:

STEP 2: NUCLEAR BONE SCAN

In some sites where subtle fractures are suspected, CT is not helpful, **and MR, although sensitive and specific, is not cost-effective.** Moreover, where stress remodeling, stress fracture, or "shin splints" are in question, a bone scan is usually diagnostic.

The bones are scanned after intravenous injection of a technetium 99m (Tc-99m)–labeled phosphate compound, usually methylene diphosphonate (MDP). In the conventional scan, images of the skeleton are obtained after 1 to 2 hours. Single-photon emission computed tomography (SPECT) technology increases the sensitivity and resolution of the study but almost doubles its cost; therefore, SPECT is reserved for solving problems in equivocal cases.

Tc-99m-MDP accumulates in bone according to several parameters, primarily bone blood flow and metabolism. Various conditions (e.g., trauma, inflammation, neoplasm, arthritis) can induce profound changes in isotope uptake. Because the scan patterns of these conditions overlap, the bone scan is not specific, but because it easily detects small changes in pharmaceutical uptake, it is highly sensitive. Thus, **a normal scan excludes a traumatic bony lesion with very high probability; an abnormal scan indicates a lesion, type often unknown.** In the patient with suspected neoplasm, this lack of specificity may be a diagnostic dilemma, but when ruling out fracture this lack of specificity is rarely perplexing; **the suspected injuries are usually in areas free of previous bone disease, and the issue is whether the site is normal or abnormal. For this purpose the bone scan excels. Increased radiopharmaceutical uptake occurs within 1 day, even in minor, undisplaced cortical fractures.**

Sports-related injuries—stress remodeling, stress fracture, periosteal avulsion, and subperiosteal hemorrhage (shin splints)—are usually defined. However, a stress injury scanned **very early in its development** is sometimes missed on a bone scan; rescanning in 1 week, if pain persists, is effective. MR is as sensitive as bone scanning for the detection of bony stress injuries and MR findings parallel the course of nuclear findings, but MR is not recommended for detecting stress injuries because of its greater cost.

SUMMARY AND CONCLUSIONS

1. Plain films are the best initial study when fracture, stress injury (remodeling or stress fracture), or "shin splints" are suspected.
2. If the initial radiographs are normal, follow-up films in 10 to 14 days are often helpful in long, tubular bones; by that time fracture healing is usually evident. (The wait is acceptable only, of course, for suspected fractures that are completely undisplaced and are under management that will prevent compounding the injury before a definitive diagnosis.)
3. When the sequelae of fracture could be life-threatening, or in certain specific anatomic regions, CT is extremely valuable, particularly for the facial bones, base of the skull, the pelvis, and the spine. Radiologic consultation is appropriate to "customize" the CT study. In the spine MR may also be necessary to visualize the spinal cord and soft tissues, depending on the clinical status.
4. If the lesion is not clarified or appropriately evaluated by CT, a bone scan is usually definitive. In most anatomic regions and populations, a negative scan excludes fracture, stress injury, or "shin splints" with virtual certainty. A positive scan, in an area free of preexisting bone disease, is diagnostic.
5. For suspected hip fracture in the elderly, the greater cost of MR is justified, assuming that initial radiographs are normal or equivocal. In this anatomic site and population, a bone scan can justifiably be skipped.

SUGGESTED READING

Berger PE, Ofstein RA, Jackson DW: MRI demonstration of radiographically occult fractures: what have we been missing? Radiographics 1989;9:407–436.

Daffner RH, Pavlov H: Stress fractures: current concepts. AJR Am J Roentgenol 1992;159:245–252.

Deutsch AL, Mink JH, Waxman AD: Occult fractures of the proximal femur: MR imaging. Radiology 1989;170:113–116.

Holder LE, Matthews L: The nuclear physician and sports medicine. In Freeman L, Weissman H (eds): Nuclear Medicine Annual 1984. New York, Raven Press, 1984, pp 81–140.

Lee JK, Yao L: Stress fractures: MR imaging. Radiology 1988;169:217–220.

Liberman CM, Hemingway DL: Scintigraphy of shin splints. Clin Nucl Med 1980;5:31.

Matin PM: Bone scintigraphy in the diagnosis and management of traumatic injury. Semin Nucl Med 1983;2:104–122.

McBryde AM: Stress fractures in runners. Clin Sports Med 1985;4:737–752.

Michael RH, Holder LE: The soleus syndrome: a cause for medial tibial stress (shin splints). Am J Sports Med 1985;13:87–94.

Mubarak SJ, Gould RN, Yu FL, et al: The medial tibial stress syndrome. Am J Sports Med 1982;10:201–205.

Norfray JF, Schlacter L, Kernahan WT, et al: Early confirmation of stress fractures in joggers. JAMA 1980;243:1647–1649.

46 Osteopenia/ Osteoporosis

INTRODUCTION

Risk factors for osteoporosis in women include postmenopausal status, late menarche, oophorectomy, low body fat, and nulliparity; for both men and women, risk factors include Caucasian or Asian origin, family history, small bones, low calcium intake, inactivity, poor calcium absorption, glucocorticoid therapy, anticonvulsant therapy, hypoparathyroidism, thyrotoxicosis, renal failure, advanced age, and heavy alcohol or tobacco use.

In strictly linguistic terms, "osteopenia" means an abnormally low amount of bone, and "osteoporosis" means porous or thin bone. To those unaware of standard World Health Organization (WHO) nomenclature, the two terms can seem to be more or less synonymous. However, WHO has defined these terms very, very specifically, and WHO definitions have become standard in virtually all diagnostic reporting. Therefore, we note that WHO defines **osteopenia** as a bone mineral density between 1.0 and 2.5 standard deviations (SD) below the mean of a young normal group and **osteoporosis** as a bone mineral density 2.5 SD or greater below the mean of a young normal group. In osteopenia, fracture risk is moderate; in osteoporosis, it is marked. **The comparison of a patient's bone mineral density to that of a young normal group is called his/her "T score," and comparison to an age-matched group is a "Z score."**

Osteoporosis is detectable on radiographs only with skeletal calcium loss of 30% to 45%. Therefore, radiographs are appropriate for **advanced** osteoporosis or its sequelae (e.g., compression fractures of the spine) but not for asymptomatic, **early** osteoporosis or osteopenia. Two different noninvasive methodologies have been developed for evaluation of early bone mineral loss: **quantitative computed tomography (QCT)** and **dual x-ray absorptiometry (DXA, pronounced "dexa").** Both of these methods are generally termed "bone mineral analysis" or "bone densitometry."

Bone densitometry has become vastly more important in recent years, because nontoxic therapy to augment bone mineral—or at least to arrest mineral loss—is readily available. Also, a growing awareness of women's health issues, the prolongation of "middle age" activities into the age brackets formerly considered "old" (e.g., jogging into the 60s or even 70s), and the initiation of antiestrogen therapy for breast cancer have all thrust bone mineral densitometry from the closet to the forefront of general medical practice.

Relative Costs: QCT, **$$**; DXA, **$$**.

▌PLAN AND RATIONALE

The efficacies of QCT and DXA are approximately equal. In most locations, DXA is more available and somewhat less expensive than QCT, because DXA machines are inexpensive, single-examination units, whereas QCT requires a CT scanner that is usually overburdened with complex diagnostic studies of other systems. The radiation dose delivered by DXA is lower than that of QCT, but this factor is considered to be of little importance for the population usually studied—patients 40 years of age or older.

STEP 1: DUAL X-RAY ABSORPTIOMETRY (DXA)

DXA measures the absorption of x-rays generated by a highly stable x-ray tube as the x-rays pass through selected portions of the body, usually the lumbar spine or hip. The technique uses a lower energy photon and a higher energy photon; absorption of the higher and lower energy photons by bone and soft tissue, respectively, is measured. Well-mineralized bone absorbs more energy than demineralized bone, and bone density can be quantified after a correction is made for soft tissue absorption.

DXA measures conglomerate bone density of the spine and hip, without separating the measurements into trabecular and cortical bone. Degenerative change of the lumbar spine with osteophyte formation can interfere with the measurement, but an alert interpreter will note this limitation on the digital images produced during the analysis and explain this limitation in the report.

Because everyone's bone mineral density declines with age, a "normal" elderly person has very fragile bones; therefore, one frequently treats the "normal" elderly, a plan that appears counterintuitive. Treatment is based upon a direct comparison of the patient's bone density to that of a young normal group, which indicates fracture risk in absolute terms—that is, **how much loss has occurred over the years, and how severe is the fracture risk.** WHO recommends treatment when the patient's bone mineral density is 1.0 SD (or greater) below the mean for a young normal comparative group (i.e., when the "T score" is less than –1.0). There is no absolute bone mineral density that triggers a treatment recommendation, because the comparative young normal database is custom fitted to each patient on the basis of ethnicity, weight, and sex.

Although no radionuclides are involved in these studies, for historical reasons **DXA is performed in nuclear medicine departments.**

Where DXA is unavailable:

STEP 1: QUANTITATIVE COMPUTED TOMOGRAPHY (QCT)

QCT is performed on a standard CT scanner but requires special software and materials of standardized density that are scanned concurrently with the patient. The computer compares the density of the patient's spine or hip with that of the reference materials. Like DXA, QCT results are reported in both absolute and relative terms. QCT of both the lumbar spine and the hip is possible, but hip measurement is considerably more complex; therefore, most often QCT is limited to the lumbar spine.

Unlike DXA, QCT can differentiate trabecular from cortical bone; in most institutions only trabecular values are reported. (Trabecular density is theoretically more important, because trabecular bone turnover is more dynamic and is a better measurement of active demineralization.)

SUMMARY AND CONCLUSIONS

1. Standard radiographs are extremely insensitive for bone mineral loss **and cannot screen for osteopenia/osteoporosis.**
2. DXA and QCT effectively evaluate bone mineral density. DXA is usually more readily available and less expensive than QCT.
3. Serial, annual bone mineral determinations are appropriate to follow the course of bone loss or the response to therapy. More frequent studies are not recommended.

ADDITIONAL COMMENTS

- Historically, the treatment for osteoporosis has involved conservative, well-established therapies, including supplemental calcium and vitamin D, weight-bearing exercise, elimination of cigarettes and excessive alcohol, and estrogens. **However, these regimens DO NOT reliably build bone mineral.** The last decade has clearly proven that oral bisphosphonate therapy, once weekly, tilts the bone resorption-deposition cycle in favor of deposition, by inactivating osteoclasts; the therapy is very rarely associated with serious side effects and has become the clinical standard. The deposition of bone mineral during bisphosphonate therapy can be objectively measured **and also correlates with fewer fractures in clinical trials.**

- Newer bisphosphonates, particularly ibandronate (Boniva), can be taken **orally once per month**—a dosing schedule that is extremely appealing to virtually all patients.

- Similar results have been reported with related compounds that are administered **intravenously, once per month.**

- Newer "designer estrogens" may provide the positive bone-protecting effects of hormone replacement therapy (HRT) with less risk.

- An entirely new compound, teriparatide (Forteo), has been developed for treatment of osteoporosis. Teriparatide was created using recombinant DNA technology; it is the first 34 amino acids of human parathyroid hormone. Administered once daily, subcutaneously, in doses of 20 µg, it is well tolerated and actually promotes formation of new bone through stimulation of osteoblasts. The drug has proven to be highly effective.

- The alert reader will have noted that both DXA and QCT address the stopping power of bone as it intercepts x-rays; thus, bone mineral density measured by these techniques is simply a function of bone mass. Clearly, microscopic bone architecture also plays a role in fracture resistance—how else could we sometimes encounter extremely osteoporotic bones that have not yet fractured? For the time being, however, analysis of bone architecture is not a clinical reality.

- A number of ultrasound-based devices have been marketed for bone mineral densitometry. None of these is discussed or recommended here because of limited availability, system-to-system variability, and a limited database for comparative purposes.

SUGGESTED READING

Lentle, BC, Prior, JC: Osteoporosis: What a clinician expects to learn from a patient's bone density examination. Radiology 2003;228:620–628.

Recker, RR: Current trends in osteoporosis. Care 2005; 14(Suppl):3–8.

Prosthesis Failure

INTRODUCTION

In our aging population, prosthetic hip and knee replacements abound. The long-term results of most prosthetic surgery are overwhelmingly favorable, but a significant number of patients develops complications, most often pain and/or limited mobility due to prosthetic **loosening or infection.**

Imaging can detect and characterize such complications; the relevant techniques are plain films, fluoroscopic arthrography, ultrasound (US)-guided aspiration, nuclear studies (bone scanning, gallium-67 [Ga-67] citrate, and technetium 99m [Tc-99m]–sulfur colloid), and, infrequently, nuclear scanning with the patient's own leukocytes labeled with one of various radionuclides: Indium-111-oxine (In-111-oxine), or Tc-99m–hexamethyl-propyleneamine oxime (Tc-99m-HMPAO).

Relative Costs: Bone scan, without SPECT, **$$**; bone scan, with SPECT, **$$$**; nuclear WBC scan with In-111-oxine, or Tc-99m-HMPAO, (depending on the radionuclide and the number of days required for complete imaging); knee films, **$**; hip films, **$**; hip arthrogram, **$$**; knee arthrogram, **$$**; Ga-67 scan, without SPECT, **$$$**; Ga-67 scan, with SPECT, **$$$**; nuclear colloid marrow scan, **$$–$$$**.

PLAN AND RATIONALE

STEP 1: PLAIN RADIOGRAPHY (PLAIN FILMS)

Plain radiographs remain the best initial study for a painful hip or knee prosthesis. They can clearly reveal many causes of pain: heterotopic bone formation, methacrylate cement fracture, bone fracture, prosthesis fracture, gross prosthesis malpositioning (from major loosening), dislocation, osteolysis, and extensive bone destruction (from major loosening or infection).

Often, plain films end the workup, but additional studies are appropriate (1) when loosening and/or infection is suspected despite a normal plain film; (2) when **the specific cause** of radiographic loosening must be characterized as infectious or mechanical; and (3) to clarify equivocal plain film interpretations—that is, "probable" or "possible" loosening/infection.

STEP 2A: FLUOROSCOPICALLY GUIDED ARTHROGRAPHY WITH JOINT ASPIRATION

The joint space is entered percutaneously, fluid is aspirated, and contrast medium is injected. The purposes of arthrography with joint aspiration are to (1) document the correct intra-articular location of the aspiration needle by visualizing contrast medium in the joint; (2) obtain joint fluid for culture, Gram stain, and white blood cell (WBC) count; and (3) diagnose loosening by filling any abnormal spaces created by loosening and/or infection with contrast medium.

If loosening with infection is proven, the imaging workup stops.

However, if loosening is documented and the joint aspirate is sterile, infection is not necessarily excluded; in fact, the sensitivity of joint fluid aspiration for infection is variable. If the orthopedic surgeon requires high presurgical confidence regarding the presence or absence of infection, further studies for infection can be helpful.

STEP 2B: ULTRASOUND (US)-GUIDED JOINT ASPIRATION

Productive US-guided taps can occur even after a "dry tap" under fluoroscopic guidance.

The joint space is visualized and any surrounding fluid collections, both intra-articular and extra-articular, are entered percutaneously and aspirated. **Aspirated fluid is sent for culture, Gram stain, and WBC count. (After antibiotic therapy has begun, fluid may be sterile, so analysis for WBCs is key as an indication of infection.)**

Uncommonly, both plain films **and** joint aspiration can miss loosening and/or infection.

In the presence of persistent pain, negative arthrography and plain films are followed by a nuclear bone scan.

STEP 3A: RADIONUCLIDE BONE SCAN

A Tc-99m-labeled phosphate compound, methylene diphosphonate (MDP), is injected intravenously; 1 to 2 hours later the entire skeleton is imaged. Additional selected high-resolution views can focus on any particular area of interest.

Most of the radiopharmaceutical ultimately accumulates in the crystalline structure of bone, in proportion to bone perfusion, which, in turn, is a function of the bone's metabolic rate. Almost all bone lesions—including old or recent trauma, acute or chronic osteomyelitis, inflammatory or degenerative arthritis, and metabolic bone disease—appear "hot," because these lesions increase bone metabolism and local blood flow. Thus, the bone scan is sensitive but **NOT SPECIFIC.**

The scan is useful for excluding significant inflammatory or mechanical disease, and a negative bone scan strongly reinforces negative plain films and arthrography. In contemporary terminology, the bone scan has a "very high negative predictive value."

If all of these imaging procedures are normal, the workup for loosening and/or infection usually ends.

If the bone scan is abnormal and the surgeon needs further confirmation, or the scan is equivocal, or when clinical evidence of infection REMAINS STRONG despite multiple previous normal studies:

Step 3b: Labeled Autologous Leukocytes (One of Various Methods), Gallium-67 (Ga-67) Citrate, or Technetium 99m (Tc-99m)–Sulfur Colloid

(See also CHAPTERS 59, Occult Bacterial Infection, and 43, Osteomyelitis, for a discussion of technique.)

Multiple algorithms have been developed for using and interpreting these studies singly or in combination **when joint/prosthesis infection remains in question.** Even among nuclear physicians the best combination is often in dispute, and the choice usually depends on local availability and experience. **Consultation with the nuclear imager at this point is mandatory.**

SUMMARY AND CONCLUSIONS

1. Plain films are the best initial study for a painful prosthesis. They may clearly reveal major prosthesis problems (e.g., cement or bony fracture, marked prosthesis malposition, gross bone destruction), ending the imaging workup.
2. If plain films are normal, **joint aspiration with arthrography is next for all patients with suspected prosthesis loosening and/or infection.** In many cases arthrography is appropriate even when the plain films reveal loosening to help exclude infection.

3. Negative plain films, arthrography, and joint aspiration **in a symptomatic patient** are typically followed by a bone scan, because **in a few cases loosening is missed by both plain films and arthrography;** a normal bone scan usually ends the workup, but an abnormal or nonspecific bone scan may require further nuclear studies.

4. For complex and equivocal cases, the nuclear physician should be consulted regarding which study or combination of further studies (labeled autologous leukocytes, Ga-67 citrate, or Tc-99m–sulfur colloid) is appropriate.

ADDITIONAL COMMENTS

- Computed tomography (CT) and magnetic resonance (MR) imaging have no clearly established roles in the evaluation of a painful prosthesis; however, they can evaluate surrounding tissues in the presence of pain. Remember, **before MR the hip prosthesis "hardware" must be confirmed as safe (see INTRODUCTION to this book for a discussion of MR and safety).**

- Increased uptake of bone-seeking radiopharmaceutical normally occurs for about 6 months after the insertion of a hip or knee prosthesis; therefore, bone scanning is not helpful until 6 months after surgery.

SUGGESTED READING

Bureau NJ, Ali SS, Chhem RK, Cardinal E: Ultrasound of musculoskeletal infections. Semin Musculoskelet Radiol 1998;2:299–306.

Cyteval C, Hamm V, Sarrabere MP, et al: Painful infection at the site of hip prosthesis: CT imaging. Radiology 2002;224:477–483.

Eustace S, Shah B, Mason M: Imaging orthopedic hardware with an emphasis on hip prostheses. Orthop Clin North Am 1998;29:67–84.

Foldes K, Balint P, Balint G, Buchanan WW: Ultrasound-guided aspiration in suspected sepsis of resection arthroplasty of the hip joint. Clin Rheumatol 1995;14:327–329.

Gelman MI, Coleman RE, Stevens PM, Davey BW: Radiology, radionuclide imaging, and arthrography in the evaluation of total hip and knee replacement. Radiology 1978;128:677–682.

Hendrix RW, Anderson TM: Arthrographic and radiologic evaluation of prosthetic joints. Radiol Clin North Am 1981;19:349–364.

Johnson JA, Christie MJ, Sandler MP, et al: Detection of occult infection following total joint arthroplasty using sequential technetium-99m HDP bone scintigraphy and Indium 111 WBC imaging. J Nucl Med 1988;29:1347–1353.

Nade S: Septic arthritis. Best Pract Res Clin Rheumatol 2003;37:183–200.

Rabin DN, Smith C, Kubica RA, et al: Problem prostheses: the radiologic evaluation of total joint replacement. Radiographics 1987;7:1107–1127.

Schneider R, Abenavoli AM, Soudry M, Insall J: Failure of total condylar knee replacement: correlation of radiographic, clinical, and surgical findings. Radiology 1984;152:309–315.

Weiss PE, Mall JC, Hoffer PB, et al: Tc99m methylene diphosphonate bone imaging in the evaluation of total hip prostheses. Radiology 1979;133:727–729.

Weissman BN: Radiology of joint replacement surgery. Radiol Clin North Am 1990;28:1111–1132.

White LM, Kim JK, Mehta M, et al: Complications of total hip arthroplasty: MR imaging—initial experience. Radiology 2000;215:254–262.

Williamson BR, McLaughlin RE, Wang GJ, et al: Radionuclide imaging as a means of differentiating loosening and infection in patients with a painful total hip prosthesis. Radiology 1979;133:723–725.

Wilson DJ: Soft tissue and joint infection. Eur Radiol 2004;14 Suppl 3:E64–E71.

48 Avascular Necrosis of the Hip

INTRODUCTION

Avascular necrosis (AVN; also called osteonecrosis or aseptic necrosis) most commonly affects the hip. Ischemic injury is probably responsible, although the exact pathophysiology is unknown. Multiple risk factors include trauma, alcoholism, sickle cell disease, steroid use, collagen vascular disease, and pancreatitis; no risk factors are apparent in many patients. Untreated AVN of the hip almost always worsens; subchondral fracture, collapse of the femoral head, and secondary arthritis result. Imaging helps to detect early hip AVN, monitor its evolution, and guide therapy.

Plain films, magnetic resonance (MR) imaging, and nuclear bone scanning have roles in the workup.

Relative Costs: Plain films of the hip, **$**; MR of the hips, unenhanced, **$$$**; bone scan, without SPECT, **$$**; bone scan, with SPECT, **$$$**.

PLAN AND RATIONALE

In the adult with suspected AVN of the hip:

STEP 1: HIP RADIOGRAPHY (PLAIN FILMS)

By the time AVN is detected on hip radiographs, the disease is usually advanced. However, hip films are appropriate in the initial workup, because they may be diagnostic and also help to exclude a hip fracture.

If hip radiographs are negative or demonstrate unilateral AVN:

Step 2: Magnetic Resonance (MR) Imaging

MR is the most sensitive imaging test for detection of early hip AVN. Even if radiographs detect unilateral AVN, MR is indicated to check for an earlier stage of AVN **on the contralateral side; 20% to 50% of AVN is bilateral.**

MR can screen asymptomatic individuals at high risk. A single series of screening coronal images is rapid and relatively inexpensive; if these are positive, additional images follow. Although some authorities advocate a bone scan before MR, **screening MR provides much more anatomic information and is more specific.** MR also determines the exact location and extent of disease, which may help the orthopedic surgeon plan therapy (see **ADDITIONAL COMMENTS**). Serial MR imaging can monitor the efficacy of therapy.

In the child with suspected idiopathic AVN (Legg-Calvé-Perthes disease):

Step 1: Hip Radiography (Plain Films)

Legg-Calvé-Perthes (LCP) disease, or idiopathic avascular necrosis of the capital femoral epiphysis, most commonly affects young males (4 to 8 years old). Plain films should be first. Findings of LCP include medial widening of the joint space, subchondral fracture, and increased density of the femoral capital epiphysis.

If hip radiographs are negative but early LCP is suspected:

STEP 2: MAGNETIC RESONANCE (MR) IMAGING

MR should follow plain films in the child with a high clinical suspicion of LCP. MR is highly accurate for detecting and staging the disease and for monitoring therapeutic response. Furthermore, MR produces anatomically detailed images of **both** hips **and can define other causes of hip pain involving both bone and soft tissue, without the need for ionizing radiation. Sedation may be required in many cases,** because scanning times are relatively long.

Despite its sensitivity, **MR occasionally is negative in strongly suspected early LCP.** A nuclear bone scan is then appropriate, if timing permits, on the same day. (In an ideal situation, the child is monitored under sedation and transferred from MR to nuclear medicine for the bone scan.) And, by performing both examinations on the same day, only one point of intravenous access is needed for both studies, decreasing patient and parental stress.

STEP 3: NUCLEAR BONE SCAN

Technetium 99m–methylene diphosphonate (Tc-99m-MDP) is injected intravenously, and 2 hours later the skeleton is scanned by a gamma camera. Tc-99m-MDP accumulates in bone in proportion to bone metabolism and blood flow. When the study is augmented by single-photon emission computed tomography (SPECT), its sensitivity is markedly increased. Compared with MR, anatomic detail is poor, and, despite its high sensitivity, the examination has a low specificity.

Unlike adults with AVN, some children with early LCP have a normal MR yet an abnormal bone scan, manifested by a focal area of decreased Tc-99m-MDP accumulation in the capital femoral epiphysis.

If the bone scan is also normal, the workup ends.

SUMMARY AND CONCLUSIONS

1. Plain films of the hips should be first in suspected AVN.
2. If hip radiographs are negative or demonstrate unilateral AVN in an adult or child, MR is appropriate. A screening MR—a single series of coronal images of both hips—is rapid and relatively inexpensive. If AVN is present, the MR findings are usually specific.
3. If hip radiographs and MR are negative yet early LCP is strongly suspected in a child, a SPECT bone scan should be considered.
4. MR more accurately stages LCP than a bone scan, defines various other soft tissue lesions, and can monitor the evolution of LCP and its response to therapy, all without the need for ionizing radiation.

ADDITIONAL COMMENTS

- Although the bone scan, particularly with SPECT, detects AVN earlier than do plain films, its false negative rate approaches 18%. By the time a bone scan is positive, even if radiographs are normal, AVN may be relatively advanced.
- Very early AVN may be missed even by MR; if an adult patient is at **very high risk** for AVN and MR is negative, a bone scan might be performed, because even **an occasional adult patient with AVN may have a falsely negative MR and a positive bone scan;** alternatively, the MR could be repeated after a short interval, especially if the hip remains painful.
- Therapy of AVN of the hip is controversial. Most authorities agree, however, that **early detection of AVN is the goal, before subchondral fracture develops.** MR can determine the extent of femoral head involvement and the exact location of disease, useful information to the orthopedic surgeon. Core decompression is a more conservative surgical

treatment for AVN than total hip replacement; although its role in treating hip AVN remains controversial, some studies have shown a much better outcome of early core decompression when less than 25% of the femoral head is affected.

- A few recent studies suggest that MR with intravenous contrast medium (enhanced) can differentiate viable from nonviable bone, increasing the specificity of MR for early AVN.
- **Although CT detects AVN of the hip earlier than do plain films, it is less sensitive than both MR and bone scanning and has no role in routine patient workup.**

SUGGESTED READING

Beltran J, Knight CT, Zuelzer WA, et al: Core decompression for avascular necrosis of the femoral head: correlation between long-term results and preoperative MR staging. Radiology 1990;175:533–536.

Coleman BG, Kressel HY, Dalinka MK, et al: Radiographically negative avascular necrosis: detection with MR imaging. Radiology 1988;168:525–528.

Collier BD, Carrera GF, Johnson RP, et al: Detection of femoral head avascular necrosis in adults by SPECT. J Nucl Med 1985;26:479–487.

Conway WF, Hayes CW, Daniel WW: Bone marrow edema pattern on MR images: transient osteoporosis or early osteonecrosis of bone? In RSNA Categorical Course in Musculoskeletal Radiology, Chicago, November 1993, pp 141–154.

Dalinka MK: Avascular necrosis-osteonecrosis. In Resnick D, Pettersson H (eds): Skeletal Radiology. NICER Series on Diagnostic Imaging. London, Merit Communications, 1992, pp 515–525.

Genez BM, Wilson MR, Houk RW, et al: Early osteonecrosis of the femoral head: detection in high-risk patients with MR imaging. Radiology 1988;168:521–524.

Goldman AB, Schneider R: Clinical pitfalls in MR imaging of the hips and pelvis. In RSNA Categorical Course in Musculoskeletal Radiology, Chicago, November 1993, pp 155–166.

Hiehle JF Jr, Kneeland JB, Dalinka MK: Magnetic resonance imaging of the hip with emphasis on avascular necrosis. Rheum Dis Clin North Am 1991;17:669–692.

Imhof H, Breitenseher M, Trattnig S, et al: Imaging of avascular necrosis of bone. Eur Radiol 1997;7:180–186.

Lafforgue P, Dahan E, Chagnaud C, et al: Early-stage avascular necrosis of the femoral head: MR imaging for prognosis in 31 cases with at least 2 years of follow-up. Radiology 1993;187:199–204.

Markisz JA, Knowles RJ, Altchek DW: Segmental patterns of avascular necrosis of the femoral heads: early detection with MR imaging. Radiology 1987;162:717–720.

Mitchell DG, Rao VM, Dalinka MK, et al: Femoral head avascular necrosis: correlation of MR imaging, radiographic staging, radionuclide imaging, and clinical findings. Radiology 1987;162:709–715.

Mitchell MD, Kundel HL, Steinberg ME, et al: Avascular necrosis of the hip: comparison of MR, CT, and scintigraphy. AJR Am J Roentgenol 1986;147:67–71.

Palmer EL, Scott JA, Strauss HW: Practical Nuclear Medicine. Philadelphia, WB Saunders, 1992, pp 150–152.

Radke S, Kirschner S, Seipel V, et al: Magnetic resonance imaging criteria of successful core decompression in avascular necrosis of the hip. Skeletal Radiol 2004;33:519–523.

Totty WG: MR imaging of the hip. In RSNA Categorical Course in Musculoskeletal Radiology, Chicago, November 1993, pp 127–140.

Vande Berg B, Malghem J, Labaisse MA, et al: Avascular necrosis of the hip: comparison of contrast-enhanced and nonenhanced MR imaging with histologic correlation. Work in progress. Radiology 1992;182:445–450.

Vande Berg BE, Malghem JJ, Labaisse MA, et al: MR imaging of avascular necrosis and transient marrow edema of the femoral head. Radiographics 1993;13:501–520.

Watson RM, Roach NA, Dalinka MK: Avascular necrosis and bone marrow edema syndrome. Radiol Clin North Am 2004;42:207–219.

Athletic/Traumatic Knee Injury

INTRODUCTION

Plain films, computed tomography (CT), and magnetic resonance (MR) imaging can define multiple causes of knee pain in the injured patient. Plain films and CT evaluate bone and, to a limited extent, soft tissue. MR is far more sensitive for soft tissue injury, "bone bruising," and some subtle osteochondral injuries.

Relative Costs: Plain films of the knee, **$**; extremity CT with three-dimensional (3-D) reconstruction, **$$$**; extremity CT with multiplanar reconstruction, **$$$**; lower extremity MR, **$$$**.

PLAN AND RATIONALE

(A) KNEE PAIN AFTER ACUTE KNEE TRAUMA

STEP 1: RADIOGRAPHY (PLAIN FILMS)

In the setting of acute knee injury, a "trauma series," including anteroposterior, oblique, patellar, and lateral knee films, is appropriate. These films assess gross bony integrity of the knee and can define a joint effusion.

If plain films are normal, the possibility of gross fracture is very low. However, if pain persists, with or without inability to bear weight, soft tissue injury should be considered, and MR is appropriate.

STEP 2: MAGNETIC RESONANCE (MR) IMAGING

Post-traumatic knee pain or decreased function often results from cartilaginous or ligamentous injury. (Although a secondary effect of such injury may be the development of a joint effusion that is apparent on plain films, plain films do not show the underling injuries themselves.) In these cases MR is invariably definitive. In fact, the development of MR has changed the entire approach to post-traumatic knee pain from "watch, rest, wait, and aspirin" to "diagnose and repair."

In some cases MR may reveal previously undetected **bony** injury termed "bone bruise"; this condition, which usually resolves spontaneously in a few weeks, involves edema within the bone marrow—a portion of the bone that is not imaged by plain films (Figs. 49-1, 49-2, and 49-3).

> **When initial plain films reveal a fracture that may require surgical repair:**

STEP 2: COMPUTED TOMOGRAPHY (CT)

CT defines the bones in exquisite detail, so that fractures can be classified and any involvement of the articular surface defined. All current scanners permit the initial "slices" to be reformatted and computer-manipulated into 3-D displays, often in multiple axes.

With CT the orthopedic surgeon can determine whether intervention is indicated. If so, CT provides a road map.

CT usually ends the workup of a knee fracture, unless significant soft tissue injury is suspected on CT and better ligamentous definition is required before surgery.

> **When initial plain films reveal a fracture and CT indicates that significant ligamentous injury may be involved:**

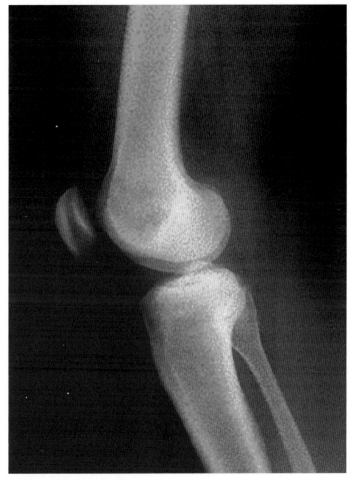

Figure 49-1. Normal lateral x-ray of the knee in a patient with recent sports injury and severe knee pain and instability.

STEP 3: MAGNETIC RESONANCE (MR) IMAGING

MR is seldom indicated in the acute setting of knee fracture, especially if the fracture is seen on plain films and subsequently studied by CT. However, in some instances the internal soft tissues of the knee, particularly ligamentous structures, should be seen in detail by the orthopedist before surgery.

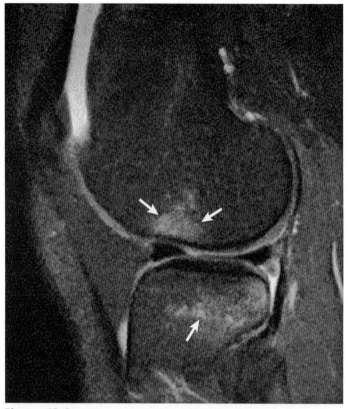

Figure 49-2. MR of the knee demonstrates bone marrow edema (*bright white, arrows*) in the lateral femoral condyle and posterior lateral tibial plateau ("T2 fat-saturated sequence"). **Marrow edema is completely invisible to traditional x-rays.** This pattern of distal femoral and proximal tibial injury is highly suggestive of prior anterior translation of the tibia (e.g., clipping injury in football).

The definition of cartilage and ligaments on MR is superb, in many cases superior to the illustrations in anatomy texts and even to cadaver photographs.

(B) Chronic Knee Pain without an Acute Incident

Step 1: Radiography (Plain Films)

The age of the patient can help define the potential cause of chronic knee pain and, therefore, the potential

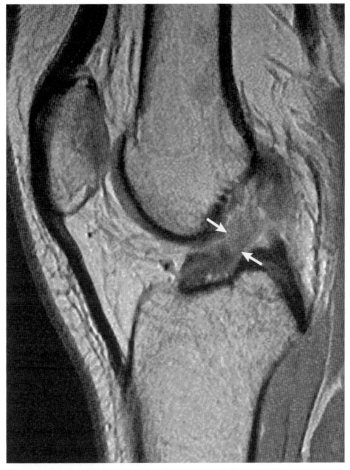

Figure 49-3. The "proton density sequence" demonstrates discontinuity (*arrows*) of the proximal one third anterior cruciate ligament fibers and thickening of the remaining fibers, **reflecting an acute anterior cruciate ligament tear. Plain films are normal, yet MR clearly demonstrates unequivocal bone marrow and ligamentous injury.**

findings on plain radiograph. In the younger adult population or skeletally immature patients, subtle osteochondral injury is more common, whereas older patients more often develop arthritic changes. In both populations, plain films are usually normal in the setting of chronic knee pain. Nonetheless, plain films should not be skipped, because they can sometimes define the cause of pain and are both inexpensive and universally available.

When plain films are normal:

STEP 2: MAGNETIC RESONANCE (MR) IMAGING

Without ionizing radiation, MR beautifully defines soft tissues, including ligament and cartilage, as well as bone marrow. Edema in the marrow, known as "bone bruise," is a clue to previous trauma and sometimes points to a previously unknown traumatic event in the patient's life and suggests other associated injuries.

Defining the articular cartilage provides information that is key to determining whether the patient would benefit from a cartilage transplant or "cartilage-producing" procedure (surgically creating holes of the bare subchondral bone to stimulate development of fibrocartilage to replace the lost original articular cartilage). In addition, demonstration of articular cartilage thinning or loss explains chronic pain.

Finally, MR can define subtle fractures in bone or cartilage that are missed on high-quality plain films. The extent and nature of these fractures determine whether they will heal spontaneously or merit surgical repair.

SUMMARY AND CONCLUSIONS

1. Plain radiographs are the first examination in the investigation of knee pain, acute or chronic.
2. CT is an excellent tool to visualize knee fractures in great detail and provide a road map for surgery.
3. MR is the tool of choice for evaluating chronic persistent knee pain when plain films are normal or for defining the ligaments and cartilage after CT but before surgery.
4. MR reveals injury or degeneration in ligaments and cartilage and better defines subtle osteochondral injury.

ADDITIONAL COMMENTS

- Almost universally, radiologists believe that musculoskeletal (MSK) imaging has become a true subspecialty, like neuroradiology or angio/interventional radiology. **Methods of MSK imaging, particularly MR, are highly specialized.** The clinician is likely to learn far more from an MSK specialist with an MR unit geared to MSK work than from a generalist.
- MR can also be useful in the setting of bony metastasis and a potential pathologic fracture (see **CHAPTER 44, Skeletal Metastases**).
- There are MAJOR contraindications to MR (see the **INTRODUCTION** to this book for a discussion).

SUGGESTED READING

Carrino JA, Schweitzer ME: Imaging of sports-related knee injuries. Radiol Clin North Am 2002;40:181–202.

El-Dieb A, Yu JS, Huang GS, Farooki S: Pathologic conditions of the ligaments and tendons of the knee. Radiol Clin North Am 2002;40:1061–1079.

Gardner MJ, Yacoubian S, Geller D, et al: The incidence of soft tissue injury in operative tibial plateau fractures: a magnetic resonance imaging analysis of 103 patients. J Orthop Trauma 2005;19:79–84.

Mohana-Borges AV, Resnick D, Chung CB: Magnetic resonance imaging of knee instability. Semin Musculoskelet Radiol 2005;9:17–33.

Roberts CS, Beck DJ Jr, Heinsen J, Seligson D: Review article: diagnostic ultrasonography: applications in orthopaedic surgery. Clin Orthop Relat Res 2002;401:248–264.

Sanders TG, Miller MD: A systematic approach to magnetic resonance imaging interpretations of sports medicine injuries of the knee. Am J Sports Med 2005;33:131–148.

Vande Berg BC, Lecouvet FE, Maldague B, Malghem J: MR appearance of cartilage defects of the knee: preliminary results of a spiral CT arthrography-guided analysis. Eur Radiol 2004;14:208–214.

Vande Berg BC, Lecouvet FE, Poilvache P, et al: Spiral CT arthrography of the knee: technique and value in the assessment of internal derangement of the knee. Eur Radiol 2002;12:1800–1810.

50 Acute and Chronic Shoulder Pain

INTRODUCTION

Shoulder pain is either acute or chronic. Acute pain usually follows trauma. Post-traumatic circumstances are highly variable (e.g., a young athlete with no underlying orthopedic issues or an older patient with underlying shoulder degeneration acutely exacerbated by trauma). Chronic shoulder pain is more common in the middle-aged athlete or older sedentary patient. Although internal articular and periarticular tissue degeneration is the most common cause, indolent malignant etiology (e.g., myeloma or metastatic disease) is always a worrisome possibility.

Relative Costs: Plain films, **$**; extremity CT with three-dimensional (3-D) reconstruction, **$$$**; extremity CT with multiplanar reconstruction, **$$$**; upper extremity MR, **$$$**; upper extremity MR arthrogram **$$$–$$$$**; upper extremity US, **$$**.

PLAN AND RATIONALE

(A) SHOULDER PAIN AFTER ACUTE TRAUMA

STEP 1: RADIOGRAPHY (PLAIN FILMS)

A "trauma series," including internal rotation, external rotation, and an axillary view ("Y" view, West Point view, Stryker's notch view), is appropriate. (These radiographic projections are universally known to radiologic technologists, and the clinician need only order a "shoulder trauma series.")

Plain films assess gross bony integrity and can suggest a dislocation by defining the position of the bones relative to each other and to the shoulder joint.

If plain films are normal, the likelihood of gross fracture is very low, and if pain spontaneously resolves, the workup ends.

> **If pain persists, with or without limited range of motion, significant soft tissue injury may be present, and MR is next:**

STEP 2: MAGNETIC RESONANCE (MR) IMAGING

Post-traumatic shoulder pain or decreased range of motion often results from ligamentous or labral (lip of the glenoid) injury; **for these, MR is the test of choice.**

Although plain films rule out most—even minor—fractures, MR can sometimes define subtle, previously undetected scapular trauma (Bankart fracture) or a "Bankart lesion" from an anterior translation of the shoulder without frank dislocation.

Moreover, because it exquisitely defines soft tissues, MR demonstrates the rotator cuff tendons, establishes if they are damaged, and determines whether surgical repair is warranted.

Finally, in a few patients shoulder pain is **causally unrelated to previous trauma,** although a temporal relationship suggests otherwise ("after this, therefore, because of this" or *"post hoc ergo propter hoc,"* as Latin scholars would say). **Some of these (especially older) patients have underlying bony malignancies, usually myelomatous or metastatic.** Although MR is certainly **NOT** the **initial** imaging test for suspected bony neoplasm (see **CHAPTER 44, Skeletal Metastases**), it is an extremely sensitive test for the neoplastic marrow infiltration that accompanies almost all metastatic bony lesions.

When plain films followed by high-quality MR are normal, the workup ends.

If MR reveals malignant marrow infiltration, the workup proceeds under the direction of medical oncology.

> **If plain films reveal a bony fracture that may require surgical repair:**

STEP 2: COMPUTED TOMOGRAPHY (CT)

CT defines the bones in exquisite detail, so that fractures can be classified and any involvement of the articular surface defined. All current scanners permit the initial "slices" to be reformatted and computer-manipulated into 3-D displays, often in multiple axes.

CT can determine whether surgery is indicated, and, if so, provides a road map.

CT usually ends the workup of a shoulder fracture, unless significant soft tissue injury is suspected on CT and better ligamentous definition is required before surgery. If so, MR may also be required (see **Step 2,** above).

(B) CHRONIC SHOULDER PAIN WITHOUT TRAUMA

STEP 1: RADIOGRAPHY (PLAIN FILMS)

Patient age can suggest potential causes of chronic shoulder pain and, therefore, potential findings on plain radiographs. In younger adults, adolescents, and children, tendinous or labral injuries are more common, whereas older patients more often develop arthritic changes or rotator cuff tendon degeneration.

Because plain films do not define soft tissues, in the younger population they are usually normal. However, in the older population, plain films often reveal degenerative arthritic joint/bone disease or even signs of **chronic** rotator cuff tear, because in the presence of a massive, **chronic** supraspinatus tendon tear, the humeral head migrates craniad, and its abnormal position is obvious on plain films.

Although they are often normal in young patients, plain films should not be skipped, because they can sometimes define the cause of pain and are both inexpensive and universally available.

When plain films are normal and the patient can tolerate MR:

STEP 2: MAGNETIC RESONANCE (MR) IMAGING OR MR ARTHROGRAM

MR demonstrates internal soft tissue and bony anatomy as well as, or better than, surgical dissection.

The specific "sequences" and views defined by the radiologist determine the quality of the MR examination; therefore, we strongly recommend that a radiologist with specific musculoskeletal (MSK) training be involved for detailed study of the shoulder.

Some radiologists prefer "MR arthrograms" to evaluate rotator cuff or labral pathology; this invasive (or "interventional") procedure involves transcutaneous puncture of the shoulder joint and installation of gadolinium-based contrast medium before MR imaging. Our view is that expert adjustment of the MR images can usually provide sufficient information, without MR arthrography.

Finally, because MR can define soft tissues, it can evaluate the shoulder for a host of conditions, including subdeltoid/subacromial bursitis and subacromial impingement associated with tendonitis; some of these conditions require surgery.

When plain films are normal and the patient cannot tolerate MR or when MR indicates the need for therapeutic injection into the joint:

STEP 2: ULTRASOUND (US)

US is ideal when MR is contraindicated (e.g., in patients with pacemakers, cochlear implants, aneurysm clips). (See **INTRODUCTION** to this book for a discussion of contraindications to MR.)

Extremity US has been used outside the United States for many years. It allows the radiologist to see the rotator cuff tendons, biceps tendon, acromioclavicular joint, and subdeltoid bursa in real time and during movement by the patient.

Finally, US is an excellent guide for needle placement and therapeutic steroid injection, especially in patients with the diagnosis of adhesive capsulitis.

SUMMARY AND CONCLUSIONS

1. Plain films are the first examination in the investigation of shoulder pain, acute or chronic.
2. CT can define shoulder fractures in great detail and provide a road map for surgery.
3. MR is the study of choice for evaluating chronic or acute-on-chronic shoulder pain when plain films are normal or for defining tendinous and labral injury.
4. MR reveals injury or degeneration in rotator cuff tendons, biceps tendon, and labrum, and clearly defines the subacromial space and adjacent subdeltoid bursa.
5. US is ideal when MR is contraindicated and can guide therapeutic injection.

ADDITIONAL COMMENTS

• Almost universally, radiologists believe that MSK imaging has become a true subspecialty, like neuroradiology or angio/interventional radiology. **Methods of MSK imaging, particularly MR, are highly specialized.** The clinician is likely to learn far more from an MSK specialist with an MR unit geared to MSK work than from a generalist.

- MSK US is **not** performed by all radiologists with subspecialty training in US or MSK. MSK US is a **subspecialty within a subspecialty,** and a clinician requesting the examination should specifically ask if a MSK-US–trained radiologist is available to perform the procedure.

SUGGESTED READING

Allen GM, Wilson DJ: Ultrasound of the shoulder. Eur J Ultrasound 2001;14:3–9.

Fritz RC: Magnetic resonance imaging of sports-related injuries to the shoulder: impingement and rotator cuff. Radiol Clin North Am 2002;40:217–234.

Griffith JF, Antonio GE, Tong CW, Ming CK: Anterior shoulder dislocation: quantification of glenoid bone loss with CT. AJR Am J Roentgenol 2003;180:1423–1430.

Haapamaki VV, Kiuru MJ, Koskinen SK: Multidetector CT in shoulder fractures. Emerg Radiology 2004;11:89–94.

Oxner KG: Magnetic resonance imaging of the musculoskeletal system. Part 6. The shoulder. Clin Orthop Relat Res 1997;334:354–373.

Tirman PF, Smith ED, Stoller DW, Fritz RC: Shoulder imaging in athletes. Semin Musculoskelet Radiol 2004;8:29–40.

Tuite MJ: MR imaging of sports injuries to the rotator cuff. Magn Reson Imaging Clin N Am 2003;11:207–219.

51 Acute and Chronic Wrist Pain

INTRODUCTION

Plain films, computed tomography (CT), magnetic resonance (MR) imaging, and ultrasound (US) are excellent tools to assess acute or chronic wrist pain. Sometimes US is an effective alternative to MR for patients who cannot tolerate MR (see **INTRODUCTION** to this book for these contraindications).

MR sometimes requires **intra-articular injection** of dilute gadolinium-based contrast medium (an MR arthrogram).

The issue of wrist pain, contrary to popular belief—even among physicians—is far more complex than the presence or absence of fracture. To a great extent, pain is a function of ligamentous injury, and its diagnosis and repair is almost a subspecialty in and of itself.

Relative Costs: Plain films of the wrist, **$**; extremity CT with three-dimensional (3-D) reconstruction, **$$$**; extremity CT with multiplanar reconstruction, **$$$**; upper extremity MR, without contrast medium (unenhanced), **$$$**; upper extremity MR arthrogram, **$$$–$$$$**; extremity US, **$$**.

PLAN AND RATIONALE

(A) ACUTE WRIST PAIN

STEP 1: RADIOGRAPHY (PLAIN FILMS)

In the setting of acute wrist pain (post-traumatic), plain radiographs are the best first test. Post-traumatic wrist films include the following views: anteroposterior, oblique, and lateral. **Plain radiographs assess gross bony status and in certain circumstances can define ligamentous instability—dorsal intercalated segment instability (DISI) or ventral intercalated segment instability (VISI).** (Although plain films do not visualize these ligaments directly, they can assess the position of carpal bones relative to each other, as an indicator of ligamentous integrity.)

> **When plain films are normal, then the possibility of bone fracture is low. However, if pain persists, with or without instability on physical examination or plain films, then further evaluation with MR is next.**

Step 2: Magnetic Resonance (MR) Imaging

Post-traumatic wrist pain often results from ligamentous injury. Although, in certain circumstances, such as DISI or VISI, ligamentous injury can be inferred from plain radiographs, **MR directly visualizes the torn ligament** (scapholunate or lunotriquetral) and associated tendon injury, if any (Figs. 51-1 and 51-2).

The "triangular fibrocartilage complex" (articular disc, meniscal homologue, extensor carpi ulnaris tendon, volar and dorsal distal radioulnar ligaments, and the ulno-lunate and ulno-triquetral ligaments) is a structure that is best defined by MR.

> **When initial plain films reveal a fracture that may require surgical repair:**

Step 2: Computed Tomography (CT)

CT defines bones in exquisite detail, so that fractures can be classified and any involvement of the articular surface defined. All current scanners permit the initial "slices" to be reformatted and computer-manipulated into 3-D displays, often in multiple axes.

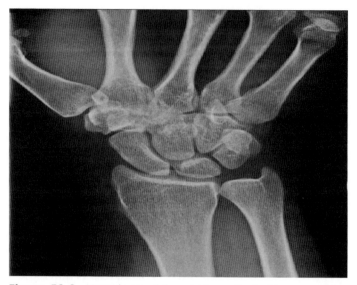

Figure 51-1. Normal x-ray of the wrist in a patient with severe wrist pain and subacute history of wrist trauma.

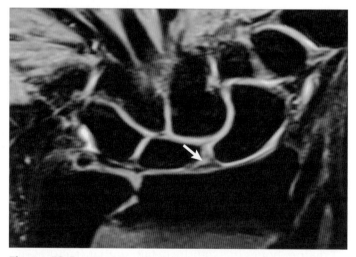

Figure 51-2. MR of the wrist demonstrates a vertical tear (*arrow*) of the scapholunate ligament. (Ligament is usually dark on this particular MR sequence; the *white triangle* indicates ligamentous disruption.) **MR reveals the cause of pain, despite the normal plain x-ray.**

Using CT the orthopedic surgeon can determine whether intervention is indicated, and, if so, CT provides a road map.

CT usually ends the workup of a wrist fracture, unless significant soft tissue injury is suspected on CT, and better ligamentous definition is required before surgery.

When initial plain films reveal a fracture and CT indicates that significant ligamentous injury may be involved:

STEP 3: MAGNETIC RESONANCE (MR) IMAGING

MR is not often indicated in the acute setting of a wrist fracture. However, in some situations associated tendinous/ligamentous injury may be clinically evident, and an internal road map of the retracted tendons is key to successful surgical repair.

(B) CHRONIC WRIST PAIN WITHOUT AN ACUTE INCIDENT

STEP 1: RADIOGRAPHY (PLAIN FILMS)

Chronic wrist pain is often, but not always, related to trauma.

Dorsal chronic wrist pain tends to be associated with chronic scapholunate ligament tears, which may result in an associated ganglion or adjacent synovitis.

Palmar chronic wrist pain tends to result from carpal tunnel syndrome (uncommonly associated with a carpal tunnel lesion).

Plain radiographs do not directly visualize soft tissue lesions; however, they are an important first step in patients with chronic wrist pain. They can demonstrate intraosseous ganglia associated with arthritis as well as erosions associated with inflammatory arthritis or pigmented nodular synovitis (PVNS). Also, plain films can diagnose carpal bone avascular necrosis (lunate or proximal pole of the scaphoid).

If plain films are definitive, the workup ends.

When plain films are normal and MR is not contraindicated:

STEP 2: MAGNETIC RESONANCE (MR) IMAGING

MR beautifully defines the detailed soft tissue anatomy of the wrist, often as exquisitely as the best anatomical text or surgical dissection.

MR is usually effective in demonstrating the cause of both dorsal and palmar (volar) wrist pain. When MR is definitive, the workup ends.

When MR is contraindicated:

STEP 2: ULTRASOUND (US)

Musculoskeletal US is **not** a first-line approach to imaging the wrist. In fact, the technique should be limited to institutions with extensive experience.

Notwithstanding the above, in expert hands, US can be invaluable for patients **with chronic wrist pain and a contraindication to MR.** US can visualize the scapholunate and lunotriquetral ligament, the triangular fibrocartilage, and the carpal tunnel. It also demonstrates tendon integrity and can differentiate normal from inflamed tendon. US can visualize bony erosions, and, with the addition of power Doppler, which evaluates blood flow, can determine if the erosions are active or inactive (see **INTRODUCTION** to this book for a discussion of Doppler US).

US is one of the few imaging modalities that sometimes allows a radiologist to diagnose and treat a patient during the same visit. If a wrist ganglion (not palpable on physical examination) is diagnosed by US, the technique can then guide needle placement into the ganglion for therapeutic drainage and steroid injection.

SUMMARY AND CONCLUSIONS

1. Plain radiographs are the first examination for wrist pain, acute or chronic.
2. CT can visualize wrist fractures in exquisite detail and provide a road map for surgery.
3. **MR is the tool of choice for evaluating soft tissue injury or underlying lesions associated with acute or chronic wrist pain, respectively.**
4. US can diagnose and help guide needle placement for treatment of chronic wrist pain, but the procedure should be performed only by an expert and is reserved for patients who cannot tolerate MR.

ADDITIONAL COMMENTS

- Almost universally, radiologists believe that musculoskeletal (MSK) imaging has become a true subspecialty, like neuroradiology or angio/interventional radiology. **Methods of MSK imaging, particularly MR and US, are highly specialized.** The clinician is likely to learn far more from an MSK specialist with an MR unit geared to MSK work than from a generalist. **This understanding by clinicians is key to successful management of wrist pain and wrist injury.**
- MR can also be useful in the setting of bony metastasis and a potential pathologic fracture (see **CHAPTER 44, Skeletal Metastases**).
- There are **MAJOR** contraindications to MR (see the **INTRODUCTION** to this book for a discussion).
- Some patients with chronic wrist pain have arthritis. In the case of inflammatory arthritis, MR after peripheral intravenous injection of gadolinium-based contrast medium (enhanced) can define active erosions and assess the response to treatment.

SUGGESTED READING

Connell D, Page P, Wright W, Hoy G: Magnetic resonance imaging of the wrist ligaments. Australas Radiol 2001;45:411–422.

Farber JM: Imaging of the wrist with multichannel CT. Semin Musculoskelet Radiol 2004;8:167–173.

Finlay K, Lee R, Friedman L: Ultrasound of intrinsic wrist ligament and triangular fibrocartilage injuries. Skeletal Radiol 2004;33:85–90.

Kiuru MJ, Haapamaki VV, Koivikko MP, Koskinen SK: Wrist injuries; diagnosis with multidetector CT. Emerg Radiol 2004;10:182–185.

Middleton WD, Teefey SA, Boyer MI: Hand and wrist sonography. Ultrasound Q 2001;17:21–36.

Oneson SR, Scales LM, Erickson SJ, Timins ME: MR imaging of the painful wrist. Radiographics 1996;16:997–1008.

Rosner JL, Zlatkin MB, Clifford P, et al: Imaging of athletic wrist and hand injuries. Semin Musculoskelet Radiol 2004;8:57–79.

52 Acute and Chronic Ankle Pain

INTRODUCTION

Plain films, computed tomography (CT), magnetic resonance (MR) imaging, and ultrasound (US) are excellent tools to assess acute or chronic ankle pain. In expert hands US can be useful for patients who cannot tolerate MR.

Subspecialty musculoskeletal (MSK) radiologists should be consulted in cases of ankle pain, because very specialized techniques are necessary; for example, **only** the hindfoot and ankle, or the midfoot or forefoot, should be included in the MR "field of view," so as to achieve the highest possible resolution. (This type of detail is beyond the ken of the clinician—and should be; clinicians have enough to worry about—so a radiologic subspecialist needs to be in the diagnostic loop.)

Relative Costs: Plain films of the ankle, **$**; extremity CT with three-dimensional (3-D) reconstruction, **$$$**; extremity CT with multiplanar reconstruction, **$$$**; lower extremity MR, **$$$**; extremity US, **$$**.

PLAN AND RATIONALE

(A) Acute or Chronic Ankle Pain, Probably Related to Trauma

Step 1: Radiography (Plain Films)

Plain radiographs are the best first step; they are inexpensive, available everywhere, and provide a gross assessment of the ankle joint and bones. Fractures, chronic arthritis, and osteochondral fracture of the talar dome are readily apparent.

Often, plain films are sufficiently specific to end the workup.

However, if pain persists, and plain films are normal, then further imaging with MR or CT is appropriate.

For patients who can tolerate MR:

STEP 2: MAGNETIC RESONANCE (MR) IMAGING

Acute ankle pain is usually associated with a known history of trauma. Contrary to expectations among laypeople and even many clinicians, **post-traumatic injury to the ankle typically results in ligamentous or tendinous injury.** MR beautifully defines the ankle ligaments (e.g., the most commonly torn anterior talofibular ligament) and tendons (e.g., commonly torn peroneus brevis or longus) (Figs. 52-1, 52-2, and 52-3).

Acute injury to the articular cartilage and subchondral bone of the talar dome usually causes **osteochondral (bone and cartilage) fracture** that MR can easily assess. MR can also establish whether the osteochondral fragment is stable or requires surgery.

For patients who cannot tolerate MR or when initial plain films reveal a bony fracture that may require surgical repair:

STEP 2 OR STEP 3: COMPUTED TOMOGRAPHY (CT)

Although plain radiographs often demonstrate a fracture, the multidimensional nature of the ankle joint is difficult to evaluate on the three basic (anteroposterior, lateral, and oblique) plain film projections normally acquired in an emergency department.

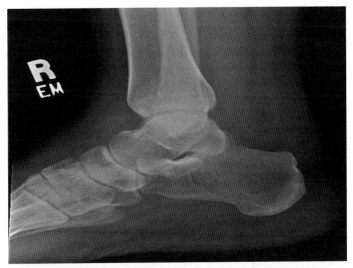

Figure 52-1. Plain x-ray of the ankle. No fracture is identified; however, posterior soft tissue swelling is present, perhaps suggesting a soft tissue/Achilles tendon injury.

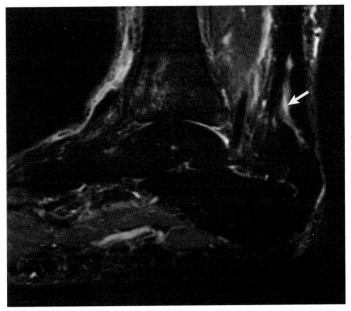

Figure 52-2. MR of the ankle in the same patient. Sagittal "inversion recovery" (*dark*) image demonstrates a tear of the Achilles tendon (*arrow*), involving more than 50% of its cross-sectional area (indication for surgery).

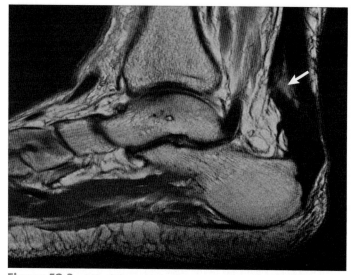

Figure 52-3. MR of the ankle in the same patient. Sagittal "proton density" (*bright*) image demonstrates the Achilles tendon tear (*arrow*). **A major tendinous injury is demonstrated by MR but invisible on plain films.**

CT provides multiplanar two- or three-dimensional (2-D or 3-D) reconstructions and defines the details of articular surfaces of the distal tibiofibular joint. CT can also demonstrate fractures of the posterior malleolus of the tibia or associated fractures of the hindfoot, which require a unique surgical approach.

CT is thus ideal for clarifying the nature of a fracture seen on plain films and for follow-up of normal plain films in the patient who has pain and cannot tolerate MR.

(B) Chronic Ankle Pain, without an Acute Incident

Step 1: Radiography (Plain Films)

Although plain films of the ankle do not directly demonstrate soft tissue lesions, they can define gross abnormalities of the associated bones or the presence of accessory ossicles.

Chronic ankle pain can be directly related to the ankle joint or referred from the surrounding joints of the hindfoot or surrounding tendons. It can also be caused by an accessory (congenital extra) ossicle of the ankle (e.g., os trigonum syndrome) or inflammation in the posterior tibialis tendon associated with an accessory navicular.

When plain films are normal and the patient can tolerate MR:

STEP 2: MAGNETIC RESONANCE (MR) IMAGING

In the setting of normal radiographs of the ankle, MR can evaluate the surrounding and directly associated soft tissues of both the ankle and hindfoot. MR defines the extensor, flexor, and peroneal tendons and ligaments in detail.

A common cause of chronic ankle and hindfoot pain in the setting of near normal plain films is tarsal coalition (partial congenital fusion). Complete talar-calcaneal or fibrous calcaneal navicular coalition can be easily demonstrated on MR, although difficult to demonstrate by plain films.

MR also demonstrates reactive changes in bone and soft tissue relating to bone marrow edema, bone inflammation, or surrounding bursitis (i.e., retrocalcaneal bursitis).

When plain films are normal and the patient cannot tolerate MR:

STEP 2: ULTRASOUND (US)

In expert hands, US can evaluate the ligamentous and surrounding tendinous structures—full thickness tendon tears to simple tendonitis. And US can demonstrate soft tissue inflammation associated with retrocalcaneal bursitis.

With power Doppler, which evaluates blood flow, US can also demonstrate inflamed tissue or active bony erosion of inflammatory arthritis (see **INTRODUCTION** to this book for a discussion of Doppler US). Finally, US can guide needle placement for therapeutic injection of tendonitis or retrocalcaneal bursitis.

SUMMARY AND CONCLUSIONS

1. Plain radiographs are the first examination in the investigation of ankle pain, acute or chronic.
2. CT can define ankle fractures in great detail, provide a road map for surgery, and reveal associated fractures missed by plain films.
3. MR is the tool of choice for evaluating soft tissue injury or underlying pathology associated with acute or chronic ankle pain, respectively.
4. US can diagnose and help guide needle placement for treatment of chronic ankle pain, and it is useful, in expert hands, for patients who cannot tolerate MR.

ADDITIONAL COMMENTS

- Almost universally, radiologists believe that MSK imaging has become a true subspecialty, like neuroradiology or angio/interventional radiology. **Methods of MSK imaging, particularly MR and US, are highly specialized.** The clinician is likely to learn far more from an MSK specialist with an MR unit geared to MSK work than from a generalist. Also, few clinicians know of the ability of the MSK radiologist **trained in MSK US** to define internal derangements and subsequently treat certain patients. **Close collaboration between the clinician and an MSK radiologist is key to the successful management of ankle pain.**
- MR can also be useful in the setting of bony metastasis and a potential pathologic fracture (see **CHAPTER 44, Skeletal Metastases**).

- There are **MAJOR** contraindications to MR (see the **INTRODUCTION** to this book for a discussion).

SUGGESTED READING

Beltran J, Shankman S: MR imaging of bone lesions of the ankle and foot. Magn Reson Imaging Clin N Am 2001;9:553–566.

Cheung Y, Rosenberg ZS: MR imaging of ligamentous abnormalities of the ankle and foot. Magn Reson Imaging Clin N Am 2001;9:507–531.

Choplin RH, Buckwalter KA, Rydberg J, Farber JM: CT with 3D rendering of the tendons of the foot and ankle: technique, normal anatomy, and disease. Radiographics 2004;24:343–356.

Dunfee WR, Dalinka MK, Kneeland JB: Imaging of athletic injuries to the ankle and foot. Radiol Clin North Am 2002;40:289–312.

Fessell DP, van Holsbeeck M: Ultrasound of the foot and ankle. Semin Musculoskelet Radiol 1998;2:271–282.

Morvan G, Busson J, Wybier M, Mathieu P: Ultrasound of the ankle. Eur J Ultrasound 2001;14:73–82.

Sofka CM, Adler RS: Ultrasound-guided interventions in the foot and ankle. Semin Musculoskelet Radiol 2002;6:163–168.

Tuite MJ: MR imaging of the tendons of the foot and ankle. Semin Musculoskelet Radiol 2002;6:119–131.

Other Injuries Usually Specific to Athletes

INTRODUCTION

Plain films are the first imaging test when assessing an athlete in pain. However, **many injuries usually specific to athletes are secondary to tendinous or ligamentous injury, which plain films miss. Therefore, magnetic resonance (MR) imaging is usually more definitive.** Occasionally ultrasound (US) is helpful (or even critical) when MR is contraindicated or for guided therapy.

Relative Costs: Plain films **$**; MR, **$$$**; musculoskeletal US, **$$**.

PLAN AND RATIONALE

(A) ATHLETE WITH SUSPECTED "TURF TOE"

"Turf toe" is an injury (sprain) to the joint capsule and connective ligamentous structures of the first metatarsal-phalangeal joint (great toe). This hyperextension injury is referred to as "turf toe" because of its frequency following high-impact flexion during football on artificial grass.

STEP 1: PLAIN RADIOGRAPHY (PLAIN FILMS)

Although "turf toe" may be a consideration in the setting of great-toe pain, plain radiographs provide a quick and broad overview of the bones and alignment of the foot to exclude other obvious injuries such as traumatic or stress fracture.

If the initial x-rays are normal, and pain is localized to the great toe, with a history of hyperflexion, then "turf toe" becomes the working diagnosis, and MR is next.

STEP 2: MAGNETIC RESONANCE (MR) IMAGING

MR is ideal for evaluating soft tissue integrity and often **the extent of** soft tissue injury. The technique beautifully defines hematoma within the bone marrow (bone bruise), joint effusion, and the capsule of the first metatarsal-phalangeal joint. **If specifically tailored MR reveals no injury, then the work up for "turf toe" ends** (see **ADDITIONAL COMMENTS** on the need for tailored MR studies).

(B) ATHLETE WITH SUSPECTED ILIOPSOAS TENDINITIS

Iliopsoas tendinitis is inflammation of the iliopsoas tendon from **primary overuse** (in a kick boxer or dancer, for example), associated bursitis (iliopsoas bursitis) **in a patient with osteoarthritis of the hip,** or direct friction in a patient with a **total hip prosthesis** (the tendon contacts the acetabular component).

STEP 1: PLAIN RADIOGRAPHY (PLAIN FILMS)

Plain films of the hip are the first step. These define osteoarthritis of the hip and exclude fracture. However, plain films are quite limited in their ability to visualize soft tissue, and if the cause of pain is not readily apparent, further imaging is required.

When MR is not contraindicated:

STEP 2A: MAGNETIC RESONANCE (MR) IMAGING

If plain films do not explain the pain, MR can demonstrate iliopsoas tendinitis and also reveal fluid or inflammation in the iliopsoas bursa (iliopsoas bursitis).

For therapy or when MR is contraindicated:

STEP 2 OR 2B: ULTRASOUND (US)

US can diagnose—and guide needle placement for treatment of—iliopsoas tendonitis with steroid and/or anesthetic injection.

(Before US, fluoroscopic guidance was used, and in many institutions it remains the guidance modality of choice, but fluoroscopy, unlike US, is for guidance only and has no role in the diagnosis of soft tissue injury.)

(C) ATHLETE WITH SUSPECTED FINGER/PULLEY INJURIES

There are five "pulleys" in the finger—three related to the joints (pulleys 1, 3, and 5) and two maintaining tendon position flush to the bone upon flexion (pulleys 2 and 4). Pulley injuries occur with forced flexion seen in rock climbers (notably in the ring or middle finger).

STEP 1: PLAIN RADIOGRAPHY (PLAIN FILMS)

Finger pain in an athlete can be caused by bone or tendon injury. Plain films define bone and may reveal small avulsion fractures associated with radiographically occult soft tissue injury.

If only a simple fracture is defined and all of the symptoms are explained, no further imaging is needed, but if a subtle fracture is present and symptoms suggest underlying significant soft tissue injury, then additional imaging is appropriate to define the extent and type of lesion.

When MR is not contraindicated:

STEP 2: MAGNETIC RESONANCE (MR) IMAGING

Evaluation of a finger pulley requires visualization of soft tissue in exquisite detail, and in this MR excels. MR defines the finger flexor tendon, the adjacent cortex, and the overlying pulley fibers. **However, if MR is not specifically tailored to evaluate a finger, the images may not identify these small structures.** Also, MR provides a "complete picture" of the region of interest and therefore can identify associated injuries of the affected digit, such as cartilage, tendon, or bone pathology.

When MR is contraindicated:

STEP 2: ULTRASOUND (US)

US demonstrates the finger flexor tendons and underlying cortex. Although it does not demonstrate pulley fibers like MR, the radiologist relies on secondary signs of pulley disruption: the tendon is free to "bow-string" upon finger flexion and the flexor tendon is volar to its normal juxta-cortical position.

SUMMARY AND CONCLUSIONS

1. Plain films are invariably the first examination in the investigation of injury to an athlete.
2. MR beautifully evaluates soft tissue injury.
3. MR also clearly defines secondary inflammatory changes (e.g., bursitis).
4. For those who cannot tolerate MR, US defines many soft tissue injuries and can guide therapeutic steroid or anesthetic injections.

ADDITIONAL COMMENTS

- **All MR units and radiologists using them are NOT equivalent.** Musculoskeletal (MSK) radiology has evolved into a separate subspecialty, like neuroradiology and angio/interventional radiology. **Almost invariably, more and better information will be provided from MSK** examinations performed by a fellowship-trained MSK radiologist using an MR unit that is specifically geared to MSK issues than from examinations performed by a generalist.

- **The key to an accurate MR diagnosis is a focus on a specific question: the more specific the clinical question, the better-tailored the MRI sequences and the more accurate the results.** Although this situation applies generally to the relationship of **all clinicians to all imagers in all circumstances, it is particularly so for MSK evaluations, because of the highly specific protocols that are designed into MR imaging of particular soft tissue injuries.**

- Note that the above algorithms do not include computed tomography (CT). Although CT is an excellent modality for evaluation of bone that should not be disregarded when there is suspicion for fracture (see **CHAPTER 45, Fracture, Stress Fracture, and "Shin Splints"**), the above scenarios are a guide when plain films are normal and the injuries primarily involve soft tissue.

Part *VI*

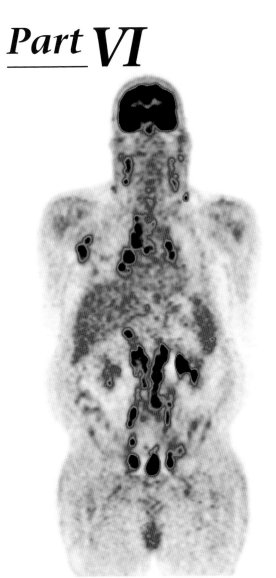

Cardiovascular

54 Coronary Artery Screening/Myocardial Ischemia

INTRODUCTION

Coronary artery disease (CAD) has been the focus of intense and growing interest over the past 20 years, because it remains the largest cause of death in the developed world. A better understanding of risk factors, new diagnostic modalities, and powerful medical, angiographic, and surgical interventions have radically changed our overall understanding of CAD in only one generation. Furthermore, the conventional workup, which had comfortably settled into the minds of internists, cardiologists, family practitioners, and nuclear imagers, has recently been challenged—to the extent that previously clear standards of practice are now the focus of bitter controversy, fueled by both honest intellectual disagreement and "turf wars" motivated by massive new and old investments in machinery and training. Moreover, the argument is increasingly made that precisely defining the status of the coronary arteries, in all but advanced and/or symptomatic patients, may provide data that no one knows how to deal with; we believe, however, that the more we know, the better off we are.

Traditionally, new **asymptomatic** patients **with a worrisome array of risk factors (high risk)** were first screened by an exercise electrocardiogram (ECG)—unless the resting ECG revealed abnormalities such as left bundle branch block or ST-T wave changes that preclude a valid exercise ECG. The consensus among cardiologists was that patients with good exercise capacity and a normal exercise ECG had an excellent cardiovascular prognosis—less than 1% mortality

349

per year over a 5-year follow-up. **Thus, such patients were usually considered unlikely to benefit from additional imaging.** Patients whose exercise ECG was equivocal or somewhat abnormal were referred for follow-up imaging, either by radionuclide methods or by a repeat exercise test with sonography (the "stress echocardiogram," or simply "stress echo"), but those with a **markedly** abnormal stress ECG often proceeded to conventional catheter coronary angiography (x-ray angiogram). **For patients with mild or questionable symptoms, the same workup applied. Asymptomatic** persons **at intermediate** risk were seldom screened by imaging. Although every specialist involved in the traditional workup realized that no test was perfect, the false-negative rates of the stress ECG and stress echo were considered acceptable.

Alas! Alert physicians have known all along that many a patient with only a few risk factors (intermediate risk) and **no** symptoms **at all** has met a sudden cardiac death, whereas others developed acute symptoms proven by x-ray angiography to result from advanced CAD, **and a goodly number of both groups had undergone NORMAL stress ECGs within a few years of their cardiac event (the "Clinton phenomenon").** This reality, and the development of new techniques in computed tomography (CT) and magnetic resonance (MR) imaging, has forced a reexamination of traditional thinking.

TECHNIQUES

STRESS ECHOCARDIOGRAPHY

The stress echo is based on the fact that myocardial ischemia—the unbalancing of myocardial oxygen supply and demand—is manifested almost immediately by decreased contractility (hypokinesis) and that this hypokinesis, which is visible on sonography, persists for at least 1 minute.

The patient is exercised on a treadmill, under the supervision of a cardiologist, according to a graded exercise routine. When exercise capacity or 85% to 90% of maximal heart rate is achieved, the patient is removed from the treadmill and imaged while supine; the images require only superficial contact between a hand-held transducer and the skin of the anterior chest wall. Pre-exercise baseline and post-exercise images in multiple planes are compared, and the left ventricular ejection fraction (LVEF) is estimated. In addition, valvular function, pericardial thickness, and myocardial thickness can be easily assessed.

For patients who are unable to exercise (e.g., due to obesity, orthopedic problems, pulmonary disease, peripheral vascular disease), pharmacologic stress is available; infusion of vasodilators (e.g., adenosine) or sympathomimetic agents (dobutamine) can unbalance myocardial oxygen supply and demand, producing ischemia manifested by hypokinesis.

NUCLEAR MYOCARDIAL PERFUSION IMAGING (MPI)

The patient is subjected to treadmill or pharmacologic stress, and one of several radiopharmaceuticals is injected intravenously. The radiopharmaceutical is rapidly extracted from the circulation by the myocardium, according to myocardial perfusion. The patient is later re-imaged at rest. When the classic pharmaceutical technetium 99m (Tc-99m)–sestamibi is used, myocardium that is under-perfused at peak stress but well perfused at rest appears as an area of transient ischemia (i.e., muscle whose marginal blood flow is unmasked by exercise), but myocardium that is poorly perfused at **both** exercise **and** rest represents scar and/or "hibernating" myocardium. ("Hibernating myocardium" refers to ischemic muscle that does not extract radiopharmaceutical from the blood or contract normally; such tissue, however, is actually viable and can often resume normal contractility and metabolism if revascularized.) Thus, nuclear MPI visualizes the myocardium itself; **perfusion is correlated directly with radiopharmaceutical uptake, rather than inferred from secondary hypokinesis. How-**

ever, the standard pharmaceutical Tc-99m–sestamibi is often unable to differentiate between dead and hibernating tissue.

A major advance in nuclear MPI is positron emission tomography (PET), which utilizes a special positron-detecting camera and the positron emitter rubidium-81. PET MPI with rubidium-81, which is a potassium analogue (same group in the Periodic Table of Elements), is more sensitive than its older technological "cousin," SPECT MPI (which uses standard pharmaceuticals such as Tc-99m–sestamibi but creates high-resolution "slices"), and it is ideal for obese patients and/or women with very large breasts, because rubidium-81's better-penetrating positrons easily overcome the attenuation of excessive soft tissue; this improved sensitivity comes at a much higher dollar cost.

A further advance in PET imaging is the **determination of myocardial viability** with the radiopharmaceutical **fluorodeoxyglucose (FDG)**; its biodistribution mimics that of glucose, so even poorly perfused (but alive) myocardium usually accumulates FDG to some extent. **Therefore, FDG-PET can often differentiate infarcted from akinetic—but viable—myocardium.**

COMPUTED TOMOGRAPHY (CT)

CT has traditionally been a sophisticated x-ray examination that produces static high-resolution cross-sectional images of the human body analogous to slices through a loaf of bread. The advent of multidetector CT (MDCT) has brought about a sea of change in this technique; image acquisition is now sufficiently fast that a **peripheral** rapid intravenous injection of contrast medium can be followed by rapid-sequence images, producing a "CT angiogram" (CTA) as the contrast medium traverses major blood vessels. This technique is now standard for the diagnosis of pulmonary emboli and for a host of other vascular problems, such as aortic aneurysm, aortic dissection, and renal artery stenosis.

Furthermore, new techniques that select portions of each image obtained during specific segments of the cardiac cycle (gating) **allow CT to visualize the beating heart and even the coronary arteries without motion blur.** (For the sake of completeness, we should mention that the technology to view a beating heart without motion blur was pioneered by "electron beam CT," a high-tech device that creates an image by exposing the patient to x-rays emanating from a stationary circular anode that is swept by a moving electron beam; these machines are inherently limited in their applications and are seldom used today.)

The generation of CT scanners installed between 2002 and 2004 was "four-slice," but scanners installed in 2005 and after will almost exclusively be faster—16-, 32-, or even 64-slice. **These scanners (16-slice and above) can effectively image the heart with sufficient speed and resolution to accurately evaluate coronary artery calcification (calcium scoring) or, after peripheral intravenous contrast medium injection, to evaluate the coronary arteries themselves for patency (CT coronary angiogram [CTCA]).** For satisfactory CTCA, commercially available "cardiac software" and a radiologist with special interest in the technique are mandatory.

Calcification in the coronary arteries occurs only in the arterial intima. Multiple studies have established that the degree of coronary arterial calcification correlates very well with coronary arterial plaque (although the correlation with arterial occlusion is much weaker). Moreover, calcification of plaque forms early, so that only very rarely does significant soft plaque exist without substantial calcification. Therefore, abundant calcification (high calcium score) may not correlate well with occlusion, but a very **LOW** calcium score has a **VERY HIGH PREDICTIVE VALUE;** in other words, **a LOW calcium score is an excellent indicator of little plaque, and the likelihood of dangerous occlusion is minimal.**

CTCA performed on a 16-slice scanner is not, to date, competitive with an x-ray angiogram in terms of resolving small coronary arterial branches. Moreover, the technique sometimes overestimates the degree of occlusion, and it is not sufficiently reliable for a percentage analysis of occlusion. An x-ray angiogram is reported as, for example, "50% occlusion" or "70% occlusion" of a coronary artery, whereas CTCA is usually reported as "mild," "moderate," or "severe" stenosis. Nonetheless, **CTCA ON A 16-CHANNEL (or greater) SCANNER IS FULLY CAPABLE OF EXCLUDING SIGNIFICANT CORONARY ARTERY NARROWING.**

Although CTCA is almost completely noninvasive, the test does require a peripheral venapuncture, the infusion of iodinated contrast medium, the ability to breath hold for 12 to 20 seconds, and a heart rate of 65 or less (usually achieved by pretreatment with a beta-adrenergic blocker). The clinician or radiologist **MUST** communicate directly with the patient before the procedure to coordinate pharmacologic pretreatment. Many institutions administer a sublingual dose of nitrate to dilate the coronary arteries immediately before scanning. It is important to understand, also, that after the coronary arteries are visualized, the contrast medium–filled chambers are seen in "cine mode"; that is, a movie is created, so that chamber wall motion can be evaluated. Although both sonography and nuclear techniques can also assess wall motion, the clarity and resolution of CT far surpass nuclear imaging and are at least equivalent to sonography. During the wall motion study, the LVEF is usually calculated.

Unlike the stress ECG, stress echo, SPECT MPI, and PET MPI, **CT directly** images the calcification of coronary arteries or, when contrast medium is infused, **visualizes the arteries themselves** (Figs. 54-1, 54-2, 54-3, and 54-4), **including remodeling of the coronary arterial wall from soft plaque, even before the plaque encroaches on the arterial lumen.** In the history of imaging, techniques that directly visualize **the root cause** of a disease ultimately dominate techniques that visualize **the effect** of a disease (e.g., CT pulmonary angiography versus nuclear ventilation/perfusion scanning for pulmonary emboli). The radiation dose

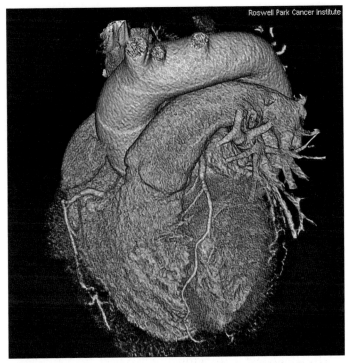

Roswell Park Cancer Institute

Figure 54-1. No, Figures 54-1, 54-2, and 54-3 are NOT photographs of a human heart or an artist's conception thereof. Incredibly, these are reconstructed 3-D renderings of "slice data" from a multidetector CT scanner. The data can easily be manipulated so that the heart is rotated and examined from any angle.

delivered by CTCA is often quoted as a major drawback; the dose varies from well below that of conventional x-ray coronary angiography to slightly more, depending upon the skill and experience of the coronary angiographer (interventional cardiologist).

MAGNETIC RESONANCE (MR) IMAGING

MR works by placing the patient in a carefully controlled high-strength magnetic field and then interrogating tissues with radiofrequency pulses (see the **INTRODUC-TION** to this book). Images are acquired in multiple

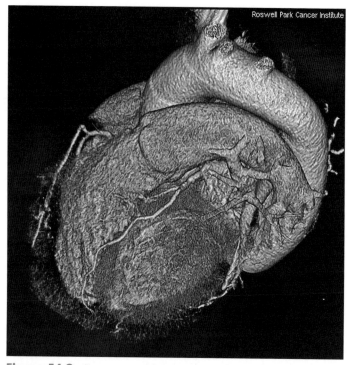

Roswell Park Cancer Institute

Figure 54-2. Reconstructed 3-D rendering of "slice data" from a multidetector CT scanner.

planes and can be viewed without degradation in multiple planes. **No ionizing radiation is required, and many examinations are feasible without contrast medium; when gadolinium-based contrast medium is used, it is safer than the iodinated contrast media of CT.**

Virtually every study of the heart that can be performed by CT can be performed by MR, although MR's visualization of coronary arteries is currently a little less accurate and invariably MR is more time consuming, expensive, and technically complex.

There are many technical limitations to MR, including the absolute contraindication of a pacemaker, but from the standpoint of this chapter three problems dominate: (1) MR scanners in most institutions are heavily occupied,

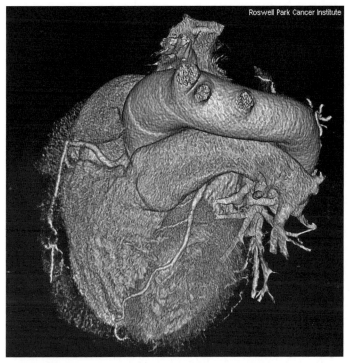

Roswell Park Cancer Institute

Figure 54-3. Reconstructed 3-D rendering of "slice data" from a multidetector CT scanner.

some "24/7," by neuroradiology and musculoskeletal cases; (2) cardiac studies are much more complex for MR than for CT; and (3) except in major medical centers and "heart centers," **most diagnostic radiology groups do not have the expertise, time, or inclination to perform cardiac MR. Therefore, for study of the coronary arteries, CT is our choice. However, MR has a unique capability that cannot be equaled by CT: the determination of myocardial viability by myocardial delayed enhancement (MDE).**

MDE is based upon the different time course of contrast medium appearance in living as opposed to infarcted myocardium after gadolinium-based contrast medium is delivered intravenously. Living myocardium (as one might expect) is rapidly perfused, and its

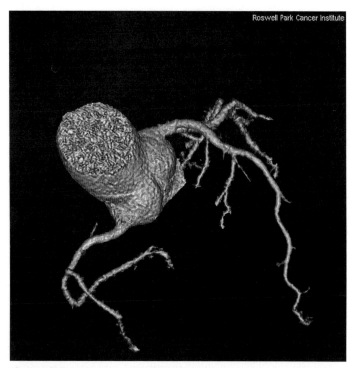

Roswell Park Cancer Institute

Figure 54-4. Electronically, data are stripped away so that only the contrast medium–filled coronary arteries remain. Remember: The contrast medium was introduced by peripheral intravenous injection, without arterial catheterization or arterial puncture of any kind.

intensity ("signal" in MR jargon) quickly increases (enhances). In contrast, infarcted myocardium is perfused only by microscopic collaterals and enhances much later. Totally dead myocardium fails to perfuse at all (a signal "black hole" or void). **The importance of estimating myocardial viability cannot be overemphasized, because, after demonstrating coronary artery closure and decreased myocardial motion distal to the closure, an interventional cardiologist or cardiac surgeon may be reluctant to intervene (angioplasty, stent, or bypass), on the ground that it is futile to revascularize a scar (or scar-to-be).**

MR for myocardial viability is the new gold standard, far surpassing SPECT MPI and probably surpassing even FDG-PET MPI. However, in **occasional** cases in which the area of probable non-viability is intermediate in size, FDG-PET can be useful for further clarification after MR.

CONVENTIONAL CATHETER CORONARY ANGIOGRAPHY (X-RAY ANGIOGRAM)

Because of its high sensitivity and specificity, conventional catheter coronary angiography remains the imaging "gold standard" for coronary artery disease, but **its expense and morbidity preclude indiscriminate use.**

A catheter is inserted via percutaneous femoral artery puncture (Judkins technique) or brachial arteriotomy (Sones technique) and passed retrograde into the proximal aorta. Contrast medium is injected into each coronary artery during rapid x-ray filming.

The coronary circulation is well visualized by the angiogram, showing atheromatous change, stenoses, and collaterals. During the same procedure, contrast medium injection into the left ventricle produces images of the chamber during the cardiac cycle: These films are useful for evaluating valvular lesions, ventricular wall motion, intraventricular thrombi, and ejection fraction. While the catheter is in place, pressure readings across the cardiac valves can be recorded. **Despite its excellent visualization of the coronary arterial lumen (which is filled with contrast medium), this technique does NOT visualize arterial walls, and it is in the arterial walls that new, soft plaque (vulnerable to rupture) is located. Thus, x-ray angiography defines narrow "pipes" that restrict flow and cause symptoms, but it does NOT demonstrate the soft plaque lesions that may rupture and precipitate acute cardiac events.**

Cardiac catheterization is an invasive procedure with uncommon but potentially serious complications. These include cardiac perforation, major arrhythmias, hemorrhage, hypotension, vascular thrombosis or dissection, cerebral embolism, stroke, subclinical stroke (perhaps more common than previously thought), myocardial infarction, and death. Moreover, the usual cautions regarding radiographic contrast medium apply.

During catheterization, the cardiologist can determine whether a lesion is amenable to angioplasty/stent.

The radiation dose delivered by x-ray angiography varies from a little lower than that of CTCA to much more, depending upon the skill and experience of the coronary angiographer (interventional cardiologist).

Relative Costs: Stress ECG, **$**; stress echo, **$$**; nuclear MPI, SPECT, **$$$**; FDG-PET myocardial viability, **$$$$$**; CT for calcium scoring (approximate), **$$$**; CTCA, **$$$**; MR for MDE, **$$$$**; catheter coronary arteriogram, **$$$$$**.

IN THE ASYMPTOMATIC PATIENT

▌PLAN AND RATIONALE

The risk factors of an **asymptomatic** patient should be determined, using the Framingham criteria, before **any** diagnostic imaging. Blood tests and a good history allow the healthcare provider to define a person's risk of an adverse cardiac event. Clearly, aggressive **medical** intervention (e.g., statins, lifestyle changes) is mandated in persons at **high** or **intermediate risk,** and in our judgment these persons also deserve an imaging screen, **even if they have no symptoms.** But, by the same token, we do not suggest imaging asymptomatic patients at **low** risk, "just because they want to be checked out." (Americans will be surprised to learn that in some developed countries such practices are considered ethical and are quite common; for example, in Japan there are multimodality imaging centers that perform screening total body CT, **and** screening total body MR, **and also** screening total body PET, sometimes all on the same client!)

IN THE ASYMPTOMATIC PATIENT AT INTERMEDIATE OR HIGH RISK

Where CT calcium scoring of the coronary arteries is established and available:

STEP 1: COMPUTED TOMOGRAPHY (CT) CALCIUM SCORING

If the calcium score is low, the likelihood of a significant plaque burden is very low, and the likelihood of significant coronary artery occlusion is very low. **Aggressive medical therapy for risk factor alteration continues,** but the imaging workup stops.

If the calcium score is intermediate or high, CTCA is the next step.

STEP 2: COMPUTED TOMOGRAPHIC CORONARY ANGIOGRAM (CTCA)

CTCA requires a 16-slice (or better) CT scanner. (It is fair to assume that a radiology practice that is experienced with calcium scoring is aware of this fact and is so equipped.)

If CTCA reveals **no** significant coronary artery narrowing, the imaging workup ends.

If CTCA reveals significantly narrowed coronary arteries but wall motion is normal, the patient may proceed to x-ray angiography (Step 3A), depending upon the pattern and severity of findings on CTCA.

If CTCA reveals narrowed coronary arteries and wall motion is abnormal, the patient proceeds (preferably) to MR for a myocardial viability study (Step 3B) or, where MR for myocardial viability is unavailable, to FDG-PET imaging for viability (Step 3C). After the

myocardial viability study, the patient may proceed to x-ray angiography, depending upon the pattern and severity of findings observed on the CTCA and the viability study.

STEP 3A: X-RAY ANGIOGRAPHY

At coronary angiography the interventional cardiologist confirms lesions demonstrated by CTCA and proceeds to angioplasty/stent, refers the patient for revascularization bypass, or recommends close observation and aggressive risk factor alteration, depending upon the pattern and extent of CAD observed.

STEP 3B: MAGNETIC RESONANCE (MR) MYOCARDIAL VIABILITY STUDY—MYOCARDIAL DELAYED ENHANCEMENT (MDE)

The demonstration of wall motion abnormality along with coronary artery narrowing should be followed by a study that can differentiate infarcted myocardium from simply "stunned" or hibernating myocardium. Furthermore, the interventional cardiologist or cardiac surgeon is often helped by an analysis of whether a lesion is subendocardial or truly transmural.

If MR reveals viable myocardium that can be salvaged, the patient may proceed to x-ray angiography.

If MR reveals no viable segments distal to narrow coronary arteries, angioplasty/stent or bypass is usually avoided. Close monitoring and medical therapy are mandatory to prevent progression of disease.

If MR is equivocal or "intermediate" (nontransmural but not subendocardial delayed enhancement), the situation may be resolved by an FDG-PET myocardial viability study (Step 3c).

STEP 3C: FLUORODEOXYGLUCOSE–POSITRON-EMISSION TOMOGRAPHY (FDG-PET) MYOCARDIAL VIABILITY STUDY

FDG-PET is an effective, but expensive, method of differentiating hibernating from nonviable myocardium, although it has recently been eclipsed by the superior spatial resolution and sensitivity of MR. When an MR study for MDE is not available, however, FDG-PET MPI is the clear choice over SPECT MPI.

If FDG-PET reveals viable myocardial tissue, the patient may proceed to x-ray angiography.

If FDG-PET reveals no viable segments distal to narrow coronary arteries, a clinical decision is made in terms of whether to proceed with angiography, knowing that nonviable areas will not benefit from revascularization. Close monitoring and medical therapy are mandatory to prevent progression of disease.

Where CT calcium scoring of the coronary arteries is not available:

STEP 1: NUCLEAR MYOCARDIAL PERFUSION IMAGING (MPI)

Although stress echo in the best hands is about as sensitive as SPECT MPI, the former test is highly operator dependent. Therefore, we suggest SPECT MPI as the initial imaging screen of the coronary arteries **when calcium scoring is not available.**

The consensus is that PET MPI with rubidium-81 is a more sensitive and accurate test than SPECT MPI, but it is also much more expensive and less available. Only 20 to 25 centers in the United States are equipped to perform this study, because rubidium-81 generators are expensive, and a very large case volume is required to support the purchase of this radiopharmaceutical/generator system. Nonetheless, it is ideal for obese patients and/or women with very large breasts; therefore, we favor rubidium-81–PET MPI as the first test in these patients.

If SPECT or PET MPI is negative in the asymptomatic patient, the imaging workup ends.

If SPECT or PET MPI is abnormal and poorly perfused myocardium is clearly viable, the patient proceeds to direct visualization of the coronary arteries. (In the context of a medical environment without available calcium scoring, there will be little likelihood of available CTCA, so the next step would be x-ray angiography, Step 3A, above.) However, if CTCA **is** available, we prefer it (see **Step 1,** below, "where CTCA is available," under B, In the Setting of Acute, Severe But Nonspecific Chest Pain in the Symptomatic Patient).

If myocardial viability remains in question after SPECT or PET MPI, then the patient proceeds to MR for a myocardial viability study by MDE (Step 3B, above). If viable segments are defined by MR, the patient may proceed to x-ray angiography (Step 3A, above). If MR for MDE is not available (this would be the usual case in a radiologic environment that did not offer calcium scoring or CTCA), then myocardial viability can be assessed by FDG-PET. If viability is established, the patient may proceed to x-ray angiography. If viability is not established, a clinical decision is made in terms of whether to proceed with angiography, knowing that nonviable areas will not benefit from revascularization.

SUMMARY AND CONCLUSIONS

1. All persons older than 40 years of age should have their risk for CAD assessed, using the Framingham criteria.
2. Traditionally, **asymptomatic** persons at intermediate or high risk for CAD have not been imaged to establish the condition of their coronary circulation. Experience has shown that asymptomatic

persons at intermediate or high risk for CAD often have undetected, advanced plaque and even major coronary artery occlusion.

3. The traditional ECG pharmacologic or exercise stress test, even with sonography, does not directly visualize the coronary arteries. **Unless there is sufficient coronary narrowing that myocardium develops an oxygen-deprived state during exercise, these tests will be falsely negative.** The same applies to radionuclide MPI, although it is probably more sensitive than a stress echo.

4. Calcium scoring correlates very well with plaque burden but less well with coronary arterial occlusion.

5. **Calcium scoring has a very high "negative predictive value";** a low calcium score is excellent evidence of a low plaque burden and makes significant coronary occlusion highly unlikely.

6. **To avoid the "Clinton phenomenon," we advocate calcium scoring in asymptomatic persons at intermediate or high risk, especially those older than 45 years of age.**

7. If calcium scoring is not available, radionuclide MPI is a viable, well-established alternative. Abnormal MPI should be followed by direct visualization of the coronary arteries; we strongly prefer CTCA, if available.

8. CTCA on a 16-channel (or better) scanner is an excellent, noninvasive method for visualizing the coronary arteries.

9. Myocardial viability in poorly moving (hypokinetic) or stationary (akinetic) segments should be determined before subjecting the patient to conventional x-ray angiography. This assessment is very well achieved by MR (which has become the new "gold standard" for myocardial viability), occasionally with follow-up by FDG-PET. In the absence of an MR study for MDE, FDG-PET is an excellent second choice for determining segmental viability.

ADDITIONAL COMMENTS

- An asymptomatic patient at **low** risk might reasonably be imaged if the patient holds a position in which a sudden cardiac event poses a danger to the public (e.g., airline pilot or president of the United States) or has a risk of CAD on the basis of other disease, such as renal failure.

- Although the above recommendations—calcium scoring as a screen, SPECT MPI over stress echo when calcium scoring is not available, CTCA as a follow-up to an intermediate or high calcium score, and MR to estimate myocardial viability—are controversial, they pale in comparison with the greatest controversy of all: **whether improving blood flow by angioplasty or stent actually prevents new ischemic events.** Although everyone agrees that improving perfusion to ischemic muscle is appropriate **for pain relief and so that a patient can resume (or begin) vigorous exercise,** a major body of opinion holds that improved vascularity is irrelevant to preventing rupture of the vulnerable, uncalcified plaque **that actually causes infarctions.** The controversy is beyond the scope of this text, but we believe that it does not bear upon the **screening** issue. Moreover, **noninvasive demonstration of plaque and/or arterial narrowing would be the best possible motivator for medication compliance and lifestyle change—and it is these processes that ultimately create positive outcomes.**

- Regarding the cost of calcium scoring in a subset of asymptomatic patients, recall that **all** government and private agencies, and all medical/scientific societies, unabashedly recommend colonoscopy **every 5 to 10 years for life in men and women older than 50 years of age, at $800 a pop!** Many of us continue to believe that our heart is as important as our colon. . .

IN THE SYMPTOMATIC PATIENT

▌ PLAN AND RATIONALE

Whether to image the symptomatic patient is not controversial; the question is: which technology to use? The imaging modality depends upon the severity **and specificity** of symptoms and associated signs.

(A) IN THE SETTING OF ACUTE CHEST PAIN

When the clinical presentation is characteristic of an acute myocardial ischemic event, with supportive ECG findings:

STEP 1: CONVENTIONAL CATHETER X-RAY ANGIOGRAPHY

At angiography, the interventional cardiologist will lyse thrombi and angioplasty/stent, if appropriate, or refer the patient for bypass.

(B) IN THE SETTING OF ACUTE, SEVERE, BUT NONSPECIFIC CHEST PAIN, WITHOUT A CONFIRMATORY ECG, AND WHEN A DECISION IS REQUIRED BEFORE DECISIVE SERUM VALUES ARE AVAILABLE

Where CTCA is available:

STEP 1: COMPUTED TOMOGRAPHY (CT) OF THE CHEST AND COMPUTED TOMOGRAPHIC CORONARY ANGIOGRAPHY (CTCA)

Because acute chest pain can result from pulmonary emboli, myocardial ischemia from coronary artery occlusion, or aortic dissection, and because CT of the chest can rule out all three with very, very high accuracy (see **CHAPTER 23, Pulmonary Embolism**), we advocate chest CT **with** CTCA. This methodology is sometimes called the "triple rule out," and so it is, but the clinician should be aware that it also excludes a large number of other causes of chest pain (e.g., pneumothorax, mediastinitis, rib fractures, and pleural-based lesions). (It goes without saying that plain chest films should precede CT, if there is time.)

If chest CTCA excludes significant coronary artery occlusion, and if the remainder of the examination is normal, many experienced clinicians stop the imaging workup and proceed to consider other causes of chest pain (e.g., esophageal lesions that are best investigated by endoscopy). However, because subsegmental emboli can be missed by CT, we would proceed to Doppler ultrasound of the legs before ending the imaging workup (see **CHAPTER 23, Pulmonary Embolism**).

Obviously, aortic dissection is referred immediately to surgery, and in the acute setting occluded coronary arteries defined by CTCA are referred to either interventional

Where CTCA is not available:

cardiology or directly to surgery, depending on the severity, pattern, and location of disease.

Where CTCA is not available, **we nonetheless suggest chest CT** to exclude pulmonary embolism, aortic dissection, and a host of other causes of acute chest pain. If these are excluded, the patient proceeds to x-ray angiography, or the imaging workup stops; this decision is entirely a clinical one.

SUMMARY AND CONCLUSIONS

1. Acute chest pain is an imaging emergency.
2. When evidence clearly indicates coronary occlusion, the patient proceeds directly to conventional catheter x-ray angiography for definitive diagnosis and therapy or for referral to surgery.

3. When evidence is mixed, we advocate CT of the chest with CTCA. **This procedure rules out the "big three" (pulmonary embolism, coronary artery occlusion, and aortic dissection) as well as a host of other etiologies of chest pain.**

4. When CTCA is **not** available, routine CT of the chest excludes many causes of chest pain but does not exclude coronary artery occlusion. Whether to delay x-ray angiography while CT of the chest is performed is a clinical decision.

ADDITIONAL COMMENTS

• Almost universally, cardiac radiologists believe that the "triple rule out" is the examination of the future in emergency departments that deal with many cases of acute chest pain. However, for purely technical reasons, this study is impossible on less than a 16-slice scanner, and, in fact, it is best performed with even faster CT scanners (32- or 64-slice units). The latter are being sold and installed as fast as they can be produced and will dominate emergency departments by 2008.

(C) IN THE SETTING OF CHRONIC OR INTERMITTENT CHEST PAIN, PERHAPS OF MYOCARDIAL ORIGIN

Although the conventional workup has involved a stress ECG, stress echo, or radionuclide MPI—depending on the availability of each study and the referral patterns in each geographic area—often related to which specialty controls patient flow and performs the examination we suggest that **direct visualization of the coronary circulation with CT is best.** Moreover, stress echo is invariably more sensitive and specific than a simple ECG stress test, and although radionuclide MPI, with the classic pharmaceutical technetium 99m (Tc-99m)–sestamibi, is similar to stress echo (sensitivity and

specificity), it is **far less operator dependent and therefore more reliable.** PET MPI with rubidium-81 is superior to sestamibi MPI and is ideal for obese patients and/or women with large breasts.
   Therefore:

Where CTCA is available:

STEP 1: COMPUTED TOMOGRAPHIC CORONARY ANGIOGRAM (CTCA) WITH A 16-SLICE (OR BETTER) CT SCANNER

If CTCA reveals no significant coronary artery narrowing, the imaging workup for CAD ends.

If CTCA reveals significantly narrowed coronary arteries and wall motion is normal, the patient proceeds to x-ray angiography. At coronary angiography the interventional cardiologist confirms lesions demonstrated by CTCA and proceeds to angioplasty/stent, refers the patient for bypass, or recommends close observation, depending upon the pattern and extent of CAD observed.

If CTCA reveals narrowed coronary arteries but wall motion is abnormal, the patient proceeds (preferably) to MR for a myocardial viability study or, where MR for myocardial viability is unavailable, for FDG-PET. Depending upon the results of the myocardial viability study, the cardiologist proceeds to x-ray angiography, refers for bypass, or recommends close observation.

Where CTCA is NOT available:

STEP 1: RADIONUCLIDE MYOCARDIAL PERFUSION IMAGING (MPI), WITH RUBIDIUM-81 PET FOR OBESE PATIENTS AND/OR WOMEN WITH LARGE BREASTS, AND WITH SESTAMIBI SPECT FOR THE REMAINDER

If radionuclide MPI is completely normal, the imaging workup for CAD almost always ends, unless symptoms cannot be traced to another system and/or worsen, in which case an entirely clinical decision is made concerning the appropriateness of x-ray angiography.

If radionuclide MPI is abnormal, and myocardial viability is established, the patient proceeds to x-ray angiography. Depending upon the pattern observed, the cardiologist proceeds to angioplasty/stent or refers the patient for bypass.

If radionuclide MPI is abnormal, and myocardial viability is questionable, the patient should proceed to MR for a viability study by MDE, if available. If MR for MDE is **not** available, then FDG-PET is an excellent second option. When either technique reveals that the poorly perfused segments are viable, the patient proceeds to x-ray angiography. If MR or FDG-PET reveal that the poorly perfused segments are nonviable, then the cardiologist makes a clinical decision regarding x-ray angiography, forearmed with the knowledge that certain segments will not benefit from revascularization.

SUMMARY AND CONCLUSIONS

1. Direct visualization of the coronary arteries by CTCA is superior to indirect methods when non-acute symptoms are very worrisome for CAD.

2. When CTCA **is not available,** we prefer radio-nuclide MPI to a stress ECG or stress echo.

3. Standard radionuclide MPI, with SPECT technology and Tc-99m–sestamibi, is clearly inferior to MPI with rubidium-81 PET. Because of its greater cost, rubidium-PET is reserved at many centers for obese patients and/or women with large breasts. However, some cardiologists believe that superior accuracy justifies its cost in **all** patients who need MPI.

4. When myocardial viability in an akinetic or hypo-kinetic segment is at issue, a myocardial viability study is preferable before an x-ray angiogram. MR is the new "gold standard," using the phenomenon of MDE. FDT-PET is an alternative.

ADDITIONAL COMMENTS

- For the sake of completeness, and to acknowledge the contribution of many thoughtful peers, we are compelled to reiterate that in the workup of chronic or intermittent chest pain possibly of myocardial origin, a substantial body of informed opinion, among cardiologists and nuclear imagers, favors a workup guided by "inducible ischemia" using treadmill exercise, stress echo, or radionuclide MPI (SPECT or PET), as opposed to a workup dominated by imaging the structure of coronary arteries (CTCA or calcium scoring).

- The rationale behind a workup based upon inducible ischemia is that the mechanical interventions (stent, angioplasty, bypass) used to manage even significant angiographic stenoses demonstrated by CTCA may be applied according to whether there is inducible ischemia (the "ischemia-guided" approach).

- Notwithstanding the above logic, our difficulty with the "inducible ischemia" workup is that a number of subjects with normal radionuclide MPI clearly have a significant calcified plaque burden, and even the strong advocates of radionuclide MPI are increasingly recommending that **their normal exams be followed by CT calcium scoring;** thus, the negative predictive value of radionuclide MPI is, in our judgment, unsatisfactory for a screen, the very essence of which is a strong negative predictive value—that is, a very, very low false negative rate.

Acknowledgment. The authors gratefully acknowledge the comments and criticisms of Sharmila Dorbala, MD, FACC, Associate Director of Nuclear Cardiology, Instructor in Radiology, Harvard Medical School, Boston, Massachusetts. Some of Dr. Dorbala's remarks have been incorporated verbatim.

SUGGESTED READING

Elgin EE, O'Malley PG, Feuerstein I, Taylor AJ: Frequency and severity of "incidentalomas" encountered during electron beam computed tomography for coronary calcium in middle-aged army personnel. Am J Cardiology 2002;90:543–545.

Executive Summary of the Third Report of the National Cholesterol Education Program (NCEP) Expert Panel on Detection, Evaluation and Treatment of High Blood Cholesterol in Adults (Adult Treatment Panel III). JAMA 2001;285:2486–2497.

Greenland P, LaBree L, Azen SP, et al: Coronary artery calcium score combined with Framingham score for risk prediction in asymptomatic individuals. JAMA 2004;291:210–215.

Greenland P, Smith SC, Grundy SM: Improving coronary heart disease risk assessment in asymptomatic people: role of traditional risk factors and noninvasive cardiovascular tests. Circulation 2001;104:1863–1867.

Khot UN, Khot MB, Bajzer CT, et al: Prevalence of conventional risk factors in patients with coronary heart disease. JAMA 2003;290:898–904.

Kim RJ, Wu E, Rafael A, et al: The use of contrast-enhanced magnetic resonance imaging to identify reversible myocardial dysfunction. N Engl J Med 2000;343:1445–1453.

Kondos GT, Hoff JA, Sevrukov A, et al: Electron-beam tomography coronary artery calcium and cardiac events: a 37-month follow-up of 5635 initially asymptomatic low- to intermediate-risk adults. Circulation 2003;107:2571–2576.

O'Malley PG, Taylor AJ, Jackson JL, et al: Prognostic value of coronary electron-beam computed tomography for coronary heart disease events in asymptomatic populations. Am J Cardiol 2000;85:945–948.

O'Rourke RA, Brundage BH, Froelicher VF, et al: American College of Cardiology/American Heart Association expert consensus document on electron-beam computed tomography for the diagnosis and prognosis of coronary artery disease. Am Coll Cardiol 2000; 36:326–340.

Raff GL, Gallagher MJ, O'Neill WW, et al: Diagnostic accuracy of noninvasive coronary angiography using 64-slice spiral computed tomography. J Am Coll Cardiol 2005;46:552–557.

Wagner A, Mahrholdt H, Holly TA, et al: Contrast-enhanced MRI and routine single photon emission computed tomography (SPECT) perfusion imaging for detection of subendocardial myocardial infarcts: an imaging study. Lancet 2003;361:374–379.

Wilson PW, D'Agostino RB, Levy D, et al: Prediction of coronary heart disease using risk factor categories. Circulation 1998;97:1837–1847.

Wong N, Sciammarella M, Arad Y, et al: Relation of thoracic aortic and aortic valve calcium to coronary artery calcium and risk assessment. Am J Cardiol 2003;92:951–955.

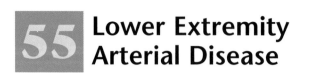

55 Lower Extremity Arterial Disease

Monica Jain, MD • Douglas Katz, MD

INTRODUCTION

Atherosclerosis is widespread in developed countries and is the most common cause of intermittent lower extremity claudication. Comorbidities include lack of mobility (due to pain), chronic ulcers, gangrene, and subsequent amputation. Lower extremity arterial compromise correlates with compromise of the coronary and/or cerebral arteries. Other conditions may simulate claudication caused by atherosclerotic disease, although the diagnosis may be evident based on physical examination.

The workup of possible lower extremity arterial disease usually begins with sonography, often followed by computed tomographic angiography (CTA) or magnetic resonance angiography (MRA). Both MRA and CTA require contrast medium administration, and each has advantages and disadvantages.

The reference standard for the evaluation of lower extremity arterial disease remains conventional catheter angiography. Traditionally, catheter angiography was performed for diagnostic purposes in each patient before planned surgery; CT/CTA and MR/MRA have recently replaced most purely diagnostic catheter angiograms, and catheter angiography is now reserved for only a few specific diagnostic cases, for those who are proceeding directly to surgery without other imaging, and for those who require transcatheter therapy—angioplasty and/or stent placement.

The plan and rationale below assume that patients are suspected of having atherosclerotic disease but are **not acutely symptomatic** (see **ADDITIONAL COMMENTS**).

Relative Costs: Sonography (US), **$$**; CT/CTA, **$$$**; MR/MRA, **$$$$;** catheter angiography with transcatheter therapy, **$$$$$$**.

PLAN AND RATIONALE

When there is equivocal evidence of peripheral vascular arterial disease:

STEP 1: SONOGRAPHY (ULTRASOUND, US)

Although it is labor intensive and operator dependent, **US of the lower extremity arteries is a good first noninvasive examination for estimating the extent of disease (if any) in the central arteries of the lower extremities.**

A variety of techniques apply: "gray-scale imaging," "color and power Doppler," and "spectral waveform analysis." (The details of this technology are best left to the sonographer and need not concern the clinician; we mention them here only for the sake of completeness.) **US of the central arteries in the thighs and calves provides an initial estimate of the extent and severity of disease,** although visualization of calf arteries may be more limited. After the legs, the aorta and iliac arteries are usually examined for aneurysm/ atherosclerotic disease, although iliac artery visualization may be limited, especially in larger patients.

When the clinical suspicion of disease is low, and US is normal, the workup ends.

When more detailed images are required, CTA or MRA is effective (Step 2, below).

When there is strong evidence of peripheral arterial disease that may be approached by transcatheter therapy or may require surgery:

STEP 1 OR 2: MAGNETIC RESONANCE ANGIOGRAPHY (MRA) OR COMPUTED TOMOGRAPHIC ANGIOGRAPHY (CTA)

For patients **who can tolerate iodinated contrast medium** (see **INTRODUCTION** to this book), we prefer CTA to MRA, based upon the following: **CT expertise is almost universally available, the examination is much less expensive than MRA, the scanning times for CTA are much shorter (a major advantage for the elderly, who are the principal victims of peripheral vascular disease), the examination is more easily performed, arterial wall calcification is better demonstrated, calf arteries are better seen, and the study is compatible with virtually all life-support systems and pacemakers.** Recent studies have shown a high level of accuracy of CTA, using multidetector scanners. Also, most patients with known or suspected peripheral arterial disease are older adults, and the concern regarding ionizing radiation is not a primary concern. However, for patients who cannot tolerate the iodinated contrast medium necessary for CTA, MRA is an effective, very well-established alternative. In fact, at many institutions it is the standard noninvasive imaging examination, despite the myriad advantages of CTA, in part because MRA has been available for a longer period of time.

The contrast medium universally used for MRA is gadolinium-based and is far less nephrotoxic than those for CTA. Arterial stenoses, occlusions, and collateral flow are well demonstrated by MRA. Usually, the abdomen and pelvis are imaged concurrently to determine the status of "inflow" to the legs (abdominal aorta and iliac arteries) and to identify aneurysms of the aorta and/or iliac arteries. In the past, technical challenges made visualization of the calf arteries difficult in some patients, but with improved technology/techniques, this has substantially improved in recent years (details are beyond the scope of this chapter).

Conventional catheter angiography involves injection of contrast medium directly into the lumen of the catheterized vessel; this produces superb resolution due to the high contrast medium concentration, but the vascular images **DO NOT** demonstrate the vessel walls. **In contrast, both MRA and CTA define the lumen and extraluminal structures/anatomy** (see **CHAPTER 54**, **Coronary Artery Screening/ Myocardial Ischemia** for a discussion of this phenomenon in terms of calcified and uncalcified coronary arterial plaque). In the legs, for example, catheter angiography shows only the residual patent lumen of a partly thrombosed aortic or popliteal artery aneurysm, **whereas MRA and CTA show both the lumen and the thrombus,** and the overall aneurysm size can be determined. (The disadvantage of both MRA and CTA, of course, is that they are diagnostic examinations only.)

If CTA or MRA reveals a surgical lesion, the diagnostic imaging workup ends, without the need for catheter angiography, unless the surgeon requires more anatomic detail as a presurgical road map; in current practice, this is relatively rare.

If CTA or MRA reveals a lesion that can be approached by transcatheter therapy, then conventional angiography (Step 3, below) follows.

When there is strong evidence of peripheral arterial disease that will require surgery:

STEP 1 OR 3: CONVENTIONAL (CATHETER) ANGIOGRAPHY

(Conventional [catheter] angiography is listed above as **Step 1 or 3** because its place in the workup sequence depends upon the index of clinical suspicion: for patients with **STRONG** evidence of peripheral arterial disease that will require surgery, conventional angiography is **Step 1,** but for patients who have already had US and CTA **or** MRA and then require a road map before surgery, it is **Step 3.**)

Although conventional angiography remains **the** reference standard for evaluation of lower extremity atherosclerotic (or other arterial) disease, it is invasive, requires an angiography team, is more expensive than any of the noninvasive exams, and may involve complications—including hematoma at the puncture site, intimal flap dissection, and arterial wall rupture. Also, the procedure requires iodinated contrast medium, and many vascular patients are also diabetics with associated renal insufficiency.

The exquisite detail of catheter angiography (high "spatial resolution") is augmented by some degree of "temporal resolution," because the movement of contrast medium down the leg vessels can be followed; current CTA and MRA technology cannot readily provide this information.

The angiogram provides an excellent presurgical road map.

SUMMARY AND CONCLUSIONS

1. US is a good first noninvasive imaging examination for peripheral arterial disease when clinical evidence is equivocal. If US is normal, the workup ends.
2. If there is a strong clinical suspicion for peripheral arterial disease, the patient can go directly to CTA or MRA, skipping US. Many patients proceed from CTA or MRA directly to surgery, if the problem that is defined cannot be approached by transcatheter therapy.
3. A conventional catheter angiogram follows if the lesions shown by CTA or MRA are amenable to transcatheter therapy or if a surgical lesion requires more detail (i.e., a presurgical road map).
4. If clinical evidence strongly indicates that there is arterial disease that will require surgery, US, CTA, and MRA can be skipped in favor of direct catheter angiography, which provides a presurgical road map, but the decision to perform initial conventional angiography rather than noninvasive

imaging should be made on a case-by-case basis (e.g., in patients with limb-threatening ischemia).

5. After US, MRA is more commonly used than CTA for peripheral arterial disease, but state-of-the-art CTA has many advantages, and we therefore recommend it, unless the patient cannot tolerate iodinated contrast medium.

6. Conventional catheter angiography, an invasive procedure, remains the reference standard for evaluating peripheral arterial disease. Therapeutic procedures can be performed at the same sitting.

ADDITIONAL COMMENTS

- If acute occlusion of a portion of the central lower extremity arterial system is suspected, due to thrombosis or embolism, there is no established role for MRA or CTA. Patients are managed either with direct surgical intervention or with conventional catheter angiography followed by interventional radiologic techniques/surgery.

- Infrequently, lower extremity arterial disease may not be related to atherosclerosis but may be due to a vasculitis or other disease. In these conditions US, MR, and CTA are less well established, compared with conventional angiography.

- Typically, US, MRA, or CTA is used for follow-up after therapy (e.g., after angioplasty), **BUT** the local metallic artifacts produced by a stent significantly limit MR and US for assessment of the lumen within the stent; if the patient can tolerate iodinated contrast medium, **CTA is the noninvasive test of choice for follow-up.** Graft patency is determined, and complications are sought.

- For patients with renal insufficiency who **need** conventional catheter angiography to guide procedures such as angioplasty and stent placement, several strategies have been devised to reduce contrast-medium–induced renal injury: (1) use of smaller amounts of contrast medium, (2) use of less nephrotoxic contrast media (see **INTRODUCTION** to this book), or (3) use of more exotic alternative contrast agents (carbon dioxide or gadolinium), and (4) judicious IV hydration.

SUGGESTED READING

Catalano C, Fraioli F, Laghi A, et al: Infrarenal aortic and lower extremity arterial disease: diagnostic performance of multi-detector row CT angiography. Radiology 2004;23:555–563.

Edwards AJ, Wells IP, Roobottom CA: Multidetector-row CT angiography of the lower limb arteries: a prospective comparison of volume-rendered techniques and intra-arterial digital subtraction angiography. Clin Radiol 2005;60:85–95.

Foshager MC, Sane SS: Evaluation of lower extremity bypass grafts with use of color duplex sonography. Radiographics 1996;16:9–25.

Jakobs TF, Wintersperger BJ, Becker CR: MDCT-imaging of peripheral arterial disease. Semin US CT MR 2004;25:145–155.

Katz DS, Hon M: CT angiography of the lower extremities and aortoiliac system with a multi-detector row helical CT scanner: promise of new opportunities fulfilled. Radiology 2001;221:7–10.

Quinn SF, Sheley RC, Semonsen KG, et al: Aortic and lower-extremity arterial disease: evaluation with MR angiography versus conventional angiography. Radiology 1998;206:693–701.

Rofsky NM, Adelman MA: MR angiography in the evaluation of atherosclerotic peripheral vascular disease. Radiology 2000;217:105–114.

Rubin GD, Schmidt AJ, Logan LJ, Sofilos MC: Multi-detector row CT angiography of lower extremity arterial inflow and runoff: initial experience. Radiology 2001;221:146–157.

Willmann JK, Mayer D, Banyai M, et al: Evaluation of peripheral arterial bypass grafts with multi-detector row CT angiography: comparison with duplex US and digital subtraction angiography. Radiology 2003;229:465–474.

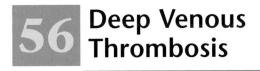

56 Deep Venous Thrombosis

Imaging plays a vital role in the evaluation of suspected deep venous thrombosis (DVT). The clinical diagnosis of DVT is notoriously unreliable, because many of the classic signs and symptoms (leg pain, swelling, redness, Homan's sign) are both insensitive and nonspecific. The insensitivity of clinical evaluation stems from the high incidence of asymptomatic cases. Myriad conditions, including cellulitis, popliteal cyst, superficial thrombophlebitis, musculoskeletal injury, postphlebitic syndrome, popliteal vessel aneurysm, and various causes of extremity edema, can mimic acute DVT on clinical examination.

Imaging for DVT is appropriate in several situations: evaluation of suspected acute DVT, follow-up of patients with known DVT, screening of high-risk patients (i.e., those with prolonged immobilization, recent surgery, lower extremity fracture, and joint replacement surgery) who are prone to the development of asymptomatic DVT, and evaluation of patients with suspected pulmonary embolism (PE) when leg symptoms are present or when imaging of the pulmonary arteries is inconclusive. Although most patients require imaging evaluation, **recent studies suggest that a negative D-dimer test, together with a low clinical suspicion of DVT, effectively excludes DVT without the need for imaging.**

Ultrasound (US) is the best initial test for suspected DVT. It is quick, readily available, uses no contrast medium or ionizing radiation, and is very accurate for

DVT above the calf. US is less accurate for calf DVT and chronic DVT. Magnetic resonance (MR) imaging, computed tomography (CT), or conventional venography (CV) may be effective when US is inconclusive or if detection of DVT in small calf veins leads to a significant change in patient management. (Most agree that DVT in smaller calf veins carries a **low** risk of PE and postphlebitic syndrome.)

Relative Costs: Pelvic US and bilateral leg US, with Doppler, **$$–$$$**; pelvic US and unilateral leg US, with Doppler, **$$–$$$**; MR venography, **$$$$;** CV, unilateral, **$$**; CV, bilateral, **$$$**.

▌ PLAN AND RATIONALE

(A) Suspected Acute DVT

Step 1: Ultrasound (US) with Color Doppler

US is the most effective noninvasive means of imaging the deep venous system **from the inguinal ligament to the popliteal trifurcation in the upper calf.** The deep veins are identified and compressed by the hand-held transducer at 1- to 2-cm intervals along the length of the thigh. Thrombi can be seen directly or inferred by failure of the vein walls to collapse under gentle compression. The procedure is often supplemented by various Doppler techniques that identify moving blood. The sensitivity and specificity of US for symptomatic DVT in the lower extremity (excluding the calf) are 95% and 98%, respectively. **US can be performed at the bedside.**

The calf veins can also be evaluated and isolated calf DVT detected, but the calf veins are not visualized completely in most patients. **Because US does not detect all calf DVT, it is prudent to perform a repeat US in 3 to 5 days if the patient's symptoms persist or worsen to detect calf clots that may have propagated proximally.**

When visualization of isolated calf DVT is considered critical and will alter treatment/ management:

STEP 1: MAGNETIC RESONANCE (MR) IMAGING/COMPUTED TOMOGRAPHIC (CT) VENOGRAPHY

MR of the deep venous system of the leg, when properly performed, is very accurate for detection of pelvic and lower extremity DVT (including calf DVT). Specific imaging sequences are performed that detect flowing blood.

CT venous-phase images performed several minutes after injection of contrast medium **into an arm vein** have also been shown to be extremely accurate for evaluation of lower extremity DVT **(see CHAPTER 23, Pulmonary Embolism, for a discussion of CT venography as the second part of a pulmonary embolism study).**

If MR venography is not available, and if there has been no pulmonary embolism study by CT (and thus no CT venography examination):

STEP 1: CONVENTIONAL CONTRAST VENOGRAPHY (CV)

CV has long been considered the reference standard for lower extremity DVT. A pedal vein is cannulated and iodinated contrast medium injected, opacifying the deep veins of the calf, thigh, and pelvis, thereby outlining DVT. Whereas CV is probably still the most accurate available test for evaluation of the calf veins, it has several significant disadvantages: it is invasive and often painful, requires intravenous contrast medium, and entails the risk of post venography thrombosis. CV is more expensive than US, is not a bedside examination (a significant consideration in debilitated patients), and suffers from flow-related artifacts or nonfilling of veins that may lead to an equivocal or inaccurate study. **Because of these factors and the preeminent role of venous US, lower extremity CV has become a rarely requested test.**

(B) SUSPECTED CHRONIC OR ACUTE-ON-CHRONIC THROMBOSIS

The imaging diagnosis of chronic DVT or acute-on-chronic DVT is difficult, largely because of postphlebitic syndrome—the anatomic/physiologic changes that occur within the venous system after clot formation. After an acute thrombus has resolved, about 50% of veins continue to exhibit abnormalities on US, because of clot organization and recanalization. Residual findings include incomplete compressibility and thickening of vein walls as well as persistent intraluminal abnormal echoes that suggest thrombus. **These residual abnormalities limit the ability of US to differentiate between acute, chronic, and acute-on-chronic DVT.**

STEP 1: ULTRASOUND (US) WITH DOPPLER

When anticoagulation is complete, a baseline US to document residual post-DVT changes is recommended, so that a significant change is more readily appreciated on subsequent studies. Serial US with Doppler is currently the best available technique.

SUMMARY AND CONCLUSIONS

1. US with Doppler is the primary imaging modality for DVT. If no clot is detected, the patient is considered to be free of significant DVT and treated conservatively. Repeat US should be performed in 3 to 5 days if symptoms persist to

exclude craniad propagation of a small venous thrombosis originating in the calf.

2. Venography using MR, CT, or contrast injection into a pedal vein should be reserved for patients with suspected lower extremity DVT, positive D-dimer, and negative US, **if detection of isolated calf DVT that may have been missed by US will alter patient management.**

3. Chronic venous thrombosis is currently best assessed by serial US, compared to a baseline study performed when anticoagulation therapy is complete.

ADDITIONAL COMMENTS

- CT venography is a technique that is often performed immediately after CT pulmonary angiography to concurrently evaluate both DVT and PE in patients with thoracic symptoms suggesting PE. A limited set of images can evaluate the deep veins of the legs, abdomen, and pelvis using the same dose of contrast medium given through an arm vein for CT pulmonary angiography (see **CHAPTER 23, Pulmonary Embolism**).

- Because of the proliferation of central venous catheters for hyperalimentation, long-term antibiotic therapy, and chemotherapy, upper extremity DVT has increased. Although CV is the accepted diagnostic reference standard for upper extremity DVT, US with Doppler evaluation, which can assess the internal jugular, subclavian, and arm veins, is also effective.

SUGGESTED READING

Cranley JJ, Canos AJ, Sull WJ: The diagnosis of deep venous thrombosis: fallibility of clinical symptoms and signs. Arch Surg 1976;111:34–36.

Fraser JD, Anderson DR: Deep venous thrombosis: recent advances and optimal investigation with US. Radiology 1999;211:9–24.

Kearon C, Julian JA, Math M, et al: Noninvasive diagnosis of deep venous thrombosis. Ann Intern Med 1998;128:663–677.

Kearon MB, Ginsberg JS, Douketis J, et al: Management of suspected deep venous thrombosis in outpatients by using clinical assessment and D-dimer testing. Ann Intern Med 2001;135:108–111.

Loud PA, Katz DS, Bruce DA, et al: Deep venous thrombosis with suspected pulmonary embolism: detection with combined CT venography and pulmonary angiography. Radiology 2001; 219:498–502.

Moser KM, LeMoine JR: Is embolic risk conditioned by location of deep venous thrombosis? Ann Intern Med 1981;94:439–444.

Wells PS, Anderson DR, Rodger M, et al: Evaluation of D-dimer in the diagnosis of suspected deep-vein thrombosis. N Engl J Med 2003;349:1227–1235.

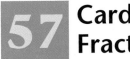

57 Cardiac Ejection Fraction

INTRODUCTION

An important measure of cardiac performance is the ejection fraction (EF)—that portion of the ventricular volume ejected by systole. Numerically, this fraction is the end-diastolic volume minus the end-systolic volume, divided by the end-diastolic volume. Although the EF has widespread applications in cardiology, it is particularly critical in cancer care, because of the potential cardiotoxicity of some anti-tumor agents.

The EF is calculated by nuclear ventriculography, x-ray cardiac angiography, computed tomography (CT), and magnetic resonance (MR) imaging, but it is usually estimated by echocardiography. Nuclear ventriculography and echocardiography are noninvasive, whereas angiography requires peripheral vascular puncture, retrograde passage of a catheter into the heart, and injection of contrast medium. CT and MR are minimally invasive, involving only a peripheral intravenous injection of contrast medium.

Although MR and CT are being used to perform more and more cardiac studies, the emphasis is on coronary artery examinations (CT) and myocardial viability (MR). Very, very few radiology departments, even in academic medical centers, have the resources and/or interest to devote CT or MR machines or manpower to the calculation of ejection fractions, especially because the standard radionuclide and sonographic methods are cheap and effective.

Relative Costs: Nuclear ventriculogram, **$$–$$$**; echocardiogram, **$$**; CT, **$$$**; MR, **$$$$**.

▌PLAN AND RATIONALE

When a precise, numerical EF is required and valvular function, pericardial disease, and myocardial thickness are not at issue:

STEP 1: THE NUCLEAR VENTRICULOGRAM

In certain patients, particularly those undergoing chemotherapy, **a quantitative determination of EF** is required to monitor cardiotoxic drug effects. The nuclear ventriculogram is well suited to this purpose.

A few milliliters of the patient's red blood cells are drawn and labeled with technetium 99m (Tc-99m). After the labeled cells have been injected and have thoroughly mixed in the circulating blood volume, the chest is imaged by a nuclear camera, which records radioactivity in the cardiac chambers during the cardiac cycle. The recording of radioactivity is correlated with multiple phases of the electrocardiogram (ECG). The computer constructs a series of individual images, each representing a slightly different phase of the cardiac cycle. The cycle—from systole through diastole—is displayed as a "movie," called a "**mu**lti-**g**ated **a**cquisition" (MUGA) study, and the EF is calculated.

By appropriate positioning, all ventricular segments except part of the left ventricular posterior wall may be imaged for an accurate assessment of regional contraction. Hypokinesis, akinesis, and dyskinesis are easily detected, and chamber size can be estimated.

Nuclear ventriculography does **not** define the cardiac valves, the pericardium, or the myocardium itself, because the blood pool, rather than the myocardium or endocardium, is visualized.

When an approximate estimate of EF is satisfactory and information regarding valvular function, the pericardium, and myocardial thickness may be useful:

STEP 1: ECHOCARDIOGRAPHY (CARDIAC ULTRASOUND OR SONOGRAPHY)

Echocardiography is a sophisticated method of cardiac imaging, useful for evaluating the motion of the cardiac valves and ventricular walls, pericardial thickness, and myocardial thickness.

In the great majority of institutions, at the time of this writing, **the ventricular EF is estimated—rather than calculated—by echocardiography.** From a practical standpoint, this estimate **usually** fulfills the clinician's requirements, but a nuclear ventriculogram remains the procedure of choice when strict quantitation is required.

Echocardiography, unlike nuclear ventriculography, **is highly operator dependent**—that is, dependent upon operator skill.

SUMMARY AND CONCLUSIONS

1. Radionuclide ventriculography and echocardiography are noninvasive methods of determining the ventricular EF.
2. When a **precise quantitation** of EF is required, particularly in the **monitoring of chemotherapy patients for cardiotoxicity,** the nuclear ventriculogram is preferable.
3. When a good estimate of the EF is satisfactory and information regarding the cardiac valves, pericardium, and myocardial thickness may be useful, echocardiography is appropriate.

ADDITIONAL COMMENTS

- Severe chronic obstructive pulmonary disease (COPD) and obesity may technically impede echocardiography, but COPD does not affect nuclear ventriculography and obesity is a minor impediment unless massive.

Therefore, **the EF in such patients is better determined by the nuclear technique.**

- The x-ray cardiac angiogram requires catheterization of the aorta and injection of radiographic contrast medium into the left ventricle. During the cardiac cycle, rapid-sequence images are generated. The EF is calculated from the change in size of the contrast medium–filled ventricle, directly measured from the images, during systole and diastole. This invasive procedure correlates well with the nuclear ventriculogram.

- Multidetector CT, with 16 or more detectors, can define the coronary arteries and wall motion, calculate an EF, and examine the pericardium. However, because of the clinical demand upon CT scanners and the radiation dose delivered, CT is not used simply to calculate an EF.

- Gated MR can define regional wall motion, anatomic and valvular lesions, the coronary arteries, pericardial disease, acute myocardial infarction, and areas of hibernating but akinetic myocardium, as well as calculate the EF—all without any radiation. Thus, MR combines the best features of nuclear imaging, CT, and echocardiography, but its higher cost and complexity have inhibited its expansion into this clinical arena.

58 Pericardial Effusion

INTRODUCTION

Although a very large pericardial effusion can be tolerated if it accumulates slowly, the rapid accumulation of pericardial fluid can quickly compromise cardiac function. Pericardial effusion can be inferred by chest radiography—although plain films are neither sensitive nor specific—and confirmed by echocardiography (sonography or ultrasound [US]), computed tomography (CT), and magnetic resonance (MR) imaging. The expense of these techniques varies significantly. In practical terms, chest films and echocardiography dominate the workup.

Relative Costs: Plain chest films, posteroanterior and lateral, **$**; chest MR, unenhanced, **$$$–$$$$**; chest CT, unenhanced, **$$$**; echocardiogram, **$$$**.

PLAN AND RATIONALE

STEPS 1 AND 2: CHEST RADIOGRAPHY (PLAIN FILMS) AND ECHOCARDIOGRAPHY (SONOGRAPHY OR ULTRASOUND [US])

A **normal cardiac silhouette on a chest film does not exclude a significant pericardial effusion, and an enlarged cardiac silhouette could reflect cardiomegaly, effusion, or both.** Thus, chest films are insensitive and rarely specific for pericardial effusion, and an additional study is necessary **following serious clinical and/or radiographic suspicion.** (An initial chest film remains mandatory, however, to exclude intrathoracic conditions that could mimic pericardial effusion and to define or characterize associated lesions.)

Echocardiography (sonography of the heart) is highly sensitive and specific for pericardial fluid; scanning over the anterior chest wall generates images of the pericardium and heart, and the quantity of fluid can be accurately estimated. **Thus, a negative echocardiogram ends the imaging workup unless there is strong clinical suspicion of a small loculated effusion** (small loculated effusions may escape detection because of limited sonographic access to certain portions of the pericardium). Echocardiography can also evaluate the heart for tamponade, an indication for urgent pericardiocentesis.

Echocardiography can be a portable, bedside examination and can guide the drainage of effusion for diagnosis and/or therapy. However, dressings and wounds from recent surgery may interfere with positioning of the sonographic transducer on the skin surface; **in such cases, or when small loculated effusions (after surgery or pericarditis) are suspected, CT or MR is appropriate.**

STEP 3: COMPUTED TOMOGRAPHY (CT) OR MAGNETIC RESONANCE (MR) IMAGING

Newer, faster multidetector CT scanners image the heart and pericardium with minimal motion artifact. CT also optimally images the remainder of the chest to evaluate other underlying pulmonary or mediastinal abnormalities. Peripheral intravenous contrast medium is generally administered to create contrast between blood in the cardiac chambers and the myocardium, and, to a lesser extent, between the myocardium and any pericardial fluid.

MR is performed with electrocardiographic "gating" to gather imaging data during selected phases of the cardiac cycle and reduce motion blur of the beating heart. MR generates highly detailed images of the heart and pericardium, but the examination is relatively time consuming and costly compared with sonography, and expertise in cardiac MR is variable. **A pacemaker contraindicates MR.**

SUMMARY AND CONCLUSIONS

1. An initial chest film is appropriate when pericardial effusion is suspected to exclude thoracic conditions that could mimic an effusion and to define or characterize associated conditions such as pulmonary edema. The chest film cannot exclude small effusions, but sizable effusions usually cause enlargement of the cardiac silhouette, which may also assume a characteristic globular (water bottle) appearance. More experienced chest radiologists can sometimes make a firm diagnosis of effusion using specific and rarely-seen signs, such as the "anterior pericardial fat pad sign."
2. Echocardiography is appropriate if there is any clinical or radiographic suspicion of pericardial effusion. It is accurate, noninvasive, quick, and portable. The procedure can localize and quantify pericardial fluid, evaluate for tamponade, and guide subsequent percutaneous drainage for diagnosis and/or therapy if necessary. However, echocardiography can miss small effusions if they are situated in an area that is not accessible to the anterior sonographic beam.
3. When strong clinical suspicion of pericardial effusion remains after a normal echocardiogram, CT or MR is appropriate.

ADDITIONAL COMMENTS

• If the routine echocardiogram is equivocal or technically limited and the patient is too ill for travel to the radiology department for CT or MR, transesophageal echocardiography is an option. This examination is unavailable in many radiology or cardiology departments and requires special expertise. The patient swallows a tiny ultrasound probe attached to a fine wire; when it reaches the retrocardiac esophagus, images produced by emitted sound waves provide an excellent "look" at the posterior cardio/pericardial region; these areas are sometimes difficult to view from the conventional anterior approach.

- With newer imaging techniques, many institutions can now perform CT or MR studies **of cardiac motion** to evaluate **the effects** of pericardial effusion or constrictive pericarditis on cardiac function.

SUGGESTED READING

Lane EJ, Carsky EW: Epicardial fat: lateral plain film analysis in normals and in pericardial effusion. Radiology 1968;91:1–5.

Rienmuller R, Groll R, Lipton MJ: CT and MR imaging of pericardial disease. Radiol Clin North Am 2004;42:587–601.

Rozenstein A, Boxt LM: Plain film diagnosis of pericardial disease. Semin Roentgenol 1999;34:195–204.

Spodick DH: Pericardial diseases. In Braunwald E (ed): Heart Disease: A Textbook of Cardiovascular Medicine, 6th ed. Philadelphia, Saunders, 2001, pp 1823–1876.

Wang ZJ, Reddy GP, Gotway MB, et al: CT and MR imaging of pericardial disease. Radiographics 2003;23:S167–S180.

Part *VII*

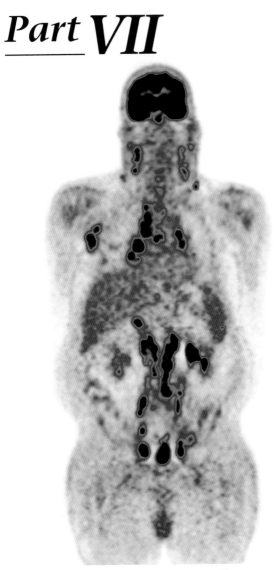

General

59 Occult Bacterial Infection

INTRODUCTION

When clinical or laboratory findings suggest occult bacterial infection, the chest, abdomen, or pelvis is usually the source. Chest radiography is the first imaging procedure. Two additional studies, computed tomography (CT) and autologous radiolabeled leukocyte (white blood cell [WBC]) scanning, may be valuable. Positron emission tomography (PET) with fluorodeoxyglucose (FDG) may have a significant role in the future.

Relative Costs: Chest films, posteroanterior and lateral, **$**; chest, abdominal, and pelvic CT, with contrast medium (enhanced), **$$$$**; nuclear WBC scanning with indium-111-oxine (In-111-oxine) or technetium 99m–hexamethylpropyleneamine oxime (Tc-99m-HMPAO), **$$$$**.

PLAN AND RATIONALE

STEP 1: CHEST RADIOGRAPHY (PLAIN CHEST FILMS)

Inflammatory disease in the chest does not necessarily produce localizing signs. Lack of physical findings or complaints related to the thorax does not exclude pneumonia or other parenchymal, pleural, or mediastinal disease. Chest radiographs (posteroanterior and lateral) are mandatory.

If chest films fail to find a source of infection, CT of the chest, abdomen, and pelvis is appropriate.

STEP 2: COMPUTED TOMOGRAPHY (CT) OF THE CHEST, ABDOMEN, AND PELVIS

Normal chest films exclude major pneumonias, **but mediastinal, hilar, and even significant parenchymal disease can be identified by CT when the chest film is normal;** therefore, although many clinicians are tempted to exclude chest CT in the subsequent workup, we recommend that it be included.

The body is scanned from the thoracic inlet to the pelvic floor. Adequate opacification of the bowel, the urinary tract, and the major blood vessels with appropriate contrast medium is essential.

If CT is even the least bit equivocal, a WBC scan may be helpful.

Even if CT is completely normal, the WBC examination is sometimes ordered, as a last resort, to screen for completely unsuspected infection in the head, neck, and extremities.

STEP 3: NUCLEAR RADIOLABELED AUTOLOGOUS LEUKOCYTE (WBC) SCAN

A WBC scan may clarify an equivocal CT by differentiating fluid-filled bowel from an abscess. Also, **the nuclear examination is a total body survey** that occasionally reveals completely unsuspected lesions in the head, neck, or extremities.

Leukocytes are harvested from 30 mL of the patient's blood and labeled with In-111-oxine or Tc-99m-HMPAO; the cells are injected intravenously and their migration to infected sites is monitored by a nuclear scan. Eighteen to twenty-four hours must elapse between injection of In-111-oxine–labeled WBCs and scanning, but scanning can begin only 2 hours after injection of Tc-99m-HMPAO– labeled WBCs.

In general, Tc-99m-HMPAO WBC scans excel for detecting lesions in the head and extremities, whereas In-111-oxine WBCs are favored for surveying the abdomen, lungs, and thorax, because some Tc-99m-

HMPAO WBCs are normally seen in the lungs, gut, and bladder, confounding scan interpretation. Nonetheless, some nuclear physicians favor early imaging with Tc-99m-HMPAO WBCs for evaluating the abdomen, because of the much briefer interval between injection and scanning. **When a radiolabeled WBC scan is contemplated, the choice of isotope should be discussed with the nuclear physician, so that options can be considered in light of the urgency of the case and probable infection source.**

SUMMARY AND CONCLUSIONS

1. Even without thoracic symptoms, chest films are crucial in the search for occult infection.
2. Most occult infections outside of the thorax are in the abdomen and pelvis; therefore, abdominal/pelvic CT is appropriate after chest radiographs. However, we recommend chest CT as well, **even after normal chest films**.
3. If CT is normal or equivocal, a total body radiolabeled WBC scan can be definitive. The proper radioisotope should be determined in consultation with the nuclear physician.

ADDITIONAL COMMENTS

- Some nuclear imagers believe that a radiolabeled WBC scan is appropriate after the initial chest film, **before chest/abdominal/pelvic CT,** on the grounds that **the WBC study is a total body scan.** Against this argument is the superior anatomic resolution of CT and the fact that a positive abdominal WBC scan is usually followed by CT to provide better anatomic definition before drainage. Thus, the choice of a WBC study versus abdominal CT is controversial; often the two are complementary. Most clinicians turn to CT first, and that, in fact, is our recommendation.

- Upright chest films in the radiology department are almost always superior to portable films, despite the time and inconvenience that they entail for the patient and nursing staff.
- Although CT is favored over ultrasound for a general abdominal survey, in some patients, such as pregnant women and young children, for whom radiation exposure should be severely limited, ultrasound is a reasonable alternative.
- Gallium-67 citrate was formerly used to scan for occult pus collections. It is inferior to labeled WBCs, and its only justifiable use for this purpose would be in patients who are agranulocytic and therefore have no WBCs to label.
- FDG-PET has been striking in osteomyelitis (see **CHAPTER 43, Osteomyelitis**). Although no studies to date have demonstrated that FDG-PET can define areas of infection outside of bone, logic suggests that possibility.

SUGGESTED READING

Kipper SL, Rypins EB, Evans DG, et al: Neutrophil-specific ^{99m}Tc-labeled anti-CD14 monoclonal antibody imaging for diagnosis of equivocal appendicitis. J Nucl Med 2000;41:449–455.

Palestro CJ, Caprioli R, Love C, et al: Rapid diagnosis of pedal osteomyelitis in diabetics with a technetium-99m-labeled monoclonal antigranulocyte antibody. J Foot Ankle Surg 2003;42:2–8.

Palestro CJ, Kipper SL, Weiland FL, et al: Osteomyelitis: diagnosis with ^{99m}Tc-labeled antigranulocyte antibodies compared with diagnosis with ^{111}In-labeled leukocytes—initial experience. Radiology 2002;223:758–764.

Rypins EB, Klipper SL: Scintigraphic determination of equivocal appendicitis. Am Surg 2000;66:891–895.

Percutaneous Guided Biopsy and Imaging-Guided Therapy

INTRODUCTION

Imaging-guided needle biopsy can be used to sample tissue from a wide variety of organs; although the tissue sample harvested is smaller than that of surgical biopsy, percutaneous guided biopsy is usually faster and safer and invariably less expensive. Furthermore, the same guidance methods that can place a needle for tissue biopsy can also place a drainage catheter for fluid collections or a **therapeutic** probe for tissue ablation of select tumors, using ethanol injection, tissue freezing (cryo-ablation), or, more recently, tissue heating by microwave or radiofrequency ablation (RFA). Also, a wide range of diagnostic and therapeutic procedures are available after the fluoroscopically guided percutaneous placement of a catheter into the vascular tree.

Guidance methods include ultrasound (US), computed tomography (CT), magnetic resonance (MR) imaging, and fluoroscopy (for vascular catheter placement).

Relative Costs: Costs vary according to the biopsy site and the guidance method; these relative costs serve as a guide: CT-guided lung biopsy, **$$$–$$$$**; CT-guided liver biopsy, **$$$–$$$$**; CT-guided deep tissue biopsy, pelvis, **$$$$**; US-guided thoracentesis, **$$**; US-guided paracentesis, **$$**; RFA of lung lesion, FDA-approval and Medicare reimbursement pending; RFA of three liver lesions, **$$$$$**; fluoroscopically guided bone biopsy, lumbar spine, **$$$**; chemoembolization of hepatic tumors, **$$$$$$**.

■ PLAN AND RATIONALE

DIAGNOSTIC

Indications

Percutaneous needle biopsy/aspiration is appropriate to (1) determine the histology of an uncharacterized mass, (2) establish whether residual tumor after therapy is viable and whether there is tumor recurrence, and (3) obtain culture material from possibly infected fluids. **The technique is ideal for patients who refuse surgery or are poor surgical risks.**

Guided biopsy is usually **an outpatient procedure** and requires no major patient preparation (only NPO). Contraindications include uncorrectable coagulopathies, a lesion that is inaccessible or inadequately visualized, and an unwillingness or inability to cooperate. **Every potential imaging-guided biopsy MUST be discussed in advance with the interventional radiologist and any prior radiographic examinations made available for review to predetermine the optimal technique and biopsy route.**

Imaging Guidance Methods

Imaging finds the target and guides the needle or catheter. Various techniques apply, depending on the lesion size and type. Although fluoroscopy was formerly used for most percutaneous biopsies of lung lesions, CT is now considered most appropriate for the thorax. CT is also the method of choice for many abdominal and pelvic lesions, particularly those that are small or deep, lie close to vital organs, or are inaccessible to US.

For many abdominal and pelvic lesions, however, US remains the method of choice. In general, US applies best to relatively large, superficial, or cystic lesions; however, some interventional radiologists achieve high diagnostic accuracy for even solid, small, deep abdominal lesions. US guidance is unsuitable for lesions obscured by overlying bowel gas or bone. Endoluminal US with a transvaginal or transrectal probe can guide biopsy in the female pelvis or the prostate.

Many lesions are amenable to fine-needle aspiration with a 20- or 22-gauge needle, but larger-bore needles that harvest a tissue core are frequently appropriate; **the decision in terms of needle type should be left to the interventional radiologist.**

Universally, interventional radiologists believe that they are the appropriate decision makers in terms of guidance method. Nothing will alienate a well-meaning clinician from an expert interventional radiologist faster than a requisition that states, "Pancreatic mass, request ultrasound-guided biopsy." **Therefore: tell the interventional radiologist what you want to find out, and respect his or her opinion as to how it can be done.**

Risks/Complications

In the chest, pneumothorax occurs occasionally but seldom requires a chest tube placed by a thoracic surgeon (interventional radiologists have become expert in placing their own small-bore chest tube under CT or fluoroscopic guidance). The risks of serious hemorrhage and/or infection depend on the type of procedure but are generally very small.

THERAPEUTIC

Indications

The indication for imaging-guided **drainage** is clear: any fluid collection that significantly impairs organ function or patient comfort is a candidate (e.g., pleural effusion that compromises respiration, ascites that causes distention, or pericardial effusion that threatens tamponade). Of course, collections of pus can be drained to promote healing and eliminate a source of sepsis.

However, the indication for **treating** (i.e., ablating or partially ablating) solid tumor is not as clear, partly because, to date, guided ablative techniques are regarded as **palliative procedures**—none are curative. As a general rule, guided therapy is reserved for unresectable lesions, lesions that resist radiotherapy/chemotherapy, lesions in which the maximum doses of radiotherapy/

chemotherapy have already been reached, or lesions in sensitive organs (e.g., the liver) that cannot tolerate the radiation required to ablate tumor. Specific indications for percutaneous guided therapy are expanding. Currently, these include ethanol ablation for unresectable hepatocellular carcinoma, RFA for unresectable liver tumors less than 5 cm in size, including metastases from certain cancers (colorectal, sarcomas, melanoma, breast), and RFA for symptomatic bone metastases. Other lesions likely to be approved for RFA in the future include tumors in the kidney, lung, adrenal gland, and prostate.

A description of the wide range of therapeutic procedures available to the interventional radiologist using vascular access with small-bore catheters is beyond the scope of this chapter but include tumor embolization and chemoembolization, thrombolysis, angioplasty and stent placement, caval filter placement, embolization of bleeding sites and vascular malformations, and placement of central venous catheters for drug administration or dialysis. Nonvascular therapeutic interventions include relief of obstructions in the biliary tree and urinary tract.

Imaging Guidance Methods

For vascular interventions, the catheter is introduced by percutaneous puncture of a peripheral vessel and fluoroscopically guided through the vascular tree to the desired location. The procedure is performed in the angiography suite of a radiology department. Contrast medium is injected intermittently to identify specific vessels. Depending upon the procedure, embolic microspheres, chemotherapeutic agents adsorbed to microspheres, thrombolytic or thrombogenic chemicals, vessel dilators (balloon devices), filters, and stents can be introduced. **Incredibly, virtually any artery in the abdomen or chest can be accessed and catheterized by this technique, leaving only a tiny femoral puncture that heals in a few days.**

Percutaneous guided tumor ablations outside of the liver are usually performed in the US or CT suite. Precise visualization of the lesion is critical to exact positioning of the needle/probe and to avoid injuring adjacent structures. Because RFA probes are disposable, and because expensive machines (e.g., a CT scanner) and personnel are occupied for a prolonged period, the procedure is expensive. Many ablations of hepatic tumor are performed in the operating room as a cooperative venture between radiology and surgery. After exposure of the liver, the US transducer is placed **directly** on the liver surface and target lesions are localized for ablation. US monitors the progress of ethanol ablation, cryotherapy, or RFA.

SUMMARY AND CONCLUSIONS

1. Percutaneous guided biopsy is an accurate, safe, established method for obtaining tissue or culture material from nearly any organ.
2. Guided therapy is a burgeoning field that allows many lesions to be addressed in a minimally invasive manner.
3. An interventional radiologist must be consulted before each procedure to optimize the biopsy route and guidance method.

ADDITIONAL COMMENTS

• MR-guided biopsy is feasible at the present time, but it is uncommon.

SUGGESTED READING

Caspers JM, Reading CC, McGahan JP, Charboneau JW: Ultrasound-guided biopsy and drainage of the abdomen and pelvis. In Rumack CM, Wilson SR, Charboneau JW (eds): Diagnostic Ultrasound. St. Louis, Mosby, 1998, pp 599–628.

Matsumoto AH, ed: Noncardiac Thoracic Interventions. Baltimore, Williams and Wilkins, 1997.

Molina PL, Mauro MA: Interventional computed tomography. In Lee JK, Sagel SS, Stanley RJ, Heiken JP (eds): Computed Body Tomography with MRI Correlation. Philadelphia, Lippincott-Raven, 1998, pp 69–105.

61 PET and PET/CT in Cancer Staging

INTRODUCTION

FDG (fluorodeoxyglucose), a glucose molecule in which one of the hydroxyl groups has been replaced by a radioactive fluorine atom, is the pharmaceutical that has brought positron emission tomography (PET)—once an obscure research tool—into the mainstream. FDG is "seen" and taken up by virtually all body tissues as if it were ordinary, unsubstituted glucose. Because tumors use more glucose than most other tissues (they metabolize and grow faster), the uptake of FDG per gram of tumor is high. Furthermore, most tumors are thought to create high-energy bonds via anaerobic metabolism (glycolysis), which is less efficient than aerobic metabolism (Krebs cycle), and to ensure the glucose supply necessary for this process many malignant cells have more glucose receptors than nonmalignant cells. However, the metabolism of FDG in a cell, malignant or benign, is incomplete; after phosphorylation the metabolic process stops, and FDG remains indefinitely in the cell. Of course, when the radioactive part of the molecule (fluorine 18 [Fl-18]) decays, it is no longer "seen" by the PET camera.

The PET camera works with positron emitters; an emitted positron invariably meets up with a tissue electron, producing an annihilation reaction, in which two 511 MeV photons traveling in opposite directions are released. Many positron emitters have extremely short half-lives, measured in seconds or minutes, and even Fl-18 is relatively short-lived (about 90 minutes).

Relative Cost: PET, **$$$$$**.

FDG-PET AND CANCER STAGING

Computed tomography (CT) remains the mainstay of cancer staging, although a few anatomic areas—notably the brain—are better imaged by magnetic resonance (MR). **Therefore, no rational clinician currently suggests that FDG-PET should replace CT and (selectively) MR in the cancer staging process.**

However, **in addition to** CT and sometimes in addition to MR, Medicare has approved FDG-PET for staging and restaging of the following cancers:

- Non–small-cell lung cancer
- Colorectal cancer
- Melanoma
- Lymphoma (Hodgkin's and non-Hodgkin's)
- Head and neck cancer
- Gastroesophageal cancer
- Certain thyroid cancers
- Re-staging and therapy response of breast cancer
- Evaluation of the solitary pulmonary nodule (see **CHAPTER 21, Solitary Pulmonary Nodule**)

Furthermore, applications for multiple myeloma and aggressive prostate cancer are pending.

WHY FDG-PET IF CT CAN COVER THE BODY FROM THE NECK TO THE PELVIC FLOOR AND MR IS EXCELLENT FOR THE BRAIN?

FDG-PET can identify lesions in the skeleton and sometimes the liver where no mass disease or tissue replacement by tumor appears on CT. Similarly, FDG accumulation in hilar or mediastinal nodes, where CT is equivocal, is often identified by FDG-PET. **The ability to "see" disease that cannot be seen by CT often "upstages" a primary tumor (i.e., changes its stage from early to advanced), drastically altering the therapeutic plan. Thus, appropriate use of PET can avoid unnecessarily aggressive surgery, can direct radiotherapy to sites that were previously** unsuspected, and can bring the medical oncologist into cases that were previously directed only to surgery. These huge effects on outcome are universally thought to justify its high cost.

FDG-PET can identify glucose metabolism in masses that remain after radiotherapy or chemotherapy, indicating living tumor, whereas CT can address only the existence of bulk tissue. Conversely, FDG-PET can establish that post-therapy mass represents only scar, without living tumor. **This ability is critical for re-staging, especially in bulky lymphomas, in which therapy may leave residual bulky scar.**

In some selected masses (e.g., solitary pulmonary nodule [see CHAPTER 21]), the negative predictive value of FDG-PET is sufficient so that low uptake of FDG changes the clinical plan from impending biopsy to observation.

Extensive studies have proven that the response of a tumor to radiation and/or chemotherapy can be better determined by a reduction in FDG uptake than by change in tumor size. This phenomenon differs from simple restaging, in which the status of a cancer is determined after a course of therapy is complete or well under way. The subtle change in FDG uptake referred to here is intended to guide chemotherapy by establishing early in the treatment course whether the administered drugs are working.

PET is a whole body, multiorgan, multisystem examination. No other single modality can generate such a global view of neoplastic disease (Fig. 61-1).

SUMMARY AND CONCLUSIONS

1. FDG-PET is a technology whose time has come. The current generation of new scanners produces clear, interpretable images that dramatically reveal areas of enhanced glucose metabolism.

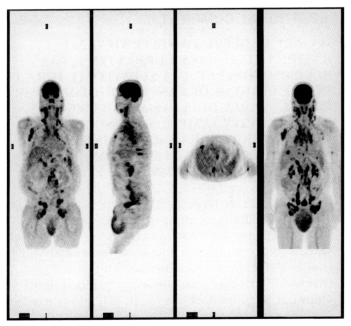

Figure 61-1. PET images of a patient with widespread lymphoma. Brain glucose utilization and excretion into the kidneys are normal; however, all other dark areas represent glucose-avid tumor: neck, axillae, mediastinum, hila, liver, spleen, and nodal chains in the abdomen and iliofemoral and inguinal regions.

2. Tumors should first be carefully staged by conventional methods, usually with CT and sometimes MR imaging of the brain.
3. For the approved tumors, unless stage IV disease is proven and further information on tumor sites would not affect outcome, **STAGING IS INCOMPLETE WITHOUT FDG-PET.**
4. Restaging with FDG-PET is particularly important in lymphomas and is proving useful in many other tumor types.
5. In the near future, quantitation of FDG uptake very likely will guide chemotherapy, in terms of determining efficacy early in the treatment course.

ADDITIONAL COMMENTS

- **WE ARE CAREFUL TO STATE THAT NO RATIONAL CLINICIAN CURRENTLY RECOMMENDS PET AS A SUBSTITUTE FOR CT IN THE STAGING OF CANCER, BUT FOR SOME PARTICULARLY GLUCOSE-AVID TUMORS, PARTICULARLY LYMPHOMA, ONCOLOGISTS ARE ON THE VERGE OF RESTAGING AFTER CHEMOTHERAPY WITH PET ALONE. HOW THIS PRACTICE PATTERN WILL EVOLVE IS UNKNOWN.**

- In this chapter we have stated that MR is primarily an anatomic modality, defining masses and addressing their vascularity and "contrast enhancement." For the sake of completeness, we note that "functional MRI" (fMRI) is an extremely sophisticated methodology that can interrogate tissue to define its blood flow almost at the microscopic level, its pH, and when coupled with MR spectroscopy (MRS) even its "signature" in terms of chemical makeup. However, this process is in its infancy and has only limited applications in current clinical oncology.

- Because FDG is the only radiopharmaceutical for PET approved by the U.S. Food and Drug Administration (FDA), the term "FDG-PET" has become synonymous—especially among clinicians—with "PET," but we recommend that each PET examination be called exactly what it is; thus, "FDG-PET" should be called "FDG-PET" rather than simply "PET." This recommendation is not for the sake of nitpicking; rather, it is motivated by recent advances in the chemistry of "molecular imaging." **New molecules labeled with Fl-18 will soon be available** (e.g., fluorinated thymidine [FLT]). **The uptake of FLT by a cell mirrors its DNA synthesis,** and the effect of chemotherapy can be more sensitively monitored by uptake of FLT (by FLT-PET) than by assessing change in tumor size (by CT) **or even glucose uptake** (by FDG-PET). Other, powerful radionuclide molecular probes are under development, including a compound labeled with copper 60 (Cu-60) that adheres only to hypoxic tissue (the most chemotherapy- and radiotherapy-resistant portion of a tumor, which is most likely to regrow and therefore merits a "boosted" radiation dose). **Thus, multiple types of PET scans will be available within 5 years, and precise terminology now will avoid confusion later. FDG-PET is only the tip of the iceberg, and the future of PET will be no less than explosive.**

- It is fair to say of PET what the late Frank Sinatra had engraved on his tombstone: **The Best Is Yet to Come.**

PET/CT

As FDG-PET established itself as a valid and useful technology for cancer staging and restaging, imagers realized that correlation of the physiologic images of FDG-PET and the anatomic images of CT was invaluable. Although side-by-side comparison is relatively effective, "fusion" programs—which place CT scans on top of PET images—were devised to match up physiologic changes with precise anatomic locations. Unfortunately, these overlay methods are usually degraded by poor matching (misregistration), because (1) the PET images are produced on one machine and the CT studies on another; (2) CT scans are created during a breath-hold, whereas PET scans are generated during quiet breathing; and (3) the position of the arms is different for the two studies (PET: arms down, CT: arms up). Voila! The solution of human ingenuity has been the dual scanner, **which combines a PET unit and a CT scanner in one machine—the "PET/CT."**

There is little doubt that images from a combined PET/CT are superior in terms of matching physiologic change to anatomic site. This superiority is manifested primarily by the increased ease of interpretation and the elimination of multiple viewings and re-viewings of comparative CT scans; moreover, some authors have reported that greater than 15% of the time PET/CT studies result in significantly different reports than separate, carefully compared PET and CT examinations, **and that these better interpretations usually change patient management.** However, there simply have not been a large number of rigorous analyses that show, one way or another, whether studies from dual PET/CT machines actually have a demonstrable effect upon the outcome of malignant disease. Indubitably, physician time and **sometimes** patient time can be saved, and in an era of human and mechanical overload this advantage should not be minimized.

Notwithstanding the above, we should emphasize that the CT that accompanies PET, generated on a dual PET/CT machine, **IS USUALLY NOT EQUIVALENT TO A FULLY DIAGNOSTIC CT AND DOES NOT SUBSTITUTE FOR THE USUAL DIAGNOSTIC CT IN THE CANCER WORKUP!!!** The reason for this apparent contradiction is that a fully diagnostic CT in oncology involves **both intravenous and oral contrast medium** (see **INTRODUCTION** to this book), whereas the CT that accompanies a PET in a PET/CT unit **usually involves neither or, in some centers, involves only dilute oral contrast medium.** (Standard doses of CT contrast medium are avoided, because they can create artifacts that interfere with accurate PET interpretation.)

SUMMARY AND CONCLUSIONS

1. PET/CT is a useful technology that makes correlation of PET and CT images better and easier to display and understand.
2. The CT that accompanies a PET in a PET/CT machine usually DOES NOT substitute for a fully diagnostic CT in the cancer workup.

ADDITIONAL COMMENTS

- For the sake of completeness we should mention that a few large medical centers are working diligently to integrate their nuclear medicine and diagnostic radiology divisions, so that a PET/CT study is **followed** by a fully diagnostic CT **while the patient is on the same table,** but these centers are few and far between. If in doubt about the practice in a particular hospital or imaging center, the clinician should ask the radiologist.
- PET/CT has been dubbed "molecular imaging" by various groups that are affiliated with hardware manufacturers; in fact, PET/CT is no more "molecular imaging" than standard PET or, for that matter, than some of the receptor-based studies (e.g., somatostatin receptor imaging or "Octreoscan") of conventional nuclear medicine. Any representation to the contrary is just so much hype.

SUGGESTED READING

Beyer T, Townsend DW, Brun T, et al: A combined PET/CT scanner for clinical oncology. J Nucl Med 2000;41:1369–1379.

Czernin J, Dahlbom M, Ratib O, Schiepers C: Atlas of PET/CT Imaging in Oncology. Berlin, Springer, 2004.

Phelps ME: PET: the merging of biology and imaging into molecular imaging. J Nucl Med 2000;41:661–681.

62 Screening for Colon Cancer and Lung Cancer and "Total Body" Screening with Multidetector CT

COLON CANCER

"Polyp detection is cancer prevention," and, without any doubt, in competent hands conventional endoscopic colonoscopy is the most sensitive and specific method of detecting premalignant polyps when they are resectable and thus curable. However, trained colonoscopists are in short supply, and as greater numbers of people seek screening colonoscopy, waiting periods have increased, and in some areas of the United States the examination is simply not available.

The number of deaths from colon cancer (more women die from this disease than from breast cancer!) has prompted various organizations to suggest alternatives that can be widely applied by less highly trained care-givers, such as sigmoidoscopy **and** testing for occult stool blood. We do **NOT** recommend this approach, because examining the sigmoid only is like doing a mammogram of one breast, and because by the time a colon lesion bleeds it is often advanced. In this context, and in view of the dread that conventional colonoscopy creates in many people, computed tomography (CT)–based "virtual colonoscopy" merits further discussion.

Virtual colonoscopy is simply a high-speed CT of the abdomen and pelvis after air has been insufflated per rectum. The distended colon can then be examined in conventional cross-sectional views, or the study can be computer-reconstructed so that the colon is seen **from**

414

the inside, as through an actual endoscope. Rapid viewing in this mode is termed "fly through."

Although many studies have indicated that "virtual colonoscopy" is slightly less sensitive than the conventional procedure, **it is also clear that as technology improves the two examinations are becoming almost equivalent diagnostically.** Clinicians need to know the following:

- The preparation for both examinations is the same, so patients cannot avoid aggressive colon cleansing by requesting the "virtual" examination. In fact, many patients (this author included) feel that the bowel preparation is the worst part of the examination.

- Although the conventional procedure is usually performed under "conscious sedation," only minimal sedation is required for the "virtual" examination, because the conventional procedure requires a scope passed from the anus to the cecum, whereas the virtual examination requires only a short rectal tube through which air is introduced, followed by a rapid abdominal CT. Nonetheless, the virtual examination is uncomfortable, and the necessary expulsion of gas per rectum after both procedures is universally considered embarrassing.

- Very rare complications of the conventional examination include colon perforation, contusion of the spleen, intramural bowel hematoma, and death from any of these. **The "virtual" examination is essentially free of complication.**

- Because of conscious sedation, the patient must be escorted home and cannot drive after conventional colonoscopy. **After a "virtual" examination the patient is awake and alert.**

- The biggest disadvantage of the "virtual" examination is that it is diagnostic only; therefore, if a suspicious lesion is defined, the patient must undergo conventional colonoscopy for biopsy/removal.

Overall, because there is a huge shortage of trained colonoscopists, we predict that the "virtual examination" will become commonplace, simply because it is a practical approach to addressing the currently neglected massive public health problem of colon screening. However, until government agencies and third-party payers are convinced of this logic, reimbursement is confined to two very limited circumstances: (1) patient with a constricting lesion that prevents passage of a scope, when the gastroenterologist or surgeon needs to "see" what is on the other side (air will pass through almost any opening, however narrow); and (2) patient with comorbid conditions that prevent conscious sedation.

LUNG CANCER

The paradigm for colon cancer and breast cancer is **find it small or before it is cancerous, remove it, and you have cured it.** Therefore, it was inevitable that when CT evolved to the point that it could reliably define tiny lesions—2 to 3 mm in diameter—at the border zone of detectability by even a high-quality chest x-ray, investigators would postulate that CT screening of a high-risk population (long-term smokers older than 50 to 55 years of age) would be appropriate and that follow-up of the screened population would show an improvement in survivability after detection and removal of small lung malignancies.

This paradigm has generated intense controversy that is beyond the scope of this book, but the essence of the issue is that although **small lung cancers can be defined by screening CT,** several complex biases influence the interpretation of screening/outcomes data; for example, a patient whose tiny cancer was discovered by CT may survive for more months between his or her CT and death than a patient whose lung cancer was discovered later in its course, but that does not prove that the patient has actually lived longer than he or she would have if he or she had not undergone the CT; **longer life after diagnosis does not necessarily equate to longer life.**

To address these issues, the American College of Radiology, through the American College of Radiology Imaging Network (ACRIN), has initiated a large, controlled, blinded study to asses the value of CT lung cancer screening in older patients with a multi–pack-year smoking history, using the only outcome that is valid— **patient mortality.** The conclusion of this ACRIN study is several years away, and, until that time, **we cannot recommend the procedure for asymptomatic persons.**

■ "TOTAL BODY" COMPUTED TOMOGRAPHY (CT) SCREENING

State-of-the-art (16- to 64-slice) CT equipment can scan an adult, head to foot, in less than 30 seconds. Therefore: why is total body screening seldom practiced, and why is it considered unethical in most practices?

All imaging screens target selected populations in whom the prevalence of disease is increased compared to the general population, and the technique of each screening test is highly specialized. Thus:

- Mammography targets women older than 40 years of age or younger women with first-order relatives who have developed breast cancer or are genetically predisposed to the disease, **and mammography produces breast images of far higher spatial resolution than that of the best total body CT.**
- MR angiography (MRA) or CT angiography (CTA) screens cerebral vessels of first-order relatives of persons proven to have a cerebral aneurysm or an arteriovenous malformation, and the contrast medium required must be injected according to specific protocols.
- Virtual colonoscopy targets adults older than 50 years of age, the colon must be prepared (just as for conventional colonoscopy), and air must be introduced per rectum, as in the classic air-contrast barium enema.
- Screening chest CT targets long-term smokers older than 50 to 55 years of age.
- Chest CT for coronary artery calcium scoring targets those older than 45 at intermediate or high risk for coronary artery disease according to Framingham

criteria, and special cardiac software is necessary to eliminate motion blur and correctly calculate calcium scores.

Thus, **you could scan a person from head to foot and miss a significant breast cancer, a large colon cancer, or a cerebral aneurysm and be unable to quantitate coronary artery calcium.** Moreover, total body CT screens of the general population, in whom the prevalence of disease is low, are a colossal waste of valuable resources **that should be directed toward populations who are more likely to benefit.** And the examinations increase radiation exposure to little end.

Conclusion: If you want to reduce your chances of dying from breast cancer, be screened with mammograms, at the appropriate age. If you have a first-order relative who has had an arteriovenous malformation or cerebral aneurysm, have your cerebral vasculature imaged (CTA or MRA, as the neuroradiologist prefers). If you don't want to develop colon cancer, undergo colonoscopy at the appropriate age. If you don't want to die from non–small cell lung cancer, **QUIT SMOKING** (or don't start to begin with). If you are older than 40 years of age, have your coronary risk assessed by the Framingham criteria (possibly followed by CT calcium scoring).

But, if you just don't want to die at all, and think that total body CT is the answer—well, you are out of luck.

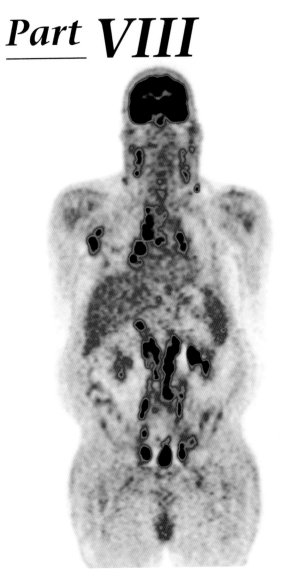

Part VIII

Breast

Breast Imaging

INTRODUCTION

The most common cancer among American women is breast cancer. In the United States more than 200,000 cases will be diagnosed in 2005, with more than 40,000 deaths. Breast cancer is the second highest cause of cancer death among American women, behind only lung cancer, and it is the leading cause of cancer death in American women between 20 and 59 years of age.

In the United States, the lifetime risk of developing breast cancer is now 1 in 8 and has been rising steadily for the past 25 years. Amidst these frightening statistics, good news is that the **mortality rate** (death per diagnosed case) has **decreased,** largely due to screening mammography. **The key to continued reduction in breast cancer mortality is early detection.**

No single method is 100% effective for detecting breast cancer; mammography detects 85% to 90% of breast cancers and is the only imaging modality that has been proven to reduce mortality from this disease. **Screening mammography decreases the death rate from breast cancer by 25% to 30%.**

The cause of breast cancer remains unknown. Major risk factors include (1) strong family history or genetic predisposition; (2) history of prior breast biopsy revealing atypical ductal hyperplasia, lobular carcinoma in situ, or atypical lobular hyperplasia; and (3) thoracic radiation. **However, most breast cancer develops in women with no identifiable risk factors.**

Mammography is applied in two distinct ways: "screening" and "diagnostic." Screening mam-

mography refers to the imaging of asymptomatic women to detect early, clinically occult breast cancers—that is, "I don't have any known problem, but it is time for my annual mammogram." **Diagnostic mammography** is the workup of a patient with clinical and/or radiographic symptoms/signs (palpable lump or thickening, nipple discharge, or further evaluation of an abnormality found on a screening mammogram)—that is, "I and/or my doctor feel and/or see a problem; what is it?"

Diagnostic mammography is perhaps better termed **"diagnostic breast imaging,"** because it often includes other imaging modalities such as ultrasound (US), magnetic resonance (MR) imaging, or galactography.

What the clinician needs to know about the "MAMMOGRAPHY QUALITY STANDARDS ACT" (MQSA) and "BREAST IMAGING REPORTING AND DATA SYSTEM" (BI-RADS):

MQSA: The Mammography Quality Standards Act of the United States Congress (1992) established regulations that **every** mammography facility (however small, however rural) and every interpreting radiologist (generalist or subspecialty-trained) must follow, with final regulations effective April 28, 1999. Under these regulations inspectors annually review each facilities' equipment, practices, and personnel (radiologists, consulting physicist, and technologists) qualifications. A passed inspection confers certification by the U.S. Food and Drug Administration (FDA), without which a radiologist **CANNOT** legally perform mammography in the United States.

BI-RADS: BI-RADS is a lexicon and reporting format for mammography developed by a panel of experts under the auspices of the American College of Radiology. The goal of the panel was to standardize the widely disparate and sometimes confusing language then current in mammographic reports. **It established a list of final assessment categories to clearly define the disposition of the patient based upon mammographic findings (i.e., what the clinician should do and what the patient needs).**

The final assessment categories are as follows:

- Category 1—negative (i.e., normal)
- Category 2—benign finding(s)
- Category 3—probably benign finding; short-interval follow-up suggested (a finding in this category should have less than a 2% risk of malignancy based on morphologic features and distribution)
- Category 4—suspicious abnormality; biopsy should be considered
- Category 5—highly suggestive of malignancy; appropriate action should be taken (a finding in this category is almost certainly malignant)
- Category 6—known biopsy-proven malignancy; appropriate action should be taken
- Category 0—need additional imaging evaluation

MQSA **MANDATES** that all mammography reports designate a final assessment category.

Relative Costs: Screening mammogram, bilateral, **$**; computer-aided detection, **.3$**; diagnostic mammogram, **$**; breast US, **$**; breast cyst aspiration, **$$**; preoperative wire localization, **$$**; galactography, **$$$**; fine-needle aspiration biopsy, **$$**; stereotactic guided core biopsy, **$$$$**; US-guided core biopsy, **$$$**; breast MR, **$$$$**; open excisional biopsy, **$$$$$**.

SCREENING MAMMOGRAPHY

PHYSICIAN AWARENESS

Because 75% of breast cancers occur in women without a known risk factor, screening mammography is recommended for all women according to age-determined guidelines. These guidelines are periodically debated and revised. **Currently, the American Cancer Society, American College of Radiology, National Comprehensive Cancer Network, American Medical Association, and the Society of Breast Imaging recommend annual mammography for the general female population beginning at age 40. Screening mammography should begin in women younger than age 40:**

- whose first-degree relative (mother, sister) has had breast cancer: begin screening mammography 10 years before the age when the relative was diagnosed, but not before age 25
- with a history of mantle radiation to the chest (i.e., for Hodgkin's disease): begin screening 8 to 10 years after radiation therapy
- with a genetic mutation for breast cancer: begin screening mammography at age 25
- with a biopsy diagnosis of atypical hyperplasia or lobular carcinoma in situ: begin yearly screening from the time of diagnosis

PATIENT AWARENESS

Women avoid annual mammography for many reasons: fear of the disease, a belief that compression views are unbearably painful, the myth that radiation from the mammogram might induce a breast cancer, and a belief (based in denial) that if they have no breast symptoms, mammography is unnecessary.

To achieve a practical result, education regarding mammography must address these issues:
- The goal of screening is to detect early, clinically **occult** breast cancers when they are likely curable and **treatable by lumpectomy (as opposed to more radical, disfiguring surgery)**.
- Most women experience tolerable discomfort (**not** pain) during the few moments of necessary compression.
- From a radiation standpoint mammography is, in fact, quite safe.

Regarding compression views, the clinician should know that **the discomfort can be minimized by scheduling mammography immediately after menstruation.** In terms of radiation safety: Extrapolation based upon induced breast cancer in populations that had received extremely high radiation doses—atomic bomb survivors, patients radiated for benign breast disease in the past, and patients who spent months to years in tuberculosis sanitariums and repeatedly underwent fluoroscopy to assess their pulmonary disease and received doses many orders of magnitude higher than those of modern mammography (100 to 1000 rads versus 0.3 to 0.4 rads)—proves that mammography is associated with a negligible risk.

THE LOGISTICS OF MAMMOGRAPHY: WHAT THE PATIENT *AND* CLINICIAN NEED TO KNOW

The "Call Back" Phenomenon: In some facilities each mammogram is interpreted **while the patient is waiting,** and if additional imaging is required it can be performed immediately. At other centers the mammogram is interpreted **after the patient has left the facility;** in these centers, patients are then contacted to return if further imaging is necessary. Typically, less than 10% of patients are called back. **A need for additional imaging does not necessarily mean that a highly suspicious lesion has been identified.** In fact, initial findings that are clarified by additional views often turn out to represent overlap of normal structure (glandular tissue). **Therefore, to avoid excess anxiety, patients should be alerted in advance to the possibility that they may be asked to return for additional views.** (At this point the alert clinician may wonder why a patient is **ever** allowed to leave a mammography facility before her mammograms are read, thus avoiding the entire "call back" scenario. The answer is logistical, operational, and financial: "Batch reading" at the end of the day is far more efficient [and possibly more accurate] than one-at-a-time mammographic interpretation while each patient waits.)

PROVIDING "OUTSIDE" FILMS FOR COMPARISON

Internal breast anatomy varies enormously, so comparison to a prior baseline is invaluable. **The clinician should therefore emphasize to the patient that prior mammograms are extremely important for comparison and that if she has had previous**

mammograms elsewhere, she should make them available to the radiologist, preferably at the time of her appointment.

The screening mammogram report assigns a BI-RADS assessment category. If the mammogram has been interpreted after the patient has left, the final assessment will typically be:

- BI-RADS 1or 2—the patient continues routine screening
- BI-RADS 0—the patient is called back for a diagnostic imaging workup of the possible abnormality

SUMMARY AND CONCLUSIONS

1. The clinician's role is to ensure that the screening study is performed, to be aware of the radiologist's interpretation and recommendation, and to act on this recommendation.

2. Patient education is key in the battle against breast cancer, on a par with elimination of tobacco in the battle against lung cancer and the implementation of screening colonoscopy to prevent colon cancer. The wise clinician does not depend upon "the government"; **personal involvement in terms of specific recommendations for screening, explaining the safety of mammography, the need for old films for comparison, and dispelling myths about pain is key.**

3. Awareness by both the clinician and the patient of mammography logistics—especially the "call back" phenomenon—will reduce anxiety and create mutual understanding that fosters better care.

ADDITIONAL COMMENTS

- Women with breast augmentation are at the same risk for breast cancer as the general population.

However, implants—especially retroglandular rather than subpectoral—can sometimes compromise mammography.

- Women with implants should be screened according to the same guidelines as those without implants.
- Mammography for women with implants includes both conventional and extra "displaced Eklund views." Thus, a typical mammogram for a woman with implants requires **a total of eight images instead of the standard four.** Before implantation, a patient should be informed that her mammogram will involve these additional views, and the clinician should be aware that a more complex examination is involved.
- Mammographic **c**omputer **a**ided **d**etection (CAD) is a technology that electronically calls attention to an area (or areas) of concern that otherwise might have been missed by the radiologist. CAD cannot differentiate benign from malignant tissue but simply identifies areas that the radiologist then evaluates.
- "Digital mammography" is analogous to digital photography; the image is electronically stored and therefore can be computer-manipulated to improve its quality at any time, without recalling the patient. **Initial studies have shown no difference in the cancer detection rate between digital and conventional mammography;** however, some studies have suggested that the call back rate is lowered with digital methodology, as one might expect. **Digital mammography is significantly more expensive than conventional film mammography.** A large prospective multicenter trial compared conventional and digital mammography in a **screening** population. Overall, there was no difference in accuracy; however digital mammography was more sensitive than conventional for detecting breast cancers in the following subgroups:
  1. women less than 50 years of age
  2. radiographically dense breasts
  3. pre- or perimenopausal

Nonetheless, we emphasize that the skill and experience of the mammographer trumps the advantages of digital technique, and we recommend against selecting a breast imaging center on the basis of digital technique alone. (Too often, installation of the "latest and greatest" technology is used in medicine as a marketing tool.)

DIAGNOSTIC MAMMOGRAPHY

Elsewhere this book describes the most cost-effective and rapid imaging workup in terms of steps that the clinician should follow, because the clinician is generally responsible for ordering tests. **Breast imaging is different: once a diagnostic mammogram has been requested, the mammographer is obliged to proceed to a diagnostic conclusion, without necessarily consulting the clinician each step of the way.** Nonetheless, we list the steps that occur in the mammographer's thought process, so that a clinician can be well informed and better able to communicate intelligently with the patient. The steps differ radically depending on the clinical presentation and/or findings on an initial study.

(A) EQUIVOCAL OR SUSPICIOUS SCREENING MAMMOGRAM

STEP 1: FURTHER MAMMOGRAPHIC EVALUATION

After a screening mammogram a few patients require further mammographic evaluation, including "spot compression" and sometimes rotated/angled and/or magnification views to determine whether a lesion is truly present and, if so, to clarify its location and characteristics. Sometimes US is also used to determine if a mass is a cyst. **Most breast imaging centers contact the patient directly** to arrange these additional studies during a "call back" visit; others do the additional diagnostic workup at the time of the original screening examination.

The diagnostic evaluation report assigns a BI-RADS final assessment category:

- BI-RADS 1 or 2—return to routine screening mammography
- BI-RADS 3—short interval follow-up (usually 6 months)
- BI-RADS 4 or 5—biopsy is recommended (see **Interventional Procedures** below)

(B) A PALPABLE ABNORMALITY

STEP 1: PHYSICAL EXAMINATION BY THE MAMMOGRAPHER

Clinicians are sometimes surprised to learn that mammographers must be expert in physical examination of the breast; the examination characterizes the location and approximate size of the abnormality.

STEP 2: IMAGING EVALUATION TAILORED TO THE PATIENT'S AGE

Patient Younger Than 30 Years of Age
US is first, to determine whether the palpable lump is a simple cyst.

If the lump is a simple cyst, the workup is complete, no intervention is required, and the woman follows routine screening mammography guidelines.

If the palpable lump is symptomatic, or if US demonstrates a complex cyst (a mass that on US is suggestive of but not fully diagnostic of a cyst), US-guided cyst aspiration follows. Unless the mass is completely resolved—both clinically and sonographically—by the aspiration, the fluid is sent for cytologic evaluation. (Cysts that are completely resolved by aspiration can be safely disregarded.)

If the mass is sonographically solid, further evaluation is required. Depending upon sonographic characteristics, further evaluation may include mammography, fine-needle aspiration biopsy (FNAB), core biopsy, excision, or short-interval follow-up. (In modern radiologic practice, the decision is made by the mammographer, in consultation with a surgeon if excision is contemplated.)

Patient 30 Years of Age and Older
A mammogram is first.

If the mammogram is negative or suggests that the mass is a cyst, US is appropriate. The workup then follows the guidelines above for the patient younger than 30 years of age.

The false negative rate of mammography is 10% to 15%, typically due to noncalcified cancers obscured by fibroglandular tissue. Therefore, a false negative mammogram is more likely to occur in the setting of dense breast tissue. (The mammographic report should make a statement concerning breast density.) **The mammographer and clinicians should inform the patient who has a palpable abnormality and a normal mammogram that the breast requires further evaluation with US and possibly a biopsy.**

(C) NIPPLE DISCHARGE

Nipple discharge is the third most common clinical breast complaint after palpable lumps and pain.

STEP 1: CHARACTERIZE THE DISCHARGE

Discharge is considered worrisome if it is from a single duct opening at the nipple and is spontaneous. Clinically suspicious discharge may be any color, but **serous or sero-sanguinous is most suspicious.**

The differential diagnosis for patients with bilateral spontaneous milky discharge (galactorrhea) includes pregnancy and an endocrine abnormality. Patients who have bilateral expressed multiduct discharge should be instructed to stop expressing and should undergo routine screening mammography.

For clinically suspicious discharge:

STEP 2: MAMMOGRAM

If the study reveals a suspicious abnormality, biopsy is appropriate. The mammographer decides upon the guidance method.

If the mammogram reveals no suspicious lesion, and the interpretation is BI-RADS 1, 2, or 3, a ductogram is indicated to see tiny lesions within the duct that have not produced a significant mammographic finding.

STEP 3: DUCTOGRAM

A ductogram is used to localize an intraductal lesion that may require biopsy.

The procedure involves cannulating the discharging duct, injecting a very small amount of radiographic contrast medium, then performing special (magnified) mammographic images. A "filling defect" (i.e., an area within the duct that is filled by a lesion and therefore not by contrast medium) or an abrupt "cut-off" of a visualized duct by an obstruction indicates a lesion. The differential diagnosis includes ductal carcinoma in situ (DCIS) and benign papilloma; differentiating between these requires biopsy. For a successful ductogram the patient must have discharge at the time of the examination, because the duct that requires cannulation is identified by expressing discharge. If the cause of the discharge is DCIS, the ductogram can be helpful in defining the extent of disease for surgical planning.

(D) BREAST PAIN

Breast pain is generally **not** a symptom of breast cancer; it is often the result of diffuse fibrocystic changes and/or hormonal influences, and **when it is diffuse**—without erythema or swelling—imaging with mammography or US is typically **not** useful.

LOCALIZED breast pain:

STEP 1: MAMMOGRAM AND/OR ULTRASOUND (US)

Either modality can sometimes define a cause of localized pain—such as a distended cyst. US-guided drainage may provide relief.

Mastitis or suspected abscess:

STEP 1: ULTRASOUND (US)

In the setting of a painful, swollen, and erythematous breast, US can detect an abscess and guide drainage.

STEP 2: MAMMOGRAPHY

Mammography is often not tolerated by patients with an acute mastitis (the breast is too tender for proper positioning).

However, if the patient does not respond to antibiotic therapy, an inflammatory breast carcinoma MUST be excluded, and mammography should be performed to rule out an underlying malignancy.

If a lesion is identified, biopsy is appropriate.

If the final assessment category for the mammogram is BI-RADS 1, 2, or 3, then skin biopsy should be considered.

(E) SUSPECTED IMPLANT(S) RUPTURE

After an implant is placed a fibrous capsule forms around it.

Intracapsular rupture is a disruption of the **implant shell** with silicone confined within the fibrous capsule.

Extracapsular rupture is a penetration of silicone **outside of the fibrous shell.**

Although mammograms can detect silicone droplets and granulomas secondary to extracapsular rupture, mammography does not define the internal structure of a silicone implant. US and MR are better able to detect subtle intracapsular rupture. Although most agree that removal of implants is indicated in the setting of extracapsular rupture, the best treatment for intracapsular rupture is unclear.

When a **saline implant** develops a tear within the shell there is a quick loss of the saline and decompression of the implant. Therefore, rupture of a saline implant is typically a clinical diagnosis.

Note that the chief indication for mammography in women with breast implants is to screen for breast cancer.

(F) MALE PATIENT WITH A PALPABLE MASS

Male breast cancer represents 1% of all breast cancers.

STEP 1: MAMMOGRAM, BILATERAL

Gynecomastia, a benign condition that presents as a clinical mass, often has a characteristic appearance on mammography.

The mammographic features of breast cancer in men are similar to those seen in women—typically a visible mass, sometimes associated with characteristically malignant calcifications.

STEP 2: ULTRASOUND (US)

US of the palpable mass can often characterize the lesion.

STEP 3: BIOPSY

The mammographer selects the guidance method. If a lesion is detected, biopsy is indicated.

INTERVENTIONAL PROCEDURES

Although mammography is a sensitive tool for the detection of breast masses, it is not highly specific. A biopsy is often required to determine whether a lesion is benign or malignant. Most biopsies can be performed percutaneously, with a special needle, guided by US or stereotactic x-ray. **The type of procedure indicated is determined by the mammographer and the procedure is performed by the mammographer.**

"Needle localization" is required before surgical excision when a mammogram or US defines a lesion that is not palpable (a commonplace event).

Guided Biopsy: FNAB uses a thin (20- to 25-gauge) needle to harvest **cellular material** for cytology. The advantages of FNAB include minimal trauma to the breast and relatively low cost. However, a significant disadvantage is that "nondiagnostic" specimen rates are significant. Also, the specimens provided by FNAB usually cannot differentiate invasive carcinoma from DCIS.

Core biopsy with an automated biopsy gun or a vacuum-assisted biopsy device provides **tissue** for **histologic** assessment rather than **cytologic** evaluation; this material is much more diagnostic than cellular material from FNAB. Core biopsy has a **low false negative rate,** approximately 2.8% (range, 0.6% to 8.2%).

Multiple studies have shown that imaging-guided core biopsy, compared with surgical biopsy, **substantially lowers the cost of diagnosis.**

- Stereotactic 14-gauge automated core biopsy can avoid a surgical biopsy in 76% to 81% of lesions, with an estimated 40% to 58% reduction in cost.
- Vacuum-assisted biopsy devices are more expensive but nonetheless remain cost-effective. One study that compared the cost of diagnosis with an 11-gauge vacuum-assisted biopsy device to that of surgery demonstrated that surgical biopsy was avoided in 75% of lesions, with a 20% reduction in the cost of diagnosis.
- US guidance, when feasible, further reduces the cost of diagnosis. One study that reviewed US-guided 14-gauge automated core biopsy found that surgical

biopsy was avoided in 85% cases, with a 56% decrease in the cost of diagnosis.

Percutaneous imaging–guided core biopsies have other advantages over surgical biopsy. The procedure is faster. A smaller amount of breast tissue is removed, so there is no breast deformity. Minimal (or no) scarring is seen on future mammograms. Recovery and healing are much faster, and **only local anesthesia is required, without "conscious sedation."**

Needle Localization: Surgical excision of a non-palpable mammographic or sonographic abnormality must be preceded by "needle localization." On the day of surgery, the patient reports to the mammographer, who inserts a needle into the lesion using mammographic or US guidance. Once the location of the needle is confirmed, a thin "hook wire" is released into the breast, and the needle is withdrawn; **this fine wire remains in the breast.** The surgeon is guided to the abnormality by this wire and by the final x-rays that show the wire in place, adjacent to or within the lesion. Specimen radiography or sonography **after the excision** is performed to confirm that the lesion has been removed.

Magnetic Resonance (MR) Imaging: MR of the breast is an adjunct to conventional breast imaging—not a replacement for mammography or US.

Breast MR requires a peripheral intravenous injection of gadolinium-based contrast medium; the "enhancement" of breast lesions after contrast medium injection markedly improves detection of lesions (i.e., they are more conspicuous). In the jargon of neuroradiologists, they have "increased conspicuity." ("Enhancement" is a complex function of lesion vascularity, perfusion, blood volume, and capillary permeability.)

Breast MR can detect breast cancers missed by conventional imaging modalities. Its sensitivity approaches 100% for invasive carcinoma, but like standard x-ray mammography, it is not highly specific. **Therefore, breast MR should be performed only in a facility that has the capability to biopsy lesions seen only by MR—that is, the capability for MR-guided biopsy.**

Current diagnostic indications for breast MR are as follows:

- Evaluation of disease extent in the patient with a known diagnosis of breast cancer
- Evaluation for residual disease after breast conservation therapy
- Differentiating scar from recurrence after breast conservation therapy
- Detecting occult primaries in patients presenting with axillary metastasis and normal conventional imaging (mammography and US)
- Follow-up after neoadjuvant chemotherapy
- Further evaluation when physical examination, mammography, and US are equivocal

Because of its high cost, relatively low specificity, and slow speed, breast MR as a general screening tool is neither practical nor recommended, but it has a potential adjunct role in the screening of women at high risk for breast cancer.

SUMMARY AND CONCLUSIONS

1. Diagnostic breast imaging is the workup of a symptomatic patient or the patient with an abnormal screening mammogram. **This workup is typically guided by the breast imager (mammographer)** and may involve additional mammographic views, US, percutaneous biopsy, and MR.
2. US is an essential tool in diagnostic breast imaging.
3. Percutaneous needle biopsy, guided by US or stereotactic x-ray, is the preferred method of biopsy of a nonpalpable abnormality. The choice of guidance method for a palpable abnormality varies and is selected on a case-by-case basis by the mammographer.
4. Breast MR is an expensive, high-sensitivity, relatively low-specificity modality for the detection of

invasive breast cancers. It is appropriate for a few specific indications that are best left to the mammographer. Recent studies suggest a possible role for MR in screening of high-risk women.

SUGGESTED READING

American College of Radiology (ACR): ACR BI-RADS—Mammography, 4th ed. In ACR Breast Imaging Reporting and Data System, Breast Imaging Atlas. Reston, Va, American College of Radiology, 2003.

Boice JD, Preston D, Davis FG, Monson RR: Frequent chest x-ray fluoroscopy and breast cancer incidence among tuberculosis patients in Massachusetts. Radiat Res 1991;125:214–222.

Breast cancer screening and diagnosis guidelines. Clinical Practice Guidelines in Oncology, vol 1. National Comprehensive Cancer Network, 2005, www.nccn.org.

Brenner RJ, Bassett LW, Fajardo LL: Stereotactic core-needle breast biopsy: a multi-institutional prospective trial. Radiology 2001;218:866–872.

Dershaw DD, Borgen PI, Deutch BM, et al: Mammographic findings in men with breast cancer. AJR Am J Roentgenol 1993;160:267–270.

Feig SA: Current issues in mammographic screening. Postgraduate course syllabus, May 2005. Society of Breast Imaging, 2005:11–18.

Hillner BE, Bear HD, Fajardo LL: Estimating the cost-effectiveness of stereotaxic biopsy for nonpalpable breast abnormalities: a decision analysis model. Acad Radiol 1996;3:351–360.

Jemal A, Murray T, Ward E, et al: Cancer statistics, 2005. CA Cancer J Clin 2005:55:10–30.

Kriege M, Brekemans CR, Boetes C, et al: Efficacy of MRI and mammography for breast-cancer screening in women with a familial or genetic predisposition. N Engl J Med 2004;351:427–437.

Lee CH: Screening mammography: proven benefit, continued controversy. Radiol Clin North Am 2002;40:395–407.

Lee CH, Egglin TI, Philpotts LE, et al: Cost effectiveness of stereotactic core needle biopsy: analysis by means of mammographic findings. Radiology 1995;195:633–637.

Lewin JM, D'Orsi CJ, Hendrick RE, et al: Clinical comparison of full-field digital mammography and screen-film mammography for the detection of breast cancer. AJR Am J Roentgenol 2002;179:671–677.

Lewin JM, Hendrick RE, D'Orsi CJ, et al: Comparison of full-field digital mammography with screen-film mammography for cancer detection: Results of 4945 paired examinations. Radiology 2001;218:873–880.

Liberman L: Percutaneous image-guided core breast biopsy. Radiol Clin N Am 2002;40:483–500.

Liberman L, Sama MP: Cost-effectiveness of stereotactic 11-gauge directional vacuum-assisted breast biopsy. AJR Am J Roentgenol 2000;175:53–58.

Liberman LL, Feng TL, Dershaw DD: Ultrasound-guided core breast biopsy: utility and cost-effectiveness. Radiology 1998;208:717–723.

Morris EA: Breast cancer imaging with MRI. Radiol Clin N Am 2002;40:443–466.

Parker SH, Burbank F, Jackman RJ: Percutaneous large-core breast biopsy: a multi-institutional study. Radiology 1994;193:359–364.

Pisano ED, Gatsonis C, Hendrick E, et al: Diagnostic performance of digital versus film mammography for breast cancer screening. N Engl J Med 2005;353:1773–1783.

Shore RE, Hildreth N, Woodward ED, et al: Breast cancer among women given x-ray therapy for acute postpartum mastitis. J Natl Cancer Inst 1998;77:689–696.

Tokunaga M, Land CE, Tokuoka S, et al: Incidence of female breast cancer among atomic bomb survivors, 1950–1985. Radiat Res 1994;138:209–223.

Warner E, Plewes DB, Hill KA, et al: Surveillance of BRCA1 and BRCA2 mutation carriers with magnetic resonance imaging, ultrasound, mammography and clinical breast examination. JAMA 2004;2:1317–1325.

Glossary

Angiography: blood vessel imaging.

Angioplasty: dilation of a narrowed blood vessel; the interventional radiologist dilates the vessel by the percutaneous transluminal approach, manipulating a special catheter introduced percutaneously. The introduction site is usually in the groin and may be distant from the vascular lesion.

Antegrade pyelogram: study of the urinary tract by injection of contrast medium into the renal collecting system by transcutaneous puncture or through a nephrostomy tube.

Arteriovenous malformation: a vascular lesion, probably congenital, composed of abnormal arteries and veins. These lesions can produce symptoms and signs characteristic of other space-occupying masses, but they also affect organ function by virtue of their abnormal blood flow.

AVM: abbreviation for *arteriovenous malformation*.

AVN: abbreviation for *avascular necrosis*.

Barium enema: a radiographic study in which barium, in suspension, is introduced per rectum under direct fluoroscopic visualization to define lesions of the colon. In most cases air is introduced after the barium to produce an "air-contrast" or "double-contrast" study. Air-contrast studies are superior for demonstrating small lesions such as polyps. This venerable study has been largely replace by direct colonoscopy and the growing popularity of "virtual colonoscopy."

BE: abbreviation for *barium enema*.

CAT scan: abbreviation for *computed axial tomography scan*; synonym for *computed tomography*; *CT* is preferred.

Cholecystokinin (CCK): a short-acting agent previously delivered intravenously to empty the gallbladder before a nuclear hepatobiliary iminodiacetic acid (HIDA) study, because an empty gallbladder fills more easily with HIDA. Most nuclear medicine departments have abandoned CCK in favor of morphine, injected intravenously **after** the common bile duct is visualized; morphine potentiates gallbladder filling by raising back pressure in the extrahepatic ducts.

Cold: a nuclear medicine term for nonradioactive.

Computed axial tomography: synonym for *computed tomography.* (See also **CAT scan**.)

Computed tomography (CT): the imaging technique that produces transaxial images of body "slices" by directing an x-ray beam through the body at many angles; the attenuation of the beam by body structures is indicated by the intensity of the beam striking special radiation detectors, which produce electrical impulses proportional to transmitted beam intensity. Computer storage and manipulation of the electrical impulses reconstruct an image that is more sensitive to small radiographic density changes than standard x-rays, is amenable to recall and optimization at any time, and is displayed in the transaxial projection as "slices" or "cuts." Newer units, called "spiral" or "helical" CT, acquire data much more rapidly and in such a way that image reconstruction and display in multiple planes, including a three-dimensional display, are feasible. The last decade has seen the introduction of multidetector-row CT (MDCT) units that create up to 128 slices concurrently. The fastest MDCT units can scan an entire thorax, abdomen, and pelvis in 12 seconds. With appropriate software, cardiac motion can be "frozen," so that the heart and coronary arteries are seen without motion blur.

Contrast material or Contrast medium: any chemical introduced into a space for the purpose of changing the radiopacity or "signal characteristics" of that space for imaging. The term most often applies to iodinated organic compounds delivered intravenously and excreted by the kidneys via glomerular filtration, but, strictly speaking, many other products, including barium and gadolinium-based compounds, are contrast media.

Contrast resolution: the ability to discern small differences in radiographic density; computed tomography is superior in contrast resolution to conventional radiography.

CT: abbreviation for *computed tomography.*

CTA: abbreviation for *computed tomographic angiography.* CTA represents the most impressive application of ultrafast CT (multidetector-row CT [MDCT]). Contrast medium is delivered by rapid peripheral intravenous infusion; as it passes through the "target" blood vessels to be imaged—neck, brain, thorax, abdomen, pelvis, or extremities—the scanner produces high-resolution, high-speed images that define blood vessel anatomy almost as well as conventional catheter angiography. **CTA has progressed to the point that catheter diagnostic angiography is becoming uncommon,** although catheter angiography is, of course, a requirement for transcatheter therapy (e.g., angioplasty or stent placement).

Diethylenetriamine pentaacetic acid (DTPA): a metal chelating agent excreted by glomerular filtration; technetium 99m–DTPA (Tc-99m-DTPA) is a common radiopharmaceutical for renal scanning.

Digitized: converted to a numerical form for computer storage or arithmetic manipulation.

Diisopropyl iminodiacetic acid (DISIDA): a chemical variant of hepatobiliary iminodiacetic acid (HIDA), the nuclear pharmaceutical used for hepatobiliary imaging.

DISIDA: abbreviation for *diisopropyl iminodiacetic acid.*

DPA: abbreviation for *dual photon absorptiometry.*

DTPA: abbreviation for *diethylenetriamine pentaacetic acid,* a nuclear renal imaging agent, when labeled with technetium 99m (Tc-99m).

Dual photon absorptiometry (DPA): a technique of estimating bone mass of the lumbar spine or hip, based on the absorption of gamma rays aimed at the anatomic area in question. Although no isotope is injected into the patient, the study is usually performed in nuclear medicine departments. The technique has been replaced virtually everywhere by DXA (DEXA).

Dual x-ray absorptiometry (DXA): a technique of estimating the bone mass of certain regions, typically the lumbar spine or hip, based on the absorption of x-rays aimed at the anatomic area in question. Although no isotope is injected into the patient, the study is usually performed in nuclear medicine departments. For technical reasons, DXA (DEXA) is superior to DPA.

DXA: abbreviation for *dual x-ray absorptiometry.*

Dye: a layperson's radiographic term loosely applied to contrast material or contrast medium.

Echocardiography: ultrasound or sonography of the heart, usually applied to the diagnosis of pericardial effusion, valvular disease, ventricular wall motion, or estimation of the ejection fraction.

Ejection fraction: that portion of the ventricular volume ejected in systole. Mathematically, the ejection fraction is the end-diastolic volume minus the end-systolic volume, divided by the end-diastolic volume.

Endorectal sonogram: sonography performed with a transducer in the rectum. This method produces superior images of the prostate and is especially useful to guide transrectal prostatic biopsy.

Endoscopic retrograde cholangiopancreatography (ERCP): an endoscopic technique involving passage of the endoscope through the mouth, esophagus, and stomach into the duodenum and then cannulation of the ampulla of Vater; contrast medium injected retrograde fills the pancreatic and bile ducts. Radiographs provide excellent ductal visualization.

Endoscopic ultrasound (EUS): ultrasound performed with a transducer in the tip of a catheter introduced into the gut—for example, the distal esophagus or duodenum.

Enhanced: images produced after infusion of intravenous contrast medium, usually referring to computed tomography or magnetic resonance imaging.

Enhanced CT: computed tomography performed during or after intravenous contrast medium infusion.

The opacification of vascular spaces, renal concentration and excretion of contrast medium, and the diffusion of contrast medium across injured capillaries into the interstitium reveal lesions that are sometimes undetectable by unenhanced CT.

Enhanced MR: Magnetic resonance imaging performed during or after intravenous infusion of gadolinium-based contrast medium. The increased "signal" from various lesions and from the vascular space is a complex function of blood flow, blood volume, and capillary permeability.

Enteroclysis: a special small bowel examination in which barium, air, water, and sometimes methylcellulose are carefully introduced into the proximal jejunum via nasoduodenal tube.

ERCP: abbreviation for *endoscopic retrograde cholangiopancreatography.*

EUS: abbreviation for *endoscopic ultrasound.*

FFDG: Fluorodeoxyglucose, the only molecule currently FDA-approved for clinical positron emission tomography (PET) imaging. Labeled with fluorine-18, FDG is taken up by actively metabolizing normal tissues (chiefly brain and heart) and **by many cancers. FDG-PET has revolutionized cancer staging.**

Gallium-67: an intermediate half-life radionuclide that accumulates in inflammatory foci and some neoplasms, notably lymphoma, after peripheral intravenous injection; uptake in both neoplastic and inflammatory lesions reduces the specificity of gallium scans, and gastrointestinal excretion sometimes obscures abdominal lesions. Gallium-67 scans for infection have been largely replaced by labeled autologous leukocyte studies, and gallium-67 studies for lymphoma have been largely replaced by FDG-PET.

Gamma camera: the standard nuclear instrument for producing images of the in vivo radiobiodistribution of previously administered pharmaceuticals; these images constitute nuclear medicine "scans."

Gamma scintigraphy: synonymous with nuclear scanning, radionuclide scans, or nuclear medicine scans. The term derives from the light flash that is produced when photons emitted by the radionuclide that is within the patient strike a crystal in the camera, known as a "scintillation."

Gantry: the physical opening or "portal" through which a patient passes for a computed tomography study.

Gastrografin: a water-soluble radiographic contrast medium usually used for gastrointestinal opacification.

Gated: images synchronized with motion of the heart (cardiac gating) or the lungs (pulmonary gating), so that the images are free from motion blur.

GFR: abbreviation for *glomerular filtration rate.*

GHA: abbreviation for *glucoheptonate.*

Guided biopsy: percutaneous needle biopsy performed under direct visualization with fluoroscopy, ultrasound, or computed tomography. Under sonographic or fluoroscopic guidance, the needle, normal structures, and the lesion are visualized during the biopsy, greatly diminishing uncertainty in needle placement and reducing risk. Tissue for cytology or histology can be harvested at less expense than by surgery.

Hepatobiliary iminodiacetic acid (HIDA): the original technetium 99m–labeled nuclear pharmaceutical for hepatobiliary imaging; after intravenous injection, the compound is cleared by the liver and excreted into the biliary tree, with visualization of the common duct, gallbladder, and duodenum. Many chemical relatives, including diisopropyl iminodiacetic acid and para-isopropyl iminodiacetic acid, are now in clinical use, but in most nuclear medicine departments, *HIDA* is the generic term for all of these.

HIDA: abbreviation for *hepatobiliary iminodiacetic acid*, also a general term loosely applied to any of its current analogues for nuclear gallbladder/biliary tract imaging.

HMPAO: abbreviation for *hexamethylpropyleneamine oxime*, a white blood cell (WBC) label when chelated to technetium 99m (Tc-99m). Leukocytes labeled with this compound are useful for imaging infection.

Hot: a nuclear medicine term for radioactive.

I-123: abbreviation for *iodine 123.*

I-125: abbreviation for *iodine 125.*

I-131: abbreviation for *iodine 131.*

Indium 111 (In-111): an intermediate half-life isotope; when chelated by oxine, In-111 is an effective leukocyte label.

Indium-111-oxine: the radiopharmaceutical used for labeling polymorphonuclear neutrophilic leukocytes for in vivo abscess localization.

Intravenous pyelogram (IVP): more correctly termed **intravenous urogram (IVU)**, a urinary tract study; radiographs of the kidneys, ureters, and bladder are obtained after intravenous injection of iodinated contrast medium that is cleared from the circulation by glomerular filtration. This venerable once-commonplace procedure has been all but replaced by computed tomography.

Iodine 131 total body metastatic thyroid carcinoma search: a method for detecting functioning metastatic thyroid cancer. The examination requires careful preparation and is most effective when endogenous thyroid-stimulating hormone levels are high, in order to stimulate radioiodine uptake by metastases.

Isodense: having the same density as surrounding tissue; in computed tomography an isodense lesion cannot be differentiated from surrounding tissue without special techniques such as enhancement with intravenous contrast medium.

Isotope imaging: synonym for *nuclear imaging.*

Isotopes: atomic species having the same atomic number (number of protons) but different atomic weights (atomic mass numbers—i.e., protons plus neutrons).

IVU: abbreviation for *intravenous urogram*; synonym for *IVP.*

KUB: abbreviation for *kidneys, ureters, bladder*; the term KUB refers to plain film of the abdomen, because a plain film was for many years the initial study for many conditions that affect the urinary tract.

Labeled leukocytes: the best current agent for localizing occult bacterial infection by nuclear methods. Both In-111-oxine and Tc-99m-HMPAO are useful as radiolabels.

Liver-spleen scan: a nuclear method of imaging the liver and spleen. Radiolabeled microcolloid particles are injected intravenously and taken up by the hepatic and splenic reticuloendothelial system. Once a mainstay for detection of hepatic metastases, the study has been superseded by computed tomography and magnetic resonance.

MAA: abbreviation for *macroaggregated albumin*, the agent for nuclear lung scanning.

Macroaggregated albumin (MAA): very small albumin particles; when labeled with technetium 99m, macroaggregated albumin particles (Tc-99m-MAA) are an excellent and inexpensive lung scanning agent, because they trap in the pulmonary capillary bed, distributing according to pulmonary arterial blood flow. Once the mainstay for detection of pulmonary emboli, this method has been largely replaced by computed tomographic pulmonary angiography.

Magnetic resonance angiography (MRA): method of MR imaging that produces good visualization of blood vessels without the need for contrast medium or catheterization. MRA, like CTA, has replaced many conventional catheter angiograms.

Magnetic resonance (MR) imaging (MRI): noninvasive technique that images body structures without ionizing radiation of any type, through analysis of signals emitted by body tissue, after the anatomic area under study is placed in a magnetic field and perturbed by pulses of radiofrequency energy.

MDCT: abbreviation for *multidetector computed tomography*.

MDP: abbreviation for *methylene diphosphonate*, the bone scanning agent.

Methylene diphosphonate (MDP): a small organic phosphate molecule; technetium 99m (Tc-99m)–MDP is the most widely used and most effective skeletal scanning agent.

MR: abbreviation for *magnetic resonance*. (See also **MRI**.)

MRA: abbreviation for *magnetic resonance angiography*.

MRI: abbreviation for *magnetic resonance imaging*. (See also **MR**.)

MUGA: abbreviation for *multigated acquisition study*.

Multigated acquisition study (MUGA): a nuclear ventriculogram created by collecting imaging data from defined portions of the cardiac cycle, by computer synchronization of the gamma camera and the electrocardiogram, so that images of the cardiac cycle can be constructed and displayed as a multiframe "movie."

Nuclear medicine: the analysis of organ structure and function by imaging the radiobiodistribution of administered radiopharmaceuticals, the determination of radionuclide levels in various body fluids, and the determination of blood levels of many chemical substances by radioimmunoassay.

Nuclear medicine imaging: that part of the broader field of nuclear medicine that consists only of imaging.

Nuclide: the current preferred term for isotope; strictly speaking, a nuclide is an atomic species, whereas a radioactive atomic species is a radionuclide.

Percutaneous angioplasty: synonym for *percutaneous transluminal angioplasty*.

Percutaneous transhepatic cholangiogram (PTC): a radiographic method of imaging the bile ducts; the liver is punctured through the abdominal wall and contrast medium is injected into a peripheral duct through a thin needle.

Percutaneous transluminal angioplasty (PTA): dilation of a narrowed, diseased blood vessel, usually by a balloon catheter. The special catheter is introduced via percutaneous puncture, usually in the groin, and threaded through appropriate vessels to the lesion.

Pericholecystic edema: fluid around the gallbladder demonstrated by ultrasound; this sign may indicate acute cholecystitis but may be mimicked by noninflammatory fluid originating elsewhere (e.g., ascites).

Pertechnetate: the term for technetium 99m (Tc-99m) in one of its common oxidation states, TcO_4^-; TcO_4^- is usually the chemical state of Tc-99m obtained from an in-house generator, and although this chemical configuration is purposely altered for the preparation of various Tc-99m–labeled radiopharmaceuticals, pertechnetate itself is excellent for imaging the thyroid gland and Meckel's diverticulum.

PET: abbreviation for *positron emission tomography*.

Positron emission tomography (PET): In clinical practice, PET is currently limited to imaging a single radionuclide, fluorine 18, incorporated into a glucose-like molecule, FDG (fluorodeoxyglucose). FDG is accumulated by rapidly metabolizing normal tissues (chiefly brain and heart) **and also MANY tumors, both primary and metastatic. FDG-PET IS THE MOST EFFECTIVE IMAGING METHOD TO DATE FOR STAGING LYMPHOMA AND CANCERS OF THE HEAD/NECK, LUNG, ESOPHAGUS, STOMACH, COLON, BREAST, AND THYROID.** Recently, FDG-PET has effectively localized some occult infections and may well secure a place in the work of fever of unknown origin.

PTC: abbreviation for *percutaneous transhepatic cholangiogram.*

QCT: abbreviation for *quantitative computed tomography.*

Quantitative computed tomography (QCT): a method of measuring bone mass of the spine with CT. The method competes with DXA (DEXA).

Radiographic density: the ability of any substance to attenuate an x-ray beam.

Radionuclide: a radioactive nuclide—that is, a radioactive atomic species.

Radionuclide imaging: synonym for *nuclear medicine imaging, nuclear scanning, nuclear imaging, scintigraphy.*

Real-time sonography: a method of continuously and instantaneously displaying sonographically visualized internal anatomy as the transducer moves across the body's skin surface. The method is analogous to viewing a subject through the viewfinder of a camera as the camera moves, as opposed to later examining single still photographs obtained one at a time. All sonography is now real time.

Red blood cell scan: a term that describes various nuclear procedures, all based on imaging the patient's radiolabeled blood pool. Imaging the cardiac blood pool produces a ventriculogram; imaging the abdominal blood pool can reveal a gastrointestinal bleed; imaging the liver with single-photon emission computed tomography (SPECT) can detect hemangiomas, and so on.

Retrograde pyelogram: study of the urinary tract by retrograde injection of contrast medium into the distal ureter via a catheter placed by a urologist after cystoscopy.

SBO: abbreviation for *small bowel obstruction*.

Signal characteristics: a term that indicates how a particular tissue or fluid appears on a magnetic resonance image.

Single-photon emission computed tomography (SPECT): an outgrowth of nuclear medicine requiring a special gamma camera that produces images of the in vivo radiobiodistribution of previously injected pharmaceuticals as "slices" of the organ under study. The slices can be in the coronal, transaxial, or sagittal projections. Conventional radionuclides (not positron emitters) are used; SPECT should not be confused with PET.

Sono: short for *sonogram*; synonym for *ultrasound*.

Sonogram (sono): synonym for *ultrasound*.

Spatial resolution: the ability to discern fine anatomic detail by imaging.

SPECT: abbreviation for *single photon emission computed tomography*.

Spiral CT: All computed tomography (CT) scanners in the United States, Western Europe, and Canada are now spiral—or, more correctly, helical. Helical CT replaced older "stop and shoot" machines, in which the patient was circled by an x-ray tube that fired a "single shot of x-rays" to generate a single "slice," after which the tube ceased firing and the stretcher moved to another location and stopped, so that another slice could be generated. **The x-ray tube of a helical machine continuously fires as the stretcher continuously moves; thus, the "track" of the beam through the patient is a continuous spiral or "helix."** The advantages of helical CT are speed, continuity of data, and tremendous flexibility in terms of slice selection for computer reconstruction. Multidetector CT (MDCT), which fires multiple beams concurrently at an array of detectors—as the patient continuously moves—represents an even greater leap forward.

Sulfur colloid: the pharmaceutical used for nuclear liver-spleen scanning when labeled with technetium 99m. Once a mainstay, this test is nearly obsolete.

Surface coil: an augmentation of standard magnetic resonance that produces superior images of a specific anatomic site (such as the knee) by applying a small metal coil over the imaged area. The coil functions as both a transmitter and a receiver of radiofrequency signals.

T1-weighted image: a magnetic resonance image in which fat is light and cerebrospinal fluid is dark.

T2-weighted image: a magnetic resonance image in which cerebrospinal fluid is light.

Tc-99m: abbreviation for *technetium 99m*.

Tc-99m-MAA: abbreviation for *technetium 99m–macroaggregated albumin*, the lung-scanning agent, now nearly obsolete.

Tc-99m-MDP: abbreviation for *technetium 99m–methylene diphosphonate*, the most common bone-scanning agent.

Technetium 99m (Tc-99m): the most clinically useful radionuclide in conventional (non-PET) nuclear imaging, with a short half-life (6 hours) and a gamma ray energy (140 KeV) almost ideal for gamma camera imaging. Technetium 99m is available around the clock in all nuclear medicine departments. The chemistry of this radionuclide allows it to be combined with molecules that are organ specific (e.g., MDP [bone-seeking], HIDA [hepatobiliary], and DTPA [renal]).

Tomography: a method for imaging slices of tissue in a given plane. Originally, the term "tomography" referred simply to a basic x-ray technique, but current technology has created computed tomography (CT), single-photon emission computed tomography (SPECT), and positron emission tomography (PET). Moreover, magnetic resonance (MR) images are tomographic.

Transaxial: the plane obtained by slicing the body perpendicular to its long (head-to-foot) axis; this plane examines the body the way one would examine a loaf of bread by slicing it.

Transrectal ultrasound: ultrasound of the prostate and seminal vesicles with a sound beam originating from an intrarectal transducer. Accurate, relatively noninvasive prostate biopsies can be performed with a special attachment to the intrarectal probe.

Transvaginal ultrasound (TVU): ultrasound of the female pelvis with a sound beam originating from an intravaginal transducer. The technique produces better images of the pelvis and adnexa than transabdominal ultrasound.

TVU: abbreviation for *transvaginal ultrasound.*

Ultrasonography: the technique of ultrasound.

Ultrasound: the method of obtaining diagnostic medical images of internal anatomy by bombarding the area of interest with an ultrasound beam and reconstructing the returning sound (echoes) into an image.

Unenhanced: without benefit of contrast medium, referring to computed tomography and magnetic resonance imaging.

Unenhanced CT: computed tomography performed without intravenous contrast medium.

Unenhanced MR: Magnetic resonance imaging performed without intravenous contrast medium.

VCUG: abbreviation for *voiding cystourethrogram.*

Ventilation scan: images of the lungs performed during ventilation with a radioactive gas to obtain information on alveolar ventilation and air trapping. In some centers, radioactive aerosol particles have been very successfully used instead of radioactive gas.

Ventriculogram: an imaging study of the cardiac ventricles designed to determine their ejection fractions and define their wall motion. Nuclear, sonographic, and angiographic methods can produce ventriculograms.

Index